Ward ethics

**Dilemmas for medical students and
doctors in training**

- Is that improper conduct?
- Was there consent?
- What does a patient have a right to know?
- Should I report that?
- What do we owe the dead and the newly dead?

These are just a few of the ethical questions that confront medical trainees daily and yet there is surprisingly
little practical guidance available to them.

Thomasine Kushner and David Thomasma have
addressed this need by compiling a series of case studies from around the world and inviting leading ethicists and clinicians to comment on them. Over 80 actual
cases cover the range of possible problems which may
be encountered by trainees on the wards, from drug and
alcohol abuse, whistle-blowing and improper sexual
conduct to performing procedures, handling authority,
disclosure, blaming, personal responses to patients, and
misrepresentation of research. The book arose from
years of listening to the real-life experiences and problems of students and trainee doctors and is an essential
guide to coping with the ethical dilemmas of those
embarking on medical careers.

Thomasine K. Kushner, Ph.D. is Clinical Professor of
Bioethics in the Joint Medical Program as well as Senior
Research Fellow in the Center for Human Rights at the
University of California, Berkeley.
David C. Thomasma, Ph.D. is Professor and English
Chair of Medical Ethics, Neiswanger Institute of Bio-
ethics and Health Policy, Loyola University Chicago
Medical Center. They are co-editors of the *Cambridge
Quarterly of Healthcare Ethics*.

Ward ethics

**Dilemmas for
medical students and
doctors in training**

edited by

Thomasine K. Kushner

and

David C. Thomasma

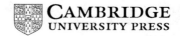
CAMBRIDGE
UNIVERSITY PRESS

CAMBRIDGE UNIVERSITY PRESS
Cambridge, New York, Melbourne, Madrid, Cape Town, Singapore, São Paulo, Delhi

Cambridge University Press
The Edinburgh Building, Cambridge CB2 8RU, UK

Published in the United States of America by Cambridge University Press, New York

www.cambridge.org
Information on this title: www.cambridge.org/9780521664523

First published 2001
Third printing 2008

Printed in the United Kingdom at the University Press, Cambridge

A catalogue record for this publication is available from the British Library

Library of Congress Cataloguing in Publication Data

Ward ethics / edited by Thomasine K. Kushner and David C. Thomasma.
    p.   ; cm.
Includes bibliographical references.
ISBN 0 521 80291 1 – ISBN 0 521 66452 7 (pbk.)
1. Medical ethics – Case studies.   2. Interns (Medicine) – Professional ethics – Case studies.
3. Residents (Medicine) – Professional ethics – Case studies.   4. Hospital care – Moral
and ethical aspects – Case studies.   I. Kushner, Thomasine Kimbrough.   II. Thomasma,
David C., 1939–
[DNLM: 1, Ethics, Medical.   2. Attitude of Health Personnel.   3. Internship and Residency.
4. Interprofessional Relations.   5. Medical Staff, Hospital.   6. Truth Disclosure.
W 50 W256 2001]
R724 W33 2001
174'2–dc21   00-050238

ISBN 978-0-521-80291-8 hardback
ISBN 978-0-521-66452-3 paperback

This book is dedicated to the physicians and future physicians who generously share their private stories here so that others may benefit.

Contents

Part I. On caring for patients   9

Section 1. Performing procedures   17

**Part II. On becoming a "team
player": searching for e*sprit
de corps* and conflicts of
socialization**   123

Acknowledgments

This book has benefited from the many helpful conversations with: Dr. William Andereck, Dr. Baruch Brody, Dr. Robert Brody, Dr. Kate Brown, Dr. Jeffrey Burack, Dr. Neal Cohen, Dr. Francesco De Martis, Dr. Elizabeth Dunn, Dr. David Holman, Dr. Andrew Jameton, Dr. Gerrit Kimsma, Dr. Tom Lequeur, Dr. Paul Rabinow, Dr. Rosamond Rhodes, Dr. Guenter Risse, Dr. Richard Selzer, Dr. Richard Smith, Dr. Alan Steinbach, Dr. Ann Stevens, and Dr. Larry Schneiderman.

Contributors

George J. Agich, Ph.D. is the F.J. O'Neil Chair in the Department of Bioethics, The Cleveland Clinic Foundation, Cleveland, Ohio.

Akira Akabayashi, M.D., Ph.D. is Professor in the School of Public Health at Kyoto University Graduate School of Medicine, Kyoto, Japan.

William Andereck, M.D. is Chair of the Ethics Committee at California Pacific Medical Center, San Francisco, California.

David Bennahum, M.D. is Chair of the Program in Medicine and the Humanities at the New Mexico School of Medicine, Albuquerque, New Mexico.

Jeffrey Burack, M.D. is Adjunct Assistant Professor of Bioethics and Medical Humanities at the University of California, Berkeley School of Public Health and Assistant Clinical Professor of Medicine at UC San Francisco.

Thomas A. Cavanaugh, Ph.D. is an Associate Professor in the Department of Philosophy, University of San Francisco, San Francisco, California.

Tod Chambers, Ph.D. is Assistant Professor of Medical Ethics and Humanities at Northwestern University Medical School.

Kate T. Christensen, M.D., F.A.C.P. is an internist and regional ethics coordinator for the Permanente Medical Group in Northern California.

Neal Cohen, M.D., M.P.H., M.S., F.C.C.M. is Professor of Anesthesia and Medicine, Vice Chairman of the Department of Anesthesia, and Director of Critical Care Medicine, University of California, San Francisco.

Pablo Rodriguez del Pozo, M.D., J.D. has an extensive academic background in bioethics, specifically issues involving justice and health. He has taught at universities in Spain and Argentina, and published in periodicals in Spain and around Latin America. In addition, he is a consultant on reform programs of Argentina's health care system.

Amnon Goldworth, Ph.D. is a philosopher and Senior Medical Ethicist at the Lucille Packard Children's Hospital at Stanford University, Palo Alto, California.

Michael L. Gross, Ph.D. is Senior Lecturer in the Department of Political Science at the University of Haifa, Israel.

John Harris is Sir David Alliance Professor of Bioethics and Research Director of The Centre for Social Ethics and Policy, University of Manchester, and a Director of The Institute of Medicine, Law and Bioethics at the Universities of Manchester and Liverpool, England.

Paul Hofmann, Dr. P.H. is Vice-President of Provenance Health Partners, Moraga, California.

Søren Holm, M.D., Ph.D. is a Senior Research Fellow in the Department of Medical Philosophy and Clinical Theory, Faculty of Health Sciences, at the University of Copenhagen, Denmark.

Marli Huijer, M.D., Ph.D. is a Family Physician and Assistant Professor of Philosophy in the Department of Philosophy and Medical Ethics at the Vrije University of Amsterdam, The Netherlands.

Kenneth V. Iserson, M.D., M.B.A. is Professor of Surgery (Emergency Medicine), Director of the Program in Bioethics, and Chair of the Bioethics Committee at the University of Arizona College of Medicine, Tucson.

Francis Kane, Ph.D. is Professor of Philosophy at Salisbury State University, Salisbury, Maryland.

Gerrit Kimsma, M.D. is a family practitioner and philosopher who lectures on family practice and medical ethics in the Departments of Family and Nursing Home Medicine and Philosophy and Medical Ethics at the Vrije University of Amsterdam, The Netherlands.

Gregory Luke Larkin, M.D., M.S., M.S.P.H., F.A.C.E.P. is the Director of Research in the Department of Emergency Medicine, Mercy Hospital and is Clinical Assistant Professor at the University of Pittsburgh School of Medicine, Pittsburgh, Pennsylvania.

Mary B. Mahowald, Ph.D. is a philosopher and Professor in the Department of Obstetrics and Gynecology, Pritzger School of Medicine, University of Chicago, and Assistant Director, Maclean Center for Clinical Medical Ethics, University of Chicago.

Richard Martinez, M.H., M.D. is Assistant Professor in the Program in Healthcare Ethics, Humanities and the Law, and in the Department of Psychiatry, at the University of Colorado Health Sciences Center, Denver, Colorado.

Guy Micco, M.D. is Chair of the Ethics Committee at Alta Bates Hospital, Berkeley, California, and a Clinical Professor in the Health and Medical Sciences Program, University of California, Berkeley.

Jean-Christophe Mino, M.P.H., M.D., Ph.D. is a researcher at the French National School of Public Health and teaches biomedical ethics at Pitie Salpetrière Medical School in Paris.

Emilio Mordini, M.D. is a psychoanalyst at the Psychoanalytic Institute for Social Research, Rome, Italy, and Professor of Bioethics at the Medical School of the University of Rome "La Sapienza."

William Nelson, Ph.D. is Ethics Education Coordinator, National Center for Clinical Ethics, Department of Veterans Affairs, and Associate Professor of Psychiatry, Dartmouth Medical School, Hanover, New Hampshire.

Ruth Purtilo, Ph.D. is Director of the Center for Health Policy and Ethics at Creighton University, Omaha, Nebraska.

Domeena Renshaw, M.D. is Professor of Psychiatry and Director of the Sexual Dysfunction Program at Loyola University, Chicago.

Rosamond Rhodes, Ph.D. is Associate Professor of Medical Education and Director of Bioethics Education at Mount Sinai School of Medicine, CUNY. She is Editor of the American Philosophical Association Newsletter on Philosophy and Medicine.

Ben A. Rich, J.D., Ph.D. is Associate Professor in the Bioethics Program at the University of California, Davis Medical Center, Sacramento, California.

Richard Selzer, M.D., formerly a Professor of Surgery at Yale University, is now a full-time writer living in New Haven, Connecticut. His books include *Rituals of Surgery, Mortal Lessons, Notes on the Art of Surgery, Confessions of a Knife*, and *Raising the Dead*.

Lawrence J. Schneiderman, M.D. is a Professor in the Departments of Family and Preventive Medicine and Medicine, School of Medicine, University of California, San Diego.

Robert L. Schwartz, J.D. is Professor of Law at the University of New Mexico, Albuquerque.

Robyn S. Shapiro, J.D. is Professor of Bioethics and Director of the Center for the Study of Bioethics at the Medical College of Wisconsin.

Jacquelyn Slomka, Ph.D., R.N. is a member of the professional staff at The Cleveland Clinic Foundation, Department of Bioethics, Cleveland, Ohio, and Assistant Professor of Clinical Medicine in the Department of Internal Medicine at The Ohio State University.

Bethany Spielman, Ph.D., J.D., M.H.A. is Associate Professor and Director of the Medical Ethics Program at Southern Illinois University School of Medicine, Adjunct Professor of Law at Southern Illinois University School of Law, and ethics consultant for Memorial Medical Center in Springfield, Illinois.

Alan Steinbach, M.D. is Associate Clinical Professor in the Division of Health and Medical Sciences, School of Public Health, University of California, Berkeley.

Carson Strong, Ph.D. is Professor of Medical Ethics in the Department of Human Values and Ethics at the College of Medicine, University of Tennessee, Memphis.

Barbara Supanich, R.S.M., M.D. is Faculty Member of the Munson Medical Center Family Practice Center in Traverse City, Michigan.

Griffin Trotter, M.D., Ph.D. is Assistant Professor of Health Care Ethics and Assistant Professor of Surgery at Saint Louis University Health Sciences Center.

Evert Van Leeuwen, Ph.D. is Professor and Chair, Department of Philosophy and Medical Ethics, Vrije University of Amsterdam, The Netherlands.

James E. Weber, D.O. is Clinical Assistant Professor in the Department of Emergency Medicine at Hurley Medical Center at the University of Michigan Medical School, Ann Arbor, Michigan.

Charles Weijer, M.D., Ph.D. is a Bioethicist and Assistant Professor of Medicine in the Department of Bioethics Education and Research, Dalhousie University, Halifax, Nova Scotia, Canada.

Harvey Weinstein, M.D. is Associate Director of the Human Rights Center and Clinical Professor in the School of Public Health, University of California, Berkeley.

David N. Weisstub, J.D. is Philippe Pinel Professor of Legal Psychiatry and Biomedical Ethics, at University of Montreal School of Medicine, Montreal, Canada.

Jonathan Wyatt, M.B., Ch.B., B. Med. Sci., F.R.C.S.(Ed.), F.F.A.E.M. is Consultant and Honorary Fellow in Forensic Medicine, Accident and Emergency Department, at the Royal Cornwall Hospital, Cornwall, England.

Prologue

Breaking the silence

Hardly a week passes that print and news media fail to herald emerging dilemmas in medicine, whether it be the future of genetic testing, human cloning, or new technologies in assisted reproduction. Consequently, the expanding world of biotechnology and the ethical problems it raises are part of common conversations everywhere, and medical trainees are apt to be more familiar with their complexities and nuances than they are with the issues that confront them daily as they struggle to become physicians.

Unfortunately, the bioethics literature does not serve the everyday needs of trainees well. Although books on bioethics have proliferated rapidly, as did the bioethics curricula for doctors in training over the past 25 years, few resources address the key ethical dilemmas that student doctors face as they enter the clinical wards. Instead, the focus is typically on the meaning and application of bioethics principles, or a variety of moral theories, with emphasis on such issues in patient care as: foregoing life-sustaining treatment, access to health care, allocation of resources, euthanasia, abortion, impaired new-borns, etc. Important as these issues are, the dilemmas posed are essentially beyond the scope of trainees' decision making and choice points whose moral struggles continue, for the most part, unnoticed and unaddressed. On the wards theories and intellectual debate, so stimulating in a classroom, are eclipsed or disappear altogether in an atmosphere of time pressures.

Patients are turned into ciphers. Even the most competent trainees feel unsure about what to do. Superiors reign supreme.

With the need for addressing these issues so apparent why has there grown a traditional "code of silence" that often prevents open discussion of the very experiences and dilemmas medical students and doctors in training find most disturbing? A senior physician offers the following explanation:

There is a sense that it is not "professional" to air our dirty laundry, and to call attention to issues that have not been addressed makes everyone uncomfortable. We are willing to talk about patient problems, but we are reluctant to open up discussions involving our own gaps in education and problems in relationships. To talk about the glitches and the screw-ups would be to admit that we are not as perfect as we are trying to portray ourselves to be.

Unattended these concerns fester, sometimes for years, and become part of the anger, disappointment, and guilt physicians later feel toward themselves and their profession.

Ward Ethics (1) is written to break the silence that surrounds the daily dilemmas faced by trainees as they try to balance learning medicine, performing procedures, and interacting with patients and colleagues. The precarious nature of the context in which the balancing takes place is highlighted by Richard Smith, editor of the *British Medical Journal*, when he reminds us that from the beginning of their training student doctors are "put through a gruelling course and exposed younger than most of their non-medical friends to death, pain, sickness, and what the great doctor William Osler called the perplexity of the soul. And all this within an environment where 'real doctors' get on with the job and only the weak weep or feel distressed." (2)

The existential reality that perplexes the soul of even the most hardy is compounded by the fact that trainees find themselves in an unsettling "one step down" position in which, because of their status, they have not yet arrived as fully independent decision-makers. Always in the shadow of their superiors, they are constantly aware of being subject to hierarchical critique, evaluation, and criticism that, if negative, can carry dire consequences for their future professional lives.

Therefore, student doctors are under a doubly heavy burden. Not only must they struggle with "What is the right thing to do?" but also "How will others judge my decision?" "How will my action, or failure to act, look in the eyes of those who hold professional power?" The words of a University of California at San Francisco medical student echo the position of many medical trainees: "No one addresses the problems of working in a power hierarchy. We are bottom feeders and we don't know how to handle it." It is precisely these often overlooked issues that *Ward Ethics* is designed to address.

Their own comments tell about the kind of help trainees are looking for: How can I maintain my own integrity and, at the same time, protect myself from negative repercussions? At what point do I go around a superior "who knows best" when I seriously question his or her ethical behavior? What methods should I use to act on my convictions in a way that is effective and constructive?

Ward Ethics came about in response to years of listening to the real-life experiences of medical students and doctors in training and their expressions of inadequacy in dealing effectively with the most perplexing questions they faced. The following chapters are based on actual cases solicited internationally from medical students, interns, residents, and now-practicing physicians, who, often for the first time, reveal cases that continue to cause them discomfort and distress, even though in some cases years have passed. The cases appear in the words of the student doctors and physicians themselves. Scenarios are presented anonymously to prevent identification of individuals and institutions involved. Although reports of actual events, none of the cases should be considered unique. All are "archetypes" in the sense that for each case included in the text, we received other similar examples of situations involving the same issues.

The authors chosen to comment on the chapters are noted international experts from the interdisciplinary backgrounds that comprise modern bioethics, e.g., medicine, law, philosophy, and health policy. They provide diversity in their areas of expertise as well as in their perspectives. The aim is not to provide "answers" but to offer readers a range of reasonable and defensible options with which to inform their own thinking and conduct. Indeed, from time to time the commentators may disagree with one another.

The plan of *Ward Ethics* is intended as analogous to an apprenticeship, the structure traditionally believed to be important for learning medicine. Readers have the opportunity to "apprentice" with bioethicists as they chart the terrain of ethical dilemmas on the wards. With their guidance, landmarks in the landscape will become recognizable. Readers will gain a sense of proportion, classification, and most of all the sense of comfort that comes from familiarity.

It is best to keep in mind, however, that different sorts of maps serve different purposes, and the negotiating tools offered here cannot be compared to the directionality and precision of the familiar cartographic map, complete with compass rose. The guideposts offered in these commentaries are more akin to maps drawn by nomadic people that focus on the critical question, "How do I get there?" Directional maps with their grids of city streets are useless in the nomad's way of life. What matters are maps indicating how travelers can arrive at the destination. Landmarks of note, events that could be expected, as well as how to negotiate the terrain are all important. Their maps anticipate questions a traveler might ask: "What have others done at this point?" "Where would that path lead?"

Similarly, commentaries on the chapters here are directed at helping readers to organize their own journey from where they are to where they want to go. They include suggestions regarding negotiating pathways and ideas when alternative

routes should be considered. The aim of the commentaries is to provide reference material to which readers may refer and by which they can measure their own decision-making process when they face similar issues on the wards – as inevitably they will.

By opening the discussion, the cases and commentaries in these chapters provide not only a much-needed public airing of issues; but also a framework for looking at the dilemmas commonly encountered in becoming a doctor. The book is thus an antiseptic to the festering sore of denial. Familiarity with the issues, and thinking in advance about the incredibly stressful situations that define life on the wards, will provide a background as trainees continue to assess "Am I on target as to my goals for working on the wards?" One physician's personal account of the goals he set for his own ward experience were: "To make this patient as well as possible, or at least not harm him; and in the process learn something so I will be able to help others." He adds, "I think unless people have those goals clearly in mind, I do not see how they can justify doing many of the things that will present themselves on the wards."

Embarking on the "ethics apprenticeship" presented in the following pages is intended to assist readers in developing a methodology for their own moral decision making. The goal is to offer a textbook that will provide trainees with a starting point and a way of directing their thinking to help untie knots in the most difficult cases they encounter. As in any good apprenticeship, skills will be developed that will serve as part of the reader's ethical tool kit:

Sensitization to issues: greater awareness in being able to identify issues that otherwise might have gone unnoticed.

Recognition of possibilities: increased skill in generating options and alternatives.

Cultivation of intellectual resources: resolve to acquire the necessary intellectual resources related to these issues and their possibilities to be able to deal with dilemmas in a more self-aware, systematic, and satisfying way.

No matter how successful the apprenticeship, not everyone will reach the same conclusions, even when using the same tools. But at least a similar language of issues and taxonomy of dilemmas will be shared, making a wider examination of the issues easier. Those outcomes alone will help to refine our moral thinking.

For the next step, Richard Smith urges, "We need to move from a culture that encourages doctors to hide distress and difficulties to one where we learn to share them and ask for help." (2) The resolve to begin the sharing and its concomitant aid in training stands as the responsible response. In the following cases, presented in the voices of those who experienced them, the distress and difficulty are apparent as well as the need for aid. The willingness of those who shared what usually remains a silent suffering is best repaid if these issues can be used for more indepth medical curricula and residency training programs. The book can also function as the basis for informative group discussions. However, medical students and doctors in training at every level will find the cases and responses important for their own use, even if there is no formal recognition of the issues in the curriculum. Faculty teaching in medical schools will gain important insights from the situations presented, should they have forgotten their own training dilemmas. They may see an earlier version of themselves in these pages and be willing to join a movement toward change.

Notes

1 It should be pointed out that the term "ward" is used here as a generic description for locations where medical trainees learn to care for real patients. We recognize that the term "ward" is frequently replaced by other terms, such as "services," "units," or "floors" and that increasingly, training encompasses not only hospitals, but also other clinical settings outside the hospital. Although the physical space may change, the interaction between mentor and apprentices as they move from patient to patient remains the main activity for care and education. The cases described here reflect that larger dimension.
2 Smith R. All doctors are problem doctors. Editorial. *BMJ* 1997;314(22):841–2.

Additional information

An important forerunner of *Ward Ethics* was an article by D.A. Christakis and C. Feudtner titled "Ethics in a Short White Coat: The Ethical Dilemmas That Medical Students Confront," *Acad Med* 1993;68(4):249–54. The content was developed for an internal medicine clerkship using cases submitted by third-year medical students during 1991–92 at a tertiary care hospital. We are grateful to these authors for the initial taxonomy of issues under which we began collecting cases. We are indebted, as well, to the other researchers, listed in the bibliography, whose work examines the perceptions and problems of student doctors.

The recognition that there is a need to examine the dilemmas presented here is beginning to grow. Workshops, presentations, small seminars, and minicourses are being developed. For example, the University of California at San Diego has presented workshops preparing students for their rotations on the ward. At Mt. Sinai School of Medicine, CUNY, students generated their own cases from their experiences for discussion, a few of which are used in this book.

Letter from a young doctor

Recently, I received the following letter from a young woman:

I am a lowly intern and I've had a long hard extraordinary week, some of it exhilarating. I haven't really slept in weeks and when I do sleep, I dream of my patients. I sent a little old lady with dead legs home to die. I told a man today he had cancer. It's late at night now, and I am worrying about them, but also I'm worrying about me. I'm so tired and lonely and I'm starting to laugh (hard) at things I shouldn't laugh at. I don't understand exactly what is happening to me – but it's happening fast . . .

Here is a person, like many of you, in dire need. She wants to be a doctor – and a good one – but her training experiences are making her question her ability, her knowledge, and why she went into this profession in the first place.

The answer to why we choose medicine is very individual. In my own case, medicine was a part of my heritage. My father was a general practitioner and from my earliest days, when we lived upstairs and he worked downstairs, I heard the cries and moans of the patients he was treating and hurting. When he died, I was only 12; I decided I would be his reincarnation. It seemed the noblest thing in the world to do – a person who could heal wounds could do anything, and I still believe it. A person who can heal a wound ought not to do anything else – that's the highest calling and the noblest profession of all. But it is easy to forget all that when you are depressed, anxious, and worried all the time; and on top of it all you are constantly being watched and criticized. It becomes a terrible struggle to continue to marvel at the human spirit and the human body and fight off that terrible demeaning laughter that comes from sleep deprivation and cynicism.

Medical students are so altruistic and humane when they start and then somewhere along the line they lose it, it's beaten out of them. My own training as a surgeon is an example. Training in surgery has traditionally been carried out "en militaire." It was awful when I was in training because the brutality was handed down from the chiefs of surgery all the way to the chief resident and the senior resident, the junior resident, the intern, the medical students, and the nurses. We learned to pass on the brutality because it had been done to us and if you quailed or if you showed any kind of fear or sense of having been embarrassed, then you lost points and you were subject to further ridicule. It was a bad way to become a doctor because it was not humane. You were brutalized emotionally, and sometimes physically, and it still goes on.

My work as a surgeon also ensured that I would be removed from normal emotions. In the operating room the patient is anesthetized in order that he or she feels no pain. In the operating room the surgeon too is in a sense anesthetized in order that he or she be at some emotional remove from the white heat of the event, the laying open of the body of a fellow human being. If you take away the purpose for which this act is being done, you have the act of an assault and battery: it is not a normal act. Surgical training takes so long, because one has to get used to the idea of taking up a knife and cutting people open. The surgeon becomes anesthetized and develops insulation against the emotions that would ordinarily accompany this act. The surgeon dons a kind of carapace, a turtle shell, to be able to do the work dispassionately without panic. No matter what the emergency, hemorrhage, perforation, etc., the surgeon must proceed calmly to the benefit of the patient who is just a little square of flesh; everything else is covered up. Machinery is all around, and in the surgeon's mind that square of flesh is

not so much another human being as a "field of activity." So, you have two anesthetized people – the patient and the surgeon.

My young correspondent already expresses concern about the possible anesthetizing of her own feelings and its effect on her compassion toward her patients. I am encouraged that today's young doctors have a very highly developed sense of compassion. When they dissect the cadaver in the anatomy lab, they keep in mind all the time that this cadaver is a sacred body; this body has a certain holiness. It is from this body that they will learn the art of healing. That reverence was missing from our training. For us, all those years ago in the 1940s, the experience prompted jokes. We shredded up the body and learned anatomy but we felt no further connection. We had no sense that cadavers had been human beings and I think there is new and marvelous awareness. In fact, today at the end of the anatomy year in medical school, many medical students have a funeral service. It is beautiful to me that this is being done. It would never have been done 50 years ago; it would have been laughed off the street.

This respect for a student's "first patient," is evidence to me of the "tendresse" that sometimes exists. I don't know if that word is translatable from the French. It means a combination of tenderness and compassion that I think has entered the profession, along with the entry of women, a great plus because until recently medicine was a male-oriented, macho profession with a dreadful foreign legion mentality. There were always a few women but not anything like what is happening now, when at least half the medical school classes are women. Perhaps they will shift the perspective of medicine so as to encompass the emotions of event.

About 10 years ago I was forced into a personal journey of discovery when a serious illness rendered me comatose and on a ventilator in the intensive care unit of the same hospital where I had practiced surgery. I fell into a coma that was to last for 23 days. As in the Biblical psalm of that number, I walked in the valley of the shadow of death. Although, I am told, my death was a certainty, I unexpectedly turned back from the other side and made a slow, year-long convalescence. I don't think that anyone can emerge from such an experience and be the same as before. I began to feel a very great love for my fellow human beings, particularly those who are afflicted, sick, and helpless as I had been. I understood what it means to be utterly helpless and at the mercy of your own fantasies and of other people's indifference or business. Everyone has priorities and you may not be high up on their list. All of that made me change. I became a person who was aware of the discomforts of my fellow human beings.

During my illness, I had been touched by what James Dickey described as "the superhuman tenderness of strangers." There is a certain natural physical revulsion for other people's wounds and diseases. Certain things we prefer not to touch. The feeling is normal and natural. We wouldn't ordinarily go up and embrace a leper. Helping others requires that we somehow overcome or become inured to this natural distaste and physical revulsion. I realize that people tended my body and perhaps did not want to touch it, because it was not a beautiful or appealing body during my illness. But they did and they saved me and made me feel comfortable and well.

I believe now that I have that full sense of what it means to overcome the revulsion, the recoiling from wounds and smells and all that degradation of the flesh. To do so is very important because without that we have no way of taking care of each other. Caregivers need to have the wisdom to see beyond the wounds of the flesh. Wounds are illuminating; they shed a light that helps you look at the human body as a kind of sacred space. Once, a long time ago, I wrote an essay called "The Exact Location of the Soul." It was a playful literary essay in which I speculated on which part of the body housed the soul. The essay became celebrated. However, now if someone were to ask me with regard to a particular person, the location of the soul, I would examine that person for a

wound because the soul would most likely be there. A wound has a voice that calls out to the wound dresser much as a faithful dog barks to bring help to his master who has fallen in the snow.

I would ask young doctors to think of wounds as illuminating. The body is unique in that the more marred, scarred, and defaced, the more beautiful the body can become. The more tumorous, oozing, and bloody the body, the more vulnerable it is, and love has a clearer avenue to express itself toward what is vulnerable and weak and afflicted.

My main message to the letter's author as well as to readers of this book is: "Never lose the emotion of events which are so often lost in medicine." Everyone will be visited with sorrow, loss, disaster, shame, and humiliation. We are all vulnerable to these aspects of the human condition – patients and doctors alike. One day it will be our child, our parent, and inevitably ourselves looking to others for compassion. Compassion for the suffering of others is sometimes forgotten when we feel persecuted and driven to the limits of our endurance, but I think it is necessary to remember that those feelings are peripheral and not the central issue of a medical career.

Oh yes, I want to tell her that I too suffered through a residency, and that I know full well what she is enduring, but it is nothing compared to the suffering of her patients. They are the ones who are heroic. The charts she writes in every day are stories of which her patients are the heroes.

Richard Selzer

On caring for patients

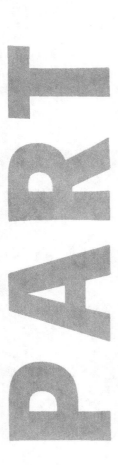

One of the essential qualities of the clinician is interest in humanity, for the secret of the care of the patient is in caring for the patient.

Francis Peabody (1)

I wouldn't demand a lot of my doctor's time; I just wish he would *brood* on my situation for perhaps five minutes, that he would give me his whole mind just once. I would like to think of him as going through my character, as he goes through my flesh, to get at my illness, for each man is ill in his own way . . . Just as he orders blood tests and bone scans of my body, I'd like my doctors to scan *me*, to grope for my spirit as well as my prostate.

Anatole Broyard (2)

When does a doctor become a doctor? We queried doctors from a wide range of specialties, age groups, and geographical locations and asked them to describe what marks the transition: What event or events must transpire in order to turn a "civilian" into a professional? Initially, they recited moments that signified "official" recognition, such as: "When I received the white coat" or "At my graduation" or "When I received my license." However, the real significance of such external signposts is captured in one doctor's story of the day he realized "the power of the white coat:"

I started the "Physical Diagnosis" class at my medical school just as I had completed most of my basic sciences courses. The class was taught by the chief of medicine, one of the best clinicians I've ever known. The first day set the format for the course. A patient was introduced and in front of the one hundred assembled medical students, the chief of medicine interviewed the patient and performed a physical exam. The patient was thanked and escorted off before he asked for the laboratory work. He then proceeded to discuss the diagnosis and a little about the disease. He was a great teacher and his presentation was incredibly illustrative.

Also on the first day of class, a noted pharmaceutical company issued all the students black bags with our names on them (I still carry mine), along with an inexpensive stethoscope, a flex hammer and a tuning fork. We were also given white coats. Thus outfitted, we were immediately able to work for attending physicians at a hospital two miles away doing pre-operative physicals and histories for $25.00 per patient. I had been making leather purses and belts to get myself through medical school and, since a leather belt took me 3 or 4 hours to make and sold for around $25.00, I thought "this is financial heaven."

At three o'clock that same afternoon, knowing nothing except what had been presented that morning in class, I got on my bicycle with my new white coat and black bag and rode across town to the hospital where they handed me a list of seven patients. I located the rooms of these seven patients, most scheduled for elective hysterectomies, introducing myself as I went, telling them I was there to do their physical exams for their surgery the next day, and asking them to remove their clothing. I had taken good notes in class and I proceeded to do all the things my professor had done in the order and fashion I had witnessed. The patients thanked me and, except for my self-conscious awkwardness when one of the patients turned out to be a young woman my own age, I felt the afternoon had gone smoothly.

Later that warm summer evening when I was riding my bicycle home, the coat tails of my new white coat flapping in the breeze and clutching my black bag, I began to think, "My God, I can't believe what I have just done. I ask people to remove their clothes, tell me their most private confidences, and examine their bodies. All the while I stand there fully clothed revealing nothing, and, instead of calling for my arrest, they thank me." It was amazing! I knew I had crossed a threshold. Inside I was different in some way. I had all the vestments and I recognized how the role worked, although I wasn't yet up to assuming the role. I didn't feel like a doctor because, even though I could convince others, I wasn't convinced myself. The experiences that day taught me I was ready to play at being a doctor, but I was still an apprentice.

All the physicians we spoke with believed that becoming a doctor by fiat, or proclamation, or external trappings counted far less than the progressive metamorphosis that transpired as they assumed increasingly more responsibility for patients. Many responded by saying that they *felt* they were physicians, "When the first patient for whom I actually had responsibility died under my care," or "When my first patient recovered from a dreaded illness." As one physician explained, "For me, it wasn't a case of one day I wasn't a doctor and the next day I was. Rather, it was a progression of markers, each one bringing me one step closer to assuming the whole, rather than the partial, professional mantle." Another commented, "When I was an intern the very first patient I saw was very sick and I remember thinking, 'This man needs a doctor!' – then saying to myself 'You can't do that anymore.'" He concluded, "You are a doctor when you realize you are IT for this patient, when you are the person who has spent time talking to the patient, who knows the most about the patient, and become the person others look to for vital information." One physician summed up the feelings of many when he explained, "There comes a time when patients become *yours*, when you can say 'This is *my* patient and not someone else's patient.' For me this happened during my residency. Colleagues recognize you as the patient's doctor and respect that relationship. At the same time, the patient looks to you as his or her doctor. You have become more than just the name on their insurance card."

The crucible, or "professional cooking pot" according to one physician's description, of this professional development is the wards where students are afforded their first opportunity to care for patients. Finally, after time spent in lectures and laboratories the reason most people cite for choosing medicine is at hand. Little wonder that memories of venturing onto the wards and becoming part of a patient's care leave an indelible impression.

Remembering his first ward experience, another physician, now teaching medical students, recounts:

Physicians have their own experiences about when they first thought of themselves as starting to care for patients. Mine came when my medical school program sent me to the hospital when I had been studying medicine for 9 months. I remember distinctly walking into the hospital and finding the room number where I was supposed to interview a patient. Within 20 minutes of our encounter, the patient had leaped out of bed, locked herself in the bathroom and was crying hysterically. Not only had I failed at filling out my 10 page write-up for my patient exam, but I had actually "broken" the patient. Inadvertently, I had asked questions in such a way that forced her to face extremely painful subjects; consequently, she felt she had to extricate herself from the situation. Eventually, the patient emerged from the bathroom, we resumed the interview, and I was able to complete my assignment; but certainly, for me, this experience raised the point right at the beginning as to what physicians are taking on when we attempt to care for patients – often, as in my case, with far less than adequate preparation and training.

First experiences of learning to care for patients form the foundation for future relations, models to be avoided or emulated. Recalling his time as a medical student at a major Mid-Western Charity Hospital, a physician says, "We participated in the care of patients much more than is typical for medical students today. For example, the hospital was so understaffed that part of the experience was emptying bed pans. If the medical students hadn't done it, it wouldn't have gotten done. This task was part of the notion of responsibility in taking care of someone and doing what needs to be done. It was an important step in my understanding of what it means to care for patients."

It is important to note that "caring for patients" is approached by medical trainees in different ways. There are those who see no special issues in doctor–patient interactions. Their response is "What's the problem here? Just learn all there is to know about the basic science, introduction to medicine, ward politics, surgical procedures – combine them all together with the proper neurological filters and you've got patient care – you are caring for patients." These trainees will approach patients with the same view reflected in the comments of a well-known hand surgeon to his colleagues as they prepared for surgery, "I would really like to have an examining room with a partition down the middle with two holes just big enough for the patients to put their hands through. I don't need anything else. The rest is just getting in the way." Although delivered in a jocular manner, his words reflect his belief that he would have been as good a surgeon, or better, if he could just focus on the hands of the patient and not have to contend with the attached person.

A similar attitude was met by a third year medical student on the obstetrics and gynecology service at a county hospital. It was his duty to see women for their yearly physical exams. These exams included taking a sexual and menstrual history and performing a Papanicolaou smear. As was the routine on most services at the institution, the student completed his task, including cardiac and pulmonary auscultation. He described one afternoon when:

Following my initial examination of a patient in for an annual exam, I presented the case to a fifth year chief resident. When I reached the point where I described my cardiac findings to him as, "the patient has an irregular heartbeat," he stopped me abruptly and asked why I was listening to patients' hearts. I told him that this was an annual exam and that, given the nature of the population we served at this clinic, we were likely to be the only medical professionals she would see over the year. He frowned and bent his left arm at the elbow and, palm flattened to the ground, positioned his hand at the epigastrium as if to indicate a transverse plane through his abdomen. Then he took his right hand, and in similar fashion, with palm upright, he placed it at the region of the mid-thigh, medially, below his inseam. He had demarcated an imaginary box and he moved his hands back and forth in gesticulation while saying, "You see this space? This is what we are interested in here. Do not listen to any more patients' hearts." He ended by chuckling and predicting I would end up in family medicine.

This chief resident's comfortable confinement of issues fails to appreciate a crucial distinction that determines focus and colors the philosophy of patient care – the distinction drawn by Francis Peabody between "care *of*" and "care *for*" with regard to patients. The first is what often preoccupies physicians in training, i.e., worrying over the details of proper medical management, its proper execution, its follow-up, and the medical skills required. These concerns dominate many of the cases in Part I as trainees are requested to perform some action about which they feel either uncomfortable or unqualified. Each time a medical trainee begins to practice a new skill, the discomfort and feelings of inadequacy naturally arise. The trainees therefore become concerned on the one hand about the proper care *of* the patients, and on the other about not appearing to resist learning new skills.

The second sense of care, caring *for* patients, involves our moral life as well as standards developed in medical ethics. It is Peabody's point that caring *for* patients makes possible the best care *of* patients. Ironically, trainees are sometimes better able to identify a quandary than are those in authority. However, by raising ethical dilemmas trainees may feel they are treading on unsure ground and challenging the moral authority of their role model professors. Granted the general assumption that the caregiver's primary obligation is to the patient, how does this principle apply to doctors in training? Where do one's loyalties lie? Maintaining one's ethical compass on the wards is enough to challenge even the most committed humanitarian.

As the cases in Part I demonstrate, physicians in training are sometimes confronted with situations in which they are required to perform activities that to them seem to be in conflict with their perceived role and commitment to patients. Once on the wards, for example, the question of "Informed Consent" arises quickly and requires careful reflection about what exactly it is that patients have a right to know. A "one size fits all" answer will not do, and varying circumstances further muddy already opaque waters. A dilemma that is far from clear involves whether or not a trainee's experience with a specific procedure, or lack of it, is relevant to a patient's granting a truly informed consent.

A special set of moral problems involves truth-telling, and the related issue of promise-keeping, where there is some conflict between the precept that one ought to tell the truth and some other prominent ethical directive. Few, if any, moral philosophers would admonish us to always "tell the truth, the whole truth, and nothing but the truth." Inevitably, there will be situations that challenge a *prima facie* duty for honesty; for example, the medical trainee may be unsure whether, and to what degree, the patient needs the information, or to what extent others are owed disclosure. To what degree is a trainee responsible for a colleague's sins of omissions or commissions with regard to the truth? What needs to be examined is: When, if ever, do circumstances and conditions justify departures from the truth?

Other specters that haunt trainees involve direct confrontations with their own lack of coping skills, either due to unanticipated events, unforeseen circumstances, or to a breakdown in receiving adequate preparation. Trainees are then faced with the dilemma of meeting the demand of their duties without "making waves," and gaining a reputation as a "difficult person" on that rotation.

A further challenge of caring for patients is the difficulty in setting individual boundaries, in situations when inappropriate advances are put forward by patients, or when trainees are confronted with patients they do not like and for whom sympathy is difficult. Temptations are part of human interactions. If caring for a patient is returned by the patient with an intimate overture, despite prohibitions, ordinary temptations can be amplified. There is also the opposite challenge of developing appropriate personal and professional boundaries in caring for patients when the overriding emotions are negative. Not all patients are likeable or even manageable. How far does the requirement to care for patients expand one's commitments into possible dysfunctional lives?

One of the most troubling issues for trainees in Part I involves the limits of compassion. Should caring have a limit? How far is too far? How much is too much? With all good intent, sensitivity, and pity towards the suffering patient medical trainees can sometimes become overinvolved to the point good care and necessary professional objectivity dissolve. Their first exposure to the tragic lives of families with compromised newborns is especially distressing for some interested in pediatrics. At what point does the virtue of compassion, a virtue in any physician, slip into the vice of excessive involvement that fails to help the patient? Without boundary preparation, guidance, and practice there is the danger that young physicians will either acquire habits of overextending themselves and therefore jeopardize the objectivity necessary for optimum care, or they will retreat and erect barriers that exclude the patient. Examples of individuals whose boundaries are either too wide or too restricted are all too familiar.

Since the cases presented in the following pages are offered by trainees themselves, it is clear that the moral instincts of doctors in training are often spot-on. These situations bothered them, and for good reason. Nonetheless, despite the best goals of medical education, the reality is that their reservations are often shunted aside and they are made to understand that their quandaries are really scruples that should not be raised – and, indeed, may interfere with the business at hand. This seems the greatest tragedy. Although medical education reports to aim at the good of the patient, the moral life of its trainees is commonly ignored.

Trainees attest that from the beginning of their life on the wards, their moral life is plagued with internal struggles, self-doubts, frustrations, disillusionments, and even despair: What is my justification? How can I take on this awesome responsibility? What right do I have to listen to, and act on, a patient's innermost confidences? Won't I make a mistake? – all the misgivings that add up to what one interviewee describes as the trainee's chronic condition – "fear and loathing on the wards." Preoccupied for so long with their scientific studies, it often comes as a surprise that, as one physician told us, "It's easy to find out the basic knowledge, information, and scientific studies. The really hard part that is pitifully neglected is what *ought* to guide our interactions with patients." Those ethical issues that arise as students and doctors in training struggle to relate to patients and not to diseases form the heart of the cases and their analyses that follow.

Notes

1 Peabody F. The care of the patient. *JAMA* 1927;877:88. Reprinted in *Connecticut Med* 1976;545:40.
2 Broyard A. Doctor, talk to me. – *New York Times Magazine,* August 26, 1990.

Performing procedures

There comes a time when neophytes, in any field, must begin to practice the theory they have been taught. Coping with insecurity is a common response to the feeling that no one is available to clarify expectations and oversee performance. What distinguishes medicine from most other fields is that, despite intentions with the highest ideal of beneficence, the danger of harming the patient is an ever-present reality. Doctors, even beginning doctors, hold the lives of patients in their trust.

The cases in this section raise the following questions: What is the responsibility of trainees when directed by supervisors to perform procedures to which patients have not clearly consented? Does a patient have the "right to know" the trainee's inexperience? What constitutes benefit to the patient as opposed to benefit to the provider?

Also, confidence and trust are at the core of the special relationship between doctor and patient. Without the assurance that intensely private information learned from or about patients will remain private, physicians cannot expect patients to tell them the truth. However, there are limits to confidentiality. How should the responsibilities of respecting privacy and confidentiality be weighed against other countervailing principles?

Further, what are the ethics of learning technical skills on patients who have recently died? Are postmortem procedures not permissible if prior consent is not obtained from relatives? Does such a requirement disregard society's interest in having an optimal number of medical care providers experienced in life-saving techniques?

The responsibility of informing

Implications of physician experience

CASE

"First time"

I was a senior fellow under the supervision of Dr. M when a situation arose regarding informed consent. Mr. W had been hospitalized 4 days earlier and was increasingly concerned that Dr. M's search to find the reason for his mysterious set of symptoms, including three consultations with colleagues, had been unsuccessful. He was convinced he had undergone almost every diagnostic procedure imaginable.

Dr. M agreed with a recommendation that a liver biopsy be performed. She carefully explained all the reasons for doing the procedure, emphasized the potentially helpful information it could produce, and described the possible complications. She also discussed what few alternatives were available and the relative advantages and disadvantages of each one, but she concluded by noting they were unlikely to produce very useful information.

Having confidence in Dr. M's clinical judgment, Mr. W stated he was willing to have the liver biopsy. At that point, Dr. M mentioned that, as her senior fellow, she would like me to perform the procedure. She informed Mr. W that she would be present during the liver biopsy, and he gave consent.

However, Dr. M did not tell Mr. W that this was the first time I would be doing this procedure, nor did he ask about my previous experience. This situation prompted a number of unasked questions in my mind:

1. Is it truly informed consent if a patient gives authorization without knowledge of the physician's competency as measured, at least in part, by past experience?
2. Is it reasonable to presume that every teaching hospital patient implicitly or explicitly consents to being treated by less experienced staff and tacitly accepts the risks and benefits of being in a teaching hospital?
3. Is it appropriate to inform a patient when a procedure is being performed for the first time? How much "practice" should be considered sufficient to make it unnecessary to acknowledge limited experience?
4. Was it my responsibility to inform the patient of my inexperience?

COMMENTARY

William Nelson and Paul B. Hofmann

Apparently Dr. M has developed a good relationship with Mr. W and is actively pursuing the diagnosis of his health care problem. However, after three consultations, a definitive diagnosis is still lacking. Dr. M accepts a suggestion from one colleague regarding the need for a liver biopsy. In seeking Mr. W's permission for a liver biopsy, Dr. M employed a predictable and common approach, one consistent with informed consent procedures in many teaching hospitals. Unfortunately, although customary and usual, this typical arrangement deserves serious reconsideration. This issue cannot be dismissed as a trivial matter; indeed, a valid consent and refusal process is one of the cornerstones of clinical ethics.

The central ethical issue being raised in this case is whether Dr. M provided adequate information to facilitate Mr. W's ability to give valid consent for the liver biopsy procedure. We believe the patient gave consent, but it was not valid. A valid consent or refusal requires that several basic criteria be satisfied. (1)

First, the patient must have decision-making capacity. This case does not present any information to suggest that the patient's decision-making capacity was a concern or was impaired to make this specific medical decision. It would seem reasonable to assume, as clinicians generally should, that this patient was competent in the absence of evidence to the contrary.

The second criterion for valid consent or refusal is the lack of coercion. Obviously coercion, undue force or pressure that would inhibit Mr. W from making an autonomous decision, is not directly present, such as, "If you do not consent to that liver biopsy, you will never be admitted to this hospital in the future."

Nevertheless, a subtle form of coercion was used. The mere framing of information can unduly influence the way a patient responds to the content. More often than not, such framing is intended to elicit a reply corresponding to what the physician has decided is the proper course of action. This is different from a physician giving his or her opinion about a procedure. If the patient is receptive, the physician can recommend a particular option and explain the rationale, but this recommendation should clearly be separated from a value-free presentation of the facts, including the risks and benefits. Ultimately, the patient's own values and desires should determine what course is taken. In our view, the manner in which Dr. M framed the information was designed to acquire an affirmative response.

Valid consent or refusal requires adequate information. On the surface, it appears that Dr. M covered all the issues. She explained the need for performing the procedure, reviewed the advantages and disadvantages of the proposed procedure and remaining alternatives, and described possible complications. Mr. W said he was willing to have the biopsy, at least partly based upon his confidence in Dr. M. It is at this point that she mentions that a senior fellow will be performing the procedure.

Conspicuous by its absence was any reference to the senior fellow's lack of previous experience in doing a liver biopsy. Withholding such information is supported by conventional wisdom because physicians in training must acquire skills to become adept professionals, and it is assumed that few patients would knowingly agree to have a novice "practice" on them. This position was defended further by emphasizing that a senior physician would be present during the procedure. Additionally, others argue that patients admitted to teaching hospitals are generally aware that physicians in training, from medical students to senior fellows, are providing direct patient care, including performing invasive procedures even though they may lack experience.

However, one study indicates that the majority of patients may not be aware that students in training are involved in their care. With specific reference to the consent issue, the study determined "that only 37 percent of all responding teaching hospitals specifically informed patients that students would be involved in their care." The authors concluded that "the ethical requirement of informed consent was incomplete." (2) We do not believe that patients inherently know who are students and which physicians are not experienced.

Unquestionably, young physicians must have an opportunity to develop and refine their skills. Most patients, however, would be reluctant to allow an inexperienced physician to perform his or her first procedure on them. Nonetheless, some patients would agree if they were assured that a senior physician would be physically present and would closely monitor the procedure. What is crucial in the ethical assessment of this case is whether useful and important information was omitted during the informed consent process. We believe it was.

Despite the presentation of customary information, under the circumstances it was not adequate. Complication rates for invasive procedures are foreseeably higher when performed by less-than-experienced physicians. When the complications are delineated in the literature, they are based on the performance of experienced physicians. For example, in a basic textbook, *Diseases of the Liver*, the authors note, "We are convinced that the procedures should be carried out only in institutions in which physicians are experienced with the technique, are aware of the risk entailed, and observe the patients closely for at least 8 hours after the procedure." (3) In view of an unequivocal recommendation to engage an experienced physician, suppressing this information is unethical. When Dr. M excluded relevant information, nondisclosure compromised Mr. W's ability to make an informed valid decision. Clinicians have an implicit obligation to preserve and enhance this basic moral and legal concept.

A fourth criterion for valid consent or refusal is understanding. The patient may be competent, the decision may be voluntary, and adequate information may be provided, but there must also be comprehension. Because hospitals are intimidating institutions, patients feel inhibited and apprehensive; therefore, they are more likely to be reticent and disinclined to ask questions for clarification, sometimes from reluctance to delay a rushing clinician or from fear of appearing obtuse. While nothing suggested Mr. W failed to comprehend what he was told, physicians must remain constantly vigilant to avoid overestimating patient knowledge. Again, the most significant concern in this case is the likely presumption on Dr. M's part that Mr. W should have understood

that a teaching hospital patient is somehow routinely, consciously, and silently supposed to allow the performance of invasive procedures by inexperienced physicians.

When a physician conceals relevant information from a patient, the decision frequently has long-term effects. If an inexperienced physician performs the procedure, the fact may become known, particularly should a complication occur. If and when Mr. W learns that crucial information was withheld, he could become very upset about the specific decision-making process and his overall confidence and trust in Dr. M could be adversely affected. Mr. W may begin to wonder what else she has not told him. When physicians, and people in general, withhold information or deceive others, such eventualities frequently appear and have the potential for producing a long-lasting negative impact. Because patients commonly share their experiences and anxieties with others, both Dr. M and the hospital could be maligned.

We are also cognizant of a closely related rationalization used to justify nondisclosure. Teaching hospitals may assert that they could not fulfill their academic or community service mission if inexperienced physicians were not permitted relatively unrestricted access to "teaching patients." This argument raises fundamental issues about the priorities of these institutions and whose goals and values should take precedence in the informed consent process. A hospital's primary mission is to provide appropriate, timely, and cost-effective patient care. While acknowledging the additional goals of education and research for teaching hospitals, these organizations should be committed first to delivering the best possible care, including the provision of honest and complete information regarding proposed procedures and treatments. Patients assume that physicians will be their advocates, and they do not expect that their needs will be subordinated to those of inexperienced clinicians. Undoubtedly, some people will be reluctant to permit a physician to perform a procedure for the first time, but such a decision is the patient's prerogative.

A hospital and physician's values and perceptions are certainly germane, but the patient must retain the prerogative to choose among the options after full disclosure. One should not rationalize that this moral concept can or should be sacrificed to serve a hospital's teaching mission.

Howard Brody tells a superb story of the medical student who "violated" the instructions of her patient's attending physician by admitting to the family that their relative was dying. (Coincidentally, this patient's terminal condition was the direct result of complications associated with a liver biopsy.) During the chief of medicine's extended reprimand of the medical student, he gave an eloquent and disturbing defense of medical paternalism. In part, he said, (4)

The masses fear sickness and death, and want the doctor to abolish those fears. The doctor who tells them that they have the power to choose in the face of sickness and death and who encourages them to choose, fills them with anguish. The message of freedom, for the millions in their desperation, is the most empty and hopeless message they can hear. They have no confidence in their own wisdom, their own resources, to pull them through. They look to the doctor to have all the power, to make all the choices, to be free to act for them.

Medical paternalism has been the subject of innumerable articles and debate. But some observers have decried the movement to unbounded patient autonomy and self-determination. (5) How much information is really required to permit fully informed consent? At a minimum, informed consent compels a description of risks and benefits of the proposed and alternative procedures. Clearly, there is greater risk to the patient if an invasive procedure is performed by a novice, regardless of supervision by a more experienced physician.

Rationalizing that complications occur infrequently and are "relatively" benign, illustrates how health professionals may unintentionally conspire to withhold relevant information from patients. From a physician's perspective, for example, minor pain and discomfort associated with a nasogastric tube might not be worth mentioning. However, speak to an Ear, Nose, and Throat specialist who has personally experienced one, and it becomes quickly apparent that his or her subsequent language in obtaining a patient's consent has been indelibly influenced.

In reviewing all these factors, we do not believe that Dr. M was justified in withholding the information that an inexperienced physician would be performing the liver biopsy. The patient should have been so informed, along with the strong reassurance that close supervision would occur, so that he could give a valid informed consent or refusal.

Recognizing this situation does raise some very complex issues, ones that many attending physicians may not have fully considered. The senior fellow should have discussed the subject with Dr. M prior to her conversation with the patient. Because the prevailing practice does not involve complete disclosure of relevant experience, the senior fellow should also have spoken with Dr. M about the hospital's current policy pertaining to informed consent procedures and suggested the policy be reviewed to determine the need for possible revisions.

Notes

1 Gert B, Nelson WA, Culver CM. Moral theory and neurology. *Ethical Issues in Neurologic Clinics* 1989;7:681–96.
2 Cohen DL, McCullough LB, Kessel RWI, Apostolidea AY, Alden ER, Heiderich KJ. Informed consent policies governing medical students interaction with patients. *J Med Educ* 1987;62:789–98.
3 Schiff L, Schiff ER. Needle biopsy of the liver. In *Diseases of the Liver*, ed. L. Schiff & E.R. Schiff, JB Lippincott, Philadelphia, 1993, p. 223.
4 Brody H. The chief of medicine. *Hastings Cent Rep* 1991;21:17–22 (p. 19).
5 Special Section: Beyond Autonomy. *Camb Q Healthc Ethics* 1995;4(1):459–62.

COMMENTARY

Robert L. Schwartz

Over the past quarter of a century most U.S. state courts have rationalized the law of informed consent, which now generally reflects the ethical principles upon which it is based. While some states still apply the anachronistic "reasonable physician" test and require only that physicians provide their patients with the information that other reasonable physicians would provide under the circumstances, a small majority of the states now apply the "reasonable patient" test in informed consent cases. Under this articulation of the physicians' duty to inform, a physician is required to provide the patient with the information that a reasonable patient would want, under the circumstances, about the proposed medical treatment and its risks, benefits, and alternatives.

A legal action for informed consent also requires that the patient prove that the failure to provide adequate information actually caused the patient's injury. Most states now interpret this causation requirement in objective terms, and they require that a patient show that a reasonable patient would not have undergone the proposed medical treatment if the information that was alleged to have been withheld had been divulged. Thus, even when a patient *can* show that a physician breached a duty to provide adequate information, an informed consent action will not be successful unless it is shown that a reasonable patient would have chosen to forgo the proposed treatment if presented with the information.

In this case, the law would first ask whether the physician breached her duty to the patient by failing to reveal that the biopsy would be performed by a physician who had never before performed one. Under the "reasonable physician" standard, the question would be whether any other reasonable physicians failed to provide this information in similar circumstances. Because this information is rarely (if ever) provided,

under this increasingly disused test there would be no obligation to provide the patient with this information.

On the other hand, under the majority "reasonable patient" rule, the question would be whether a reasonable patient would want to have this information in order to make a decision about whether to have the proposed liver biopsy. Most of us have little difficulty concluding that this information would be relevant to our decision to have the biopsy performed as proposed – at least as long as we have the option of having another, more experienced physician perform it – and thus the failure to provide this information would be a breach of the physician's duty to adequately inform the patient. In either case, if we were to conclude that a reasonable patient would choose to undergo the liver biopsy as proposed even if the missing information about the senior fellow's experience were to have been provided, then the physician will not be liable for failure to obtain informed consent because the patient would not be able to prove that the physician's breach actually caused any injury to the patient.

Here the plaintiff's case is bolstered by speculation about why Dr. M did not provide Mr. W with the information about the senior fellow's experience. She wanted him to have the biopsy (perhaps because she believed it to be in his best interest) and she wanted her senior fellow to develop experience in doing this kind of medical work, but she feared that Mr. W would withhold his consent if she provided this information. That is, she knew that this information would be material to this reasonable patient. Here the physician's interest in the therapeutic value of the treatment is tempered, at least, by her independent and potentially conflicting interest in training her fellow. Where the physician has such a potential conflict of interest, it is especially important that the patient be given all of the information that he would deem important in consenting to a treatment. It would hardly be surprising under these circumstances, for the patient to feel defrauded if he later found out that such information was withheld. Dr. M's actions are not so different from the "ghost surgery" that was common 25 years ago, when surgeons would get consent to do surgery that would actually be performed by a substitute surgeon whose identity was never revealed to the patient. The law has now soundly rejected the propriety of ghost surgery, even when the substitute surgeon is competent to perform the work.

The fact that this procedure was being performed at a teaching hospital is not relevant to the outcome of the informed consent analysis. Patients admitted to teaching hospitals do not understand that they will be the subject of trial and error by students, and any general consent to being used as a teaching prop is probably itself illegal. In any case, such a consent does not supplant a specific consent given to a particular treatment. It may be that indigent patients, who are often treated at teaching hospitals, do not have the option of choosing to have the procedure performed by another, more experienced physician. This is a problem with our increasingly finance-dependent two (or more) tiered health care system, but it does not change the obligation of the physician to obtain informed consent. An indigent patient may not be able to find another physician to do the biopsy, but he still has the option of forgoing the biopsy altogether or of trying to convince Dr. M, or another experienced physician, to do it herself.

The application of the doctrine of informed consent to patients in teaching hospitals need not be an impediment to teaching and learning, or to good patient care. Instead of figuring out how much information she could keep from her patient, Dr. M would have better served her patient and her student by honestly and openly providing the patient with information about the senior fellow's experience. Dr. M also could have informed Mr. W that she would be present through the entire procedure, that she would direct the medical treatment, and that she would actively participate with the senior fellow in performing the biopsy. She could have explicitly addressed the question of whether his inexperience put the patient at risk, and how she intended to protect him from that risk. Patients are as altruistic as physicians, overall, and they are likely to be willing to participate in medical training as long as they are assured that there is adequate backup present, and that their own risks are minimized. Until a physician has enough experience performing a procedure so that a reasonable patient would not consider the physician's inexperience to be material in deciding whether to undergo that procedure, the patient is entitled to know of that inexperience and any protection or supervision that will be provided by the physician's supervisors, colleagues, or teachers.

Finally, the responsibility to assure that a properly informed consent has been obtained falls squarely on the physician doing the procedure that is the subject of the consent. Thus, if the senior fellow will be doing the biopsy, the senior fellow has the obligation to make certain that the patient has been explained the material risks and benefits of that treatment and understands the alternatives. This does not mean that the physician performing the procedure must personally provide the information to the patient or obtain the patient's formal consent; those duties can be delegated to another physician, a nurse, a consent team, or anyone else competent to explain the risks, benefits, and alternatives of the proposed care and evaluate the capacity of the patient to give consent. In this case, most of the information appears to have been provided, appropriately, by Dr. M. If any necessary information has not been provided to the patient, however, or if the process is otherwise legally deficient, responsibility will lie at the door of the senior fellow, who is the one who will actually do the biopsy.

COMMENTARY

Neal Cohen

This case presents a number of interesting and challenging ethical issues regarding informed consent, medical staff privileges, and responsibilities for physician education and training. Some of the questions posed are more easily addressed than others. The issues of informed consent relative to medical student, resident, and fellow training, for example, are similar to other concerns regarding informed consent and have been addressed in many educational settings. Those issues related to physician credentialing and competence, as well as those related to delivery of innovative services, are more complex. In the era of managed care in the United States, the challenges posed by the case presented are even greater. In an effort to limit physician panels, payers are now requiring a minimum level of experience in order to credential practitioners and reimburse them for procedures. At the same time, primary care providers often find themselves in the position of having to perform diagnostic and therapeutic procedures for which they may have little or no recent training or for which their training was obtained in the distant past.

First, the ethical issues posed relate to the responsibility to inform the patient of the level of experience of the provider and disseminate sufficient information to the patient so that he or she can make an educated decision about proceeding. With sufficient information, patients can determine for themselves the level of risk they are willing to take and the potential benefits they might gain. There is the suggestion that the majority of patients would decline to have a procedure performed by an "inexperienced" physician. In many cases, I think this is correct. On the other hand, many patients agree to undergo innovative treatments such as fetal surgical procedures, repair of congenital heart abnormalities, and transplantation, all of which are innovative and represent evolving technology and

experience. Under these circumstances, providing a clear indication of the physician's experience with the procedure to be performed, its risks, benefits, and alternatives can be challenging. Many times the specific procedure performed has never been done before, either by the physician caring for the patient or, in some cases, by anyone. The extent to which patients and their families understand this is variable. Nonetheless, patients frequently agree to proceed.

With respect to the educational issues raised by the case, many of the concerns expressed are dealt with in teaching hospitals on a daily basis. The case as presented does not sufficiently emphasize the importance of supervision and teaching of residents and fellows. The fact that the senior fellow performed the procedure is not as important as the need to have appropriate supervision, guidance, and direction. The patient was not consenting to a procedure performed by the fellow, but was relying on the clinical judgment and experience of Dr. M. Most patients cared for in teaching hospitals understand the value of care provided in that setting and the role they play in educating medical students and physicians in training. They depend, however, on the judgment and experience of the attending physicians, not only in performing procedures, but also in supervising trainees and ensuring that the procedures they perform are done in ways to minimize complications.

Some of the concerns expressed relating to informed consent in teaching hospitals must also be addressed by not only emphasizing the role trainees will play in the clinical service to be provided, but also the risks and complications of procedures performed in that institution, one in which trainees participate. The risks and complications may in fact be less in a teaching hospital than in a community hospital. For example, is the risk greater when a procedure is performed by a senior fellow supervised by an experienced attending physician in a teaching hospital than when performed by a private practitioner who has done the procedure, such as a liver biopsy, only once a year? For a patient to make an informed decision, he or she must not only be made aware of the experience of the physician holding the needle, but also of the additional support, teaching, and guidance that are used to ensure that the procedure is done correctly.

The issues of competence and experience of trainees are not the only clinical issues raised by this case. Equally important is the credentialing process for physicians in general. In the United States, accrediting agencies, both federal and state, are mandating that the credentialing process include an assessment of recent experience. The Joint Commission on Accreditation of Healthcare Organizations (JCAHO) has emphasized that credentials committees must document that they have assessed competence related to each clinical privilege. In the case of liver biopsy, for example, the credentials committee and clinical chair must assess not only the complication rate, but must also determine a sufficient number of biopsies were performed to ensure the expertise of the provider. This monitoring requirement becomes complicated when a sufficient number of procedures may have been done in the past, but the recent experience is limited. Should a physician who has performed only one liver biopsy in the past 12 months maintain the privilege to do so? Does it matter that the physician has successfully performed hundreds of the procedures in the past? Should a general surgeon who has not performed a pediatric hernia repair since his training maintain credential to do so? How is competence ensured in this situation? What should a patient or family be told about the skills and experience of the physician?

Finally, in the era of managed care, payers are also playing a role in defining who should perform procedures and the level of experience necessary to maintain specific privileges. For a variety of reasons, managed care organizations are attempting to limit their panel of physicians. This policy reduces a patient's options to select the most experienced provider. In a capitated payment system, primary care providers have a financial incentive to perform procedures themselves that they might in the past have referred to other more experienced specialists.

In summary, this brief case presents many ethical issues in addition to those related to the challenges regarding informed consent in an educational institution. At the same time, as we acknowledge the difficulties inherent in the informed consent process, we cannot lose sight of our responsibility to ensure that patients have the information necessary to make educated decisions. The challenge to the clinician is to determine how much information the patient requires to be well informed.

Special vulnerabilities

CASE

"Who was really benefiting from the multiple exams?"

We were in a rural hospital in India, the chief of medicine, two junior doctors, three first year interns and myself, an American medical student of Indian extraction. The patient was an 80-year-old man, who spoke no English, and had come to the clinic from the countryside. The chief of medicine was performing a rectal exam to rule out prostate cancer when he said, "Wow! This is big." "Get your gloves on and feel this!" One by one all seven of us followed the chief and inserted our fingers into his rectum. I don't know if any of the others were as disturbed by this event as I was.

I saw an elderly man, embarrassed by what he was being subjected to, and to whom nothing had been explained. He was a man whose life had encompassed the history of British colonialism with all its social consequences. The medical system had been set up by the British and even today physicians are seen as vestiges of this strict hierarchy. Physicians, even non-British ones, are viewed as the seat of power, not to be questioned or trusted, but always obeyed. I knew I needed the experience in the procedure, but no one had explained anything to the patient, much less asked for his consent. Who was really benefiting from the multiple exams?

CASE

"Hey, you want to drain an abscess?"

In surgery clinic one afternoon, I was waiting to get another patient when the chief resident came into the consult room and said, "Hey, you want to drain an abscess?" "Sure," I replied, anxious to get some experience in a procedure I would have to know how to do and also anxious not to alienate my chief. As we walked into the room, the chief said, "I'll guide you through the whole thing, this one is very superficial, it shouldn't be a problem." We entered the room and he began to describe the procedure to me: lots of local anesthetic and then a small incision to drain the pus, then pack with gauze.

Before we began the patient was already thanking us and telling us how much the abscess hurt. The more the patient spoke, the more I realized that she was developmentally delayed. She was a woman in her 30s but her speech suggested a person in her early teens. The chief described the procedure to her and she again expressed her thanks. At this time I realized the abscess was on the patient's left breast about 2 inches from the nipple. The chief continued to describe the procedure as I gathered the equipment. Together we anesthetized the area; after which he turned to me and said, "Now make an incision about 2 cm long" as he outlined the place. I made a superficial incision that was not deep enough. He put his hand over mine and made a deeper one. The pus drained and we packed the wound with gauze. Again, the patient thanked us and vowed never again to place her wallet in her bra. We reassured her that a reoccurrence was unlikely.

Several areas trouble me: Considering the pa-

tient came to the hospital by herself (although on the advice of her mother) should she be considered sufficiently competent to consent? Also, did the patient need to know that I had never drained an abscess on an awake patient? I admit I was less willing to express my reservations knowing that if I refused I would miss learning a skill I needed to have. I may have been overly excited to finally have the opportunity to do something with my hands after many days in the operating room of just holding a retractor and not being spoken to.

CASE

"Medically correct, but an ethical catastrophe"

I was an intern in a French hospital. One of the patients in the ward was an HIV-infected man in a very bad condition. He was in septic shock and the question was raised as to whether care should be withdrawn. The attending was a man who was very taciturn and seldom engaged in the team discussions. On this occasion he waited until lunch time when the nurses and interns were away and he withdrew all support. Then he left. There had been no discussion, no informed consent. When we returned the patient was dead. At that moment, the patient's family arrived and the rest of us, house staff and nursing staff, had to cope with a very bad situation.

This attending believed that doctors must be able to make life and death decisions and assume responsibility for "playing God." He was convinced that he acted in the patient's best interest. Although I did not take issue with his medical conclusion, the way the situation was mishandled created an ethical catastrophe.

I talked to the head of the unit about what happened, but he shrugged off any need for further discussion. This incident was a major trauma for several of us who lived through it. Although I still felt unsettled, I recovered after a few days, but one of the nurses took a month to get over her upset. I still remember that incident with pain and remorse for us as well as the family. What could we have done to prevent similar horrific repeats in the future?

CASE

"I was not supposed to be there"

The morning after my weekend shift in the Dutch hospital where I was training, I went to the emergency room to drink coffee with the nurses and the residents before I went home. While I was there a man was brought in by ambulance. He was short of breath and had low blood pressure. After eliminating a number of possibilities, the resident called for the surgeon who determined that the patient might have burst an aneurysm. He was taken with some speed for an ultrasound. The patient very soon developed bradycardia and needed to be resuscitated.

During the resuscitation, without anyone noticing, the door of the echo room was opened and to everyone's surprise the patient's wife was standing nearby watching the procedure. I was given the assignment to remove her and remain with her while everyone else was occupied with the resuscitation. As we walked back to the emergency room she pressed me asking what was going on. I did not think I had the authority to respond fully to her questions even though I thought she deserved and needed answers. I was not part of the team caring for her husband, I was not even supposed to be there. I found myself talking "around" her questions, leaving the answers somewhere in the middle.

What was my authority? What should I have done?

COMMENTARY

Amnon Goldworth

The lack of information or consent is of significance in the four cases under discussion.

Informed consent is a type of authorization by which a patient permits or disallows a medical intervention. The process of achieving informed consent is an expression of individual autonomy. The validity of this process depends on an adequate comprehension of the material facts in which the decision to consent or to withhold consent is unimpeded by external interference or inhibiting emotional factors. Informed consent in the United States began in the late 1950s in recognition that the competent patient was an autonomous being whose judgment about personal medical treatment deserved attention and respect.

In the case, "Medically correct, but an ethical catastrophe," the catastrophe is the lack of communication between the attending physician and his colleagues and the failure to obtain informed consent from family members. The attending physician decided unilaterally to withdraw the medical support needed by the patient to continue to live out of the conviction that, as a physician, he must be able to make a life and death decision without involving others. The resulting death of the patient surprised and traumatized members of the medical staff and the patient's family.

The paternalistic behavior of the attending physician was morally wrong on several counts. He was "convinced that he acted in the patient's best interest." But, there is no evidence that he had made any effort to learn anything about his patient's personality, history, interests, and values, or to determine his wishes, whether expressed verbally or in written form, in anticipation of his death. There is no evidence that the attending physician had sought information from those on the hospital staff or from family members who might have enlarged his understanding of the patient. The best interest of his patient was determined by the physician projecting his own interests and values on the patient. There was no awareness that the interests and values of one individual may not necessarily be the same as the interests and values of another. Any such differences, if recognized, might have indicated that the withdrawal of support was premature.

From the description of the case, it is fair to assume that the patient could have been alive when his family came to visit him. If he was conscious at the time, this would have afforded an opportunity for final farewells. Even if he was comatose, there were family rituals that could have preceded his approaching death.

The intern asked what could be done to prevent a repetition of the events of the case. As stated in the case, "the question was raised as to whether care should have been withdrawn." Given his taciturn nature and his paternalistic outlook, this question was not discussed by the attending physician. One cannot order a person to change his personality or to automatically stop believing in the paternalistic responsibilities of the physician. But one can adopt policies or procedures that legitimate and thus facilitate the discussion of the withdrawal of treatment with colleagues, the patient, family members or surrogates when the patient is incompetent. In addition, valid informed consent should be required of the patient or surrogate. The adoption of such policies and procedures would discourage and perhaps stop physicians from playing God and by so doing prevent ungodlike moral mistakes.

I assume that the events in the case "Hey, you want to drain an abscess?" took place in an American teaching hospital. I also assume that this hospital's "Condition of Admission" form contains a statement indicating that because of its teaching role, patients can expect to be examined and treated by junior staff members under the tutelage of experienced physicians. By accepting this condition of admission, a patient has implicitly consented to possible encounters with relatively inexperienced medical personnel. However, where risky procedures are involved, the patient should be explicitly informed that some portion of the procedure will be performed by a novice under the control and careful supervision of an experienced physician. The patient may refuse to consent to this arrangement which may require that he or she obtains the services of a physician at a nonteaching facility.

Although all medical interventions involve some measure of risk, draining an abscess is not considered a particularly risky procedure. Thus, no specific reference to staff in training was called for. Nor was there a need for informed consent which might have revealed the in-training status of some participating members of the medical staff.

Some might complain that the implicit consent based on the content of the admission form is questionable since few people read these forms carefully. But, in this instance, the issue was irrelevant. Even if the patient had read the document with care, one could not be sure that she was sufficiently competent to understand what it said.

When consent is required, whether explicit or implicit, the patient must be competent. The fact that the patient had been able to come to the hospital by herself was not a sufficient sign of competency. Nor was her mother able to consent without first being informed of the teaching status of the hospital.

In the final analysis, it was the responsibility of the chief resident to obtain consent from the patient's mother or some other surrogate prior to draining the abscess. This step would have avoided compromising the junior staff member who was eager to learn, anxious to avoid alienating his chief but also worried about the immorality of practicing on a possibly incompetent patient.

In the abscess case just discussed, the training provided therapy for the patient. What the junior staff member learned to do provided a medical benefit to her. In the case "Who was really benefiting from the multiple exams?" the 80-year-old man did not benefit from more than one rectal examination. Those exams that followed for instructional purposes were nontherapeutic. They violated Kant's dictum that it is morally wrong to use human beings, who are deserving of moral respect, solely as means by which to satisfy the interests of others, even when these interests will serve some useful purposes in the future. Of course, if this dictum were obeyed to the letter, there would not be any nontherapeutic medical practices. But, individuals do voluntarily consent to invasive procedures with the full knowledge that they are not therapeutic. And such behavior is generally acknowledged to be morally legitimate.

To become a physician, one must learn by acquaintance as well as by description: by hands-on experience as well as by lectures, demonstrations, and books. In this instance, the rectal probing constituted learning by acquaintance. But this was not explained to the patient. In England, informed consent is required for research subjects but not for patients in a clinical setting because it is assumed that the physician can be trusted to do whatever is in the best interest of the patient. In India, which is based on the British system of medicine, physicians are not even trusted, "but always obeyed."

Even if no formal process of informed consent existed, the chief of medicine could have forewarned his patient about the multiple rectal examinations and explained the value of these examinations as part of medical education. He might even have attempted to elicit the cooperation of the patient in this educational exercise. If successful, this would have provided the 80-year-old man, perhaps for the first time in his life, with a sense of being respected by those in power and a corresponding feeling of empowerment. But these small efforts on the part of the chief of medicine would require a large change in the network of social and political relationships that constitutes the culture of India. Kant's dictum and related moral precepts can only be implemented where the moral worth of each and every individual is fully recognized by law and custom.

When informed consent as a requirement for medical treatment was introduced in the United States, there was skepticism concerning its validity. Critics argued that, in many circumstances, the ordinary individual who lacked medical sophistication, was not capable of understanding the information he or she needed for genuine con-

sent. This was answered by those who pointed out that it was not necessary to have the kind of sophisticated knowledge that the skeptic believed was required. Information of material interest to the patient or patient surrogate sufficient for the purposes of valid informed consent could successfully be communicated. However, the process of informed consent cannot be initiated or advanced where reliable communication is not possible. This condition obtains in emergencies where immediate medical intervention must be taken, or where those who can provide accurate information are not available.

In the case "I was not supposed to be there," both of these circumstances were present. The patient was receiving emergency care and his wife, who was present, was in the company of a trainee who may have appeared to be an appropriate authority, but was not.

The trainee was given the task of removing the wife from the echo room and remaining with her because this seemed to be the most reasonable option under the circumstances. But, it probably created the mistaken impression that the trainee had both the authority and expertise to communicate responsibly in response to the wife's questions.

The trainee should have clarified the true situation to the wife, particularly, that her right and need to have answers would be satisfied by a member of her husband's health care team as soon as this was possible. Any effort on the part of the trainee to "second guess" what was happening to the patient might lead to miscommunication and consequent confusion, embarrassment, and anger for all the interested parties.

COMMENTARY

George J. Agich

These cases of "special vulnerabilities" illustrate two parallel concerns, namely, the vulnerability of patients and their families on the one hand and the vulnerability of caregivers, specifically, medical students and health professionals on the other. Although three of these cases occur in the countries of India, France, and the Netherlands, we should resist the attempt to attribute these morally problematic behaviors to cultural variation. The first case involves an 80-year-old man who speaks no English and who comes to the clinic from the countryside. The student is an American of Indian extraction who is given the opportunity to perform a rectal exam. The student reports that seven individuals followed the invitation of the chief of medicine to insert their fingers into the patient's rectum with no information provided to the patient and certainly no consent. The student is highly disturbed seeing the man embarrassed and discomforted by the examination. Although the student partly attributes the behavior of the chief of staff to the British Colonial medical system, the ethical phenomenon in this case is the fact that the patient is not treated with due respect; his body is turned into an occasion for exhibiting a specific and unusual pathological finding. Although the student understands that physicians in the Indian system are always authorities who must be obeyed, he/she is morally troubled.

I would argue that the ethical issue is less a matter of consent than it is a matter of failing to respect this patient's vulnerability. In doing so, not only is the patient's vulnerability not appreciated, but the student him/herself is drawn into performing a physical examination in a way that denies rather than reinforces the physician's position as an empathetic caregiver.

The issue of consent is present as well in the second case in which a medical student is allowed to drain an abscess. In this case the chief resident offers appropriate support to the student lacking experience in performing the procedure on a nonsedated patient, and the procedure goes well. However, the procedure is complicated by the patient's obsequious gratitude. She is described as a developmentally delayed woman in

her early 30s. Her gratitude highlights the students' own inexperience. The question explicitly raised involves whether the patient is sufficiently competent to consent, but is consent the real issue? It is clear that there is no evidence of any sort of coercion, so one can only imagine that the student raises the question of consent as a way to express other, possibly deeper, disquietude about the case. This is also a vulnerable patient who has a therapeutic procedure performed to drain an abscess performed by a novice, though without difficulty. The case reminds us that most, if not all clinical skills are learned with the cooperation of patients. Without patients physicians would not be trained to practice their art; hence, they are a necessary partner in the process of medical education. It is a partnership about which medical ethics has been remarkably silent. The patient in this particular case, however, is perceived to be more vulnerable than most patients, because of her developmental disability. Is this true?

The patient clearly wants treatment, is compliant with the procedure, and expresses gratitude. There is no hint of coercion or untoward pressure. At most, the patient is not told that the student has no experience in draining the abscess, though is evidently aware that directions are being proffered by the chief resident. The case thus illustrates not a case of treatment without competent consent, but the inextricable interdependence of patient and learner. Certainly, some of the student's reservations and questioning involve a keen awareness of his/her inexperience. Ideally, experience should be gained from patients who consent to be the object of medical learning. Confronted by a patient who wants to be relieved of the discomfort associated with the abscess and is willing to have the procedure performed underscores for the student his own dependence upon the patient. That dependence is a paradoxical corollary of the power that the student has over the patient. In this case and in the first case, the patient is characteristically an object of a medical regard. Whereas in the first case, the patient is simply an occasion to display pathology which thus involves a dehumanization of the patient, in the second case, the patient receives a genuine and direct benefit. Both of these cases suggest that we need to cultivate in medical students less an ability to raise typical ethical questions about medical practice than a certain attitude of respect toward patients and a gratitude for the privilege of learning and practicing medicine on other human beings. The potential vulnerability of all patients makes this gratitude an essential ingredient in the character development of the good physician. Both cases remind us that the patient should never be taken for granted. Even if explicit consent is not always required, because consent is not a feature of the local cultural practice in the first case or because consent is presumed in the patient's willingness to receive treatment in the second case, the student needs to be aware of his/her dependence upon the patient and that respect for the patient should involve informing the patient. In contemporary American medical ethics, the primacy of the patient is captured in the rather austere notion of patient rights which stresses that the dependency relationship runs in the other direction, namely, patient dependence on physician. The legal and political concept of consent misses some of the primacy of the rich existential role that the patient and his/her suffering plays in medicine.

The third case illustrates that even justified withdrawal of life support can be ethically problematic if done with insufficient attention to process. In this case an attending physician in a French hospital withdraws life support on an HIV-infected man in septic shock. There is no doubt that the patient would not survive, but there was no discussion and no consent. Furthermore, the withdrawal occurs when the nurses and interns are away, making it feel illicit since it was conducted out of view. Yet, if we have learned anything about withdrawal of life support, it is that attention to process is critically important for ethically sound decision making.

It is, of course, significant that the family is not involved in the decision making. But a word of caution is appropriate here. Too often, physicians educated in and sensitive to patient rights leave difficult withdrawal of life support decisions to family members. I am not questioning the legitimacy of patient and surrogate decision making, but suggesting that in situations in which interventions do not afford the patient any prospect of benefit, making the family decide can be cruel. In this case, it is commendable that the physician is willing to assume responsibility for what is in effect a clinical decision, namely, that interventions have reached their limit of effectiveness. In such situations, a professional judgment is properly made, but the actions should not be carried out in the unilateral fashion of the case. Families should be informed of the judgment and the decision to withdraw futile interventions. Although the responsibility for the decision rightly belongs to the physician, the physician unfortunately did not effectively communicate with family or other caregivers thereby creating a crisis of credibility and motive. In this instance, the nursing and resident staff are shocked at the physician's action. Not only must they deal with the death of a patient, but with their own and the family's shock at the abruptness of the decision. When life support is not clinically effective withdrawal can be justified. However, death is an important human experience that should be approached openly and supportively and not with the suddenness of a vengeful God. The attending physician's action forces the nursing and resident staff to deal with the aftermath of a decision made retrospectively and denies their prospective and concurrent role in addressing family psychosocial needs and process. This distorts the process of grieving and creates moral distress. Situations that cause moral distress can only be prevented by realizing that the medical decision is itself contextually situated. Sensitivity to family needs as well as nurses and other caregivers is an integral component of a fully responsible and ethically sound handling of cases of withdrawal of life support based on medical futility.

The final case could have occurred in any hospital. The emergent bradycardia caused the team to provide appropriate resuscitation efforts. Even though the primary focus of attention is on the patient needing resuscitation, the presence of the patient's wife was duly noted. It was appropriate that the medical student was asked to attend to the wife, yet understandable that the medical student found him/herself in a difficult situation. This case illustrates an, unfortunately, often-forgotten aspect of ethics in medicine, namely, that medical ethics does not replace ordinary ethics. The first question asked, namely, "What was my authority?" is remarkably out of place. Circumstances provided the student with "authority," because the proper response was not professional, but human. The second question, "What should I have done?" is more apt. Here the important point is that there is no recipe that could reliably guide action even though there are some guiding points. A sensitive individual would identify the wife's shock and concern, validate it, and explain to the best of one's knowledge what was transpiring. Such an explanation should honestly include: "I don't fully know or understand what they are doing." Medical facts in the course of resuscitation are so dynamic that it would be absurd to try to provide those to the wife, even if one were able. Rather, the wife needs to know that her husband is receiving appropriate and urgent care. Beyond that, the wife's immediate emotional reaction should be addressed through a process of active listening. Making sure the wife knows of your concern is critically important and to do that one must empathize with her concern.

This case illustrates that too often medical interventions are regarded as procedures or actions within the proper scope of authority of the physician or health professional. As a result, situations that demand something other than a specifically professional response, as the human empathic response demanded in this situation, can be set aside or denigrated. The case suggests that the virtues required to be a good physician rest upon rather than replace the virtues associated with being a good person. One can only hope that the medical student in this situation responded as a person and learned that ethically justified responses cannot always be defined in terms of rules or principles. Dynamic situations exist that confront the ability of anyone's quick application of a rule or principle. For this reason, physicians need to fall back on basic human affects and responses such as compassion and consolation.

2

Treating despite discomfort and self-doubt

CASE

"Aren't you done yet?"

The only surgery I was able to do as a third year medical student involved a deltoid abscess on a patient who was an IV drug user. He had suffered a number of traumatic accidents and infections. The patient had been "skin popping" and injecting heroin directly into his skin, because his veins were no longer accessible. Abscesses are a common result of this practice.

A first year resident supervised me during the surgery, but I was very aware that I probably would not have been allowed to do the surgery if the patient had been a member of the Hospital Board instead of this black man who was clearly a medical "train wreck." I was also hounded by the nurses and anesthesiologist who thought I was taking too long. They were all after me to "hurry up" and kept asking "Aren't you done yet?"

I was sweating because this was my first surgery and the rest of the team just wanted to get out of there.

CASE

"Have you ever done a lumbar puncture?"

We were doing an evaluation for headaches on an elderly gentleman. The patient was alert and could hear everything that was being said. The neurosurgical resident asked, rather casually I thought, "Have you ever done a lumbar puncture?" I told him I had.

The resident set the patient up and then left the room. I was in a very awkward position. In no way did I feel ready to do a lumbar puncture unsupervised.

CASE

"The emergency department at 4:00 a.m."

At 4:00 a.m. a young Latin-American male who had just been stabbed in the chest came to the Emergency Department with a pneumothorax. The Emergency physician contacted the attending thoracic surgeon, described the situation and asked him for advice. The surgeon (perhaps influenced by the time of night) instructed the ER physician to call the surgical intern – me. I was to examine the patient, work him up, put in a chest tube, follow him and discharge him as I saw fit.

I felt uncomfortable being told to put in the chest tube, not having done the procedure in a long time and not being supervised by a staff person. On the other hand, I was aware that I was expected to be able to do this procedure, and certainly if I told the emergency department physician that I did not feel competent, his regard for me as a professional would suffer.

CASE

"Operating without experience"

Eighteen months after leaving medical school I got a job as a trainee surgeon ("senior house officer") in a rural part of the United Kingdom. Apart from assisting at major operations and suturing a few skin wounds in Accident and Emergency, I had little previous surgical experience. On my first day, I did an outpatient clinic in the morning, then went to another hospital at lunch time in order to join a consultant surgeon for an afternoon operating list. I arrived early, got changed and took my place in the operating theater. Two patients (both were middle-aged men) were already prepared for surgery: one was anesthetized awaiting a circumcision for his phimosis, the other was expecting a rigid sigmoidoscopy and banding of his hemorrhoids. The consultant surgeon had not yet arrived. Having no previous experience of either procedure, I waited. The consultant surgeon was really quite late. I waited some more. A message came from the surgeon asking me to start, saying he would join me in theater. I waited some more. Finally, under a large amount of pressure from the theater staff, I conceded and agreed to start. I felt less daunted by the prospect of a sigmoidoscopy – I had seen some done previously and felt I could do less damage, so slowly set about the task, hoping that the surgeon would arrive. He did not. I am sure I made a mess, but at least it was hidden inside and would hopefully heal up and be sorted out by someone else later. The list was proceeding very slowly. The first patient was still anesthetized and awaiting his circumcision. I had never even seen one before, but was pressured into starting. The surgeon had still not arrived. I made an excuse and disappeared to the changing room, where I retrieved a pocket-sized manual from my bag and took it quickly into the lavatory to scan the relevant pages. Armed with new knowledge, I started the circumcision, but got slightly confused about how much foreskin to cut away, but luckily got some advice from the anesthetist. Somehow, I muddled through and was even persuaded to start another case before the surgeon arrived.

In a short space of time I came to accept this lack of supervision as almost "normal." The following week I did an orchidectomy for a young man with testicular cancer, assisted by a foreign medical student who had never been in theater before. She had no idea about usual sterile procedures and had to change her gloves six times. On this occasion, however, I felt relatively protected, as the consultant surgeon was operating in the theater next door and I was able to go through and ask for occasional advice.

COMMENTARY

Marli Huijer

The situations as described are not regularly encountered by Dutch medical students. Sometimes a self-confident student boasts about the interventions he or she was allowed to perform, but this almost always happened under supervision. Students also report that they have been sent to the Emergency room to be the first to check on a patient, but usually the resident arrived shortly afterwards. When asked about failures, they rather complain more about not being allowed to carry out any responsibility than about a lack of supervision. Nevertheless, Dutch students, like the students in the cases, encounter many situations in which they feel discomfort and self-doubt.

The differences needed in the approach to specific patients, as mentioned in the cases, seem also to be less frequent in the Netherlands. The rather homogeneous population, continuously striving for an equal distribution of income, and guaranteed equal access to health care services make any differences in approach more subtle, and less visible. But that does not prevent Dutch students from making distinctions between different patients, for example because they feel more attracted to some rather than other patients.

All these cases involve feelings. The interns and residents tell us about sweating, about being in an awkward position, and about feeling uncomfortable. Despite this discomfort and self-doubt they still treated the patients and committed this fact to writing. None of them explains what exactly was the moral dilemma they experienced. The cases are presented as situations in which the students had been manipulated without any possibility of escape. They acted like actors do in a theater pressed by a director, submitting to the direction of the play, the rest of the team, and the public, to start the show. Their moral sense was overruled by these pressures. They performed, although they felt uncomfortable. Did they have any alternative? To answer this question, we have to explore exactly what moral problem is wrapped up in the students' and residents' feelings.

One can draw several conclusions from these cases:

1 The interns and resident were aware they had little or no experience with the interventions they had to perform.
2 The interns and resident knew their inexperience could inflict harm to the patient.
3 The interns and resident were aware that they probably would not have been allowed to do these interventions if the patients had been members of the Hospital Board.
4 After some time, the interns and resident accepted the lack of supervision as something "normal."
5 Despite feelings of discomfort and self-doubt, all students and the resident still decided to go ahead with the procedure.

Awareness of inexperience

Medical students are always aware that their medical knowledge and skills are limited. They experience daily how they are forced to remain silent on questions that physicians, nurses, or patients pose. To be able to learn, they have to acknowledge and accept the limits of their knowledge and skill without shame or fear, and ask for explanations as soon as they do not understand anything. On the other hand, they do not want, and are not allowed, to come across as stupid or clumsy. They want to be taken seriously by colleagues and patients. Medical students perma-

nently balance the tension between the demand to look like a professional and the demand to be honest about the limits of their present knowledge and skills. The ambivalence of the medical students' position is outlined well in an imaginary conversation described by Sukol:

Patient: Have you ever done this procedure before?
Medical student: I am a student doctor. I have never done this particular procedure, but I have seen it done a number of times and have done other similar ones. I am comfortable doing this now, and I want you to be comfortable too. If you would feel better, I can have a resident or a staff physician supervise me or even do the procedure, but I will leave that up to you. Why don't you give it some thought, and I'll be back in a little while. (1)

Not surprisingly, Sukol never witnessed a conversation like this. Despite their lack of knowledge and practice, medical students like to be approached as real professionals. They want to meet the expectations of others, formulated in one of the cases in this way:

If I told the Emergency room physician that I did not feel competent, his regard for me as a professional would suffer.

Inflicting harm

The conversation described by Sukol is not only unusual because of the students' wish to be approached as professionals, but also because of the patients' preference for an experienced doctor. If patients had the choice between a skilled physician and an inexperienced medical student, the majority would opt for the first. Giving in to this preference would mean that no student could ever become a skilled professional. To be sure of future experienced physicians, patients therefore have to be subjected to the less-practiced hands of medical students and residents. However, this utilitarian approach which aims at the greatest well-being of the greatest number of patients in the present and future, should not take priority over the bioethical principle of nonmaleficence, that is, the obligation not to inflict evil or harm. The medical student's inexperience ought not to inflict harm on the individual patient. In the case descriptions, the interns and resident appear not to be sure that the lack of practice and of supervision might be disadvantageous to the patient. "I am sure I made a mess," writes the trainee surgeon, "but at least it was hidden inside and would hopefully heal up and be sorted out by someone else later." Neither the interns, nor the resident intend to inflict harm on the patients by treating them, but at the same time they are not in the position to delegate the interventions to be performed to others. The only hope they have is that when they perform as well as possible they will not inflict harm on the patient.

Valuing patients differently

A complicating factor is the students' awareness that they were allowed to do the intervention partly because the patient involved was valued less than, for example, a member of the Hospital Board! Drug use, race, social status, age, and unconsciousness appear to be factors that make it easier for the supervisors to retreat and shift the responsibility to the intern or resident. For the interns and resident, on their part, these factors made them more inclined to accept the responsibility; it is easier to cover up the consequences of any medical failure when patients are unconscious during the performance or when they have a general difficulty in voicing their interests.

Getting accustomed to the strange

In the case descriptions, the feelings of discomfort do not start off a set of arguments that support or undermine the decisions made. Instead of this, the state of affairs is reluctantly accepted as "normal." This is especially evident in the case of the trainee surgeon: "In a short space of time I came to accept this lack of supervision as almost normal." It took him a week to become accustomed to the lack of supervision. In comparison with the foreign medical student who had to

change her gloves six times, he already felt relatively protected. The process in which the unusual becomes accepted as normal is called "the process of socialization": "A process that transforms the strange, the unusual, the disconcerting, and even the abhorrent into something normal, familiar, usual, reassuring." (2)

Options

The difference in approach to different patients combined with the risk of inflicting harm on them gives the students and resident a feeling of discomfort and self-doubt, but it does not prevent them from treating. Do medical students and residents have any alternative to treating despite discomfort? Do we have to view students and residents as no more than cog wheels in an automatic medical process? Are their options limited to (a) keep on turning or (b) stop completely? Or do they have a third option of "voice"? (3) Could it be that medical students and residents themselves are, in fact, influential actors in the medical theater, with their moral responses included as an important contribution to the events?

In medical ethics, students are generally approached as persons who develop their own opinions and attitudes toward the moral experiences and dilemmas they encounter. To be able to voice their feelings and opinions, and build consistent moral reasoning, students are taught to investigate the values relevant for the case, to analyze which value has priority over others, to map the possible strategies, and to argue why they choose a certain strategy. Students and residents have to be able to weigh up the conflicting values that arise in medical dilemmas.

To explore the conflicting values that arise in the case descriptions, it is useful to recall the five frequently conflicting goals common to all medical students as described by Hundert et al.: (2)
1 To learn medicine.
2 To be part of a team.
3 To care for patients.
4 To perform well.
5 To get good grades.

In the case of medical students, these five values are easily recognized. In none of them has priority been given to care for patients. Getting good grades, being part of a team, learning medicine and performing well were valued more than the care for patients.

Ethics education can help students to weigh the different values and to determine which value, in theory, has priority. If the feelings of discomfort and self-doubt turn out to be caused by the undervaluation of the patient's care and if this is in contrast with what students in theory prefer, the next step is to explore why they cannot put their opinions and values into practice. Ethics education can play an important role in teaching students how to voice the opinions, values, and priorities they have in clinical education and hopefully to have their values respected.

Notes

1 Sukol RB. Teaching ethical thinking and behavior to medical students. *JAMA* 1995;273:1388–9.
2 Hundert EM, Hafferty F, Christakis D. Characteristics of the informal curriculum and trainees' ethical choices. *Acad Med* 1996;71(6):624–42.
3 Hirschman, AO. *Exit, Voice and Loyalty: Responses to Decline in Firms, Organizations, and States.* Harvard University Press, Cambridge, 1970.

COMMENTARY

William Andereck

A few months ago I was talking with a group of medical residents. My topic was "Telling bad news." In the course of our discussion, I asked the residents if they could give me an example of having to tell a patient bad news. One woman spoke up. She had been on call a few weeks earlier when she was called by the radiologist from CT to inform her that late that afternoon her new admission had been diagnosed with widely metastatic cancer. The resident immediately called the attending physician and presented the information. The attending then told her that he was tied up at another hospital and would not be able to return until morning. Since the patient was quite anxious for the X-ray results, he suggested that the resident inform the patient herself.

Like the doctors in training in the previous cases, our resident was left hanging, unprepared for the task ahead and appropriately anxious. But the resident also had confidence in her ability to meet challenges. Medical school training had been a series of successfully met challenges. Despite the anxious feelings there is a practiced ability to put them aside and "get the job done." So our resident gathered herself, made herself as familiar with the patient as the chart would allow, and went into the patient's room.

The introduction was brusque and uncomfortable, more focused on explaining the attending's absence than anything else. After a short, but very uncomfortable pause, the resident told him the findings on the CT scan most certainly represented some form of malignant cancer which had spread to liver, lung, and lymph nodes. The man was devastated and he began to cry. Our resident, until only a few minutes ago a perfect stranger, could only put her hand on his shoulder and wonder to herself, "What in the hell have I just done?" The whole experience was new to her and her only frames of reference were melodramas she had seen on TV. At this point she realized that she really did not have a clue as to what to expect or how to respond. After a few minutes the man composed himself, thanked her for letting him know the findings, and then asked to be left alone.

It was clear, as she related the story, that the incident still troubled her. She was still questioning the best way to have told the man his diagnosis. What she was seeking from me were techniques for patient interaction and insights into how to offer information in a sensitive and understandable way. I was much more interested in the sense of responsibility that made her agree to deliver bad news to a total stranger in the first place, and why she had not listened to that inner voice that was surely screaming, "Don't do it!"

"See one, do one, teach one." This was the anthem for medical education in the 70s and 80s. The sheer volume of medical need in an under-served population like the metropolitan county hospital in which I trained, made it easy to as-sume as much clinical responsibility as desired. Procedures such as a lumbar puncture were taught, demonstrated, and often performed for the first time, on the same day. As a result, many of the doctors who trained during this period have seen themselves thrust into uncomfortable circumstances similar to the situations described here. All the while asking themselves the ques-tion, "What is going on here?" In retrospect, one can see that the problem with each of these cases is that the situation has evolved from "see one, do one," to "do one, see one." What is it about our-selves that allows us to act without proper train-ing or supervision, and how does the medical education process promote such irresponsible behavior?

Responses to being put in a situation like one of those described above would be heavily in-fluenced by factors unique to the role of student or resident, as well as factors related to the under-lying personality of the trainee. The characteristi-cs of the student role include a level of insecurity based on a lesser degree of knowledge and experi-ence. Desire for acceptance and recognition from one's teachers promotes within the student a willingness to please and to avoid conflict. The desire for acceptance demonstrated by most incoming trainees makes it unlikely that anyone would suffer the loss of face necessary to admit their incapability or even their concerns. Like-wise, doctors in training are motivated by a desire to help their patients and thus open to "do every-thing they can." A genuine desire to help a pa-tient in need may be the prime motivator to move a resident to handle a new situation. In most cases everything goes successfully and with a good outcome, but even these successful scen-arios can leave scars on the individuals caught up in them.

In addition to the perspective inherent in the student role, there are a number of personal traits or characteristics that would influence an individ-ual's response to having responsibility thrust on them. Personal aggressiveness and willingness to take risk are two traits that are expressed in vari-able degrees within the physician population. A particularly aggressive individual, or one comfort-able with risk-taking activities might be more willing to assume the care expected with less trepidation, than someone uncomfortable with risk taking or less confident of their skills.

Beyond the influences of being in the student role or the personal characteristics that govern one's actions, it is important to reflect on the factors unique to the process of medical educa-tion that might promote a willingness to act with-out proper training or supervision. In fact, it should be noted that, until recently, such issues were not really discussed or seen as ethical prob-lems in physician training. What has occurred that now makes us open to exploring such activ-ity?

The medical training model that characterizes my experience, as well as that of most of my col-leagues, is what I would call the "military model." Developed after World War II by veterans accus-tomed to a hierarchical, male-dominated system of command, the culture of medicine demanded toughness and attention to detail as essential characteristics in young physicians. Expectations were set and met without question. We never thought much about the fact that five medical students were the closest thing to a doctor the 40 or so patients in the endocrine clinic would see that day as we presented our findings and dis-cussed therapy with the attending in a separate room. The characteristic most positively rein-forced was the "no problem, I can handle it" attitude.

Roundsmanship and "pimping" were the rit-uals of clinical education, felt to toughen the sleep-deprived trainee and improve their per-formance under stress. Questioning authority was the road to ruin in medicine. Individuals expected to perform unsupervised surgery would never think to refuse, except in the most egregious circumstances. Rookie surgeons were routinely hazed. Most surgical residents were eager for every case they could get, regardless of supervision. Some even sought out the less skilled surgeons so that they might have a greater hand in the operation. Surviving a night of multiple "hits," as medical admissions are now called, was the badge of valor and bragging rights were earned about how many patients you evaluated.

Perhaps things are beginning to change. The degree of tolerance for open expression of divergent ideas and emotional feelings has increased in our society since I and many of my colleagues were in training. It is not that medicine has changed within a vacuum. In fact, I would contend that our profession has unsuccessfully resisted the trend. Nevertheless, coincident with this societal shift, the days of the "military model" of training are waning. Medicine has had to open its mind to how we train our young physicians and now recognize some of the ethical difficulties students of medicine face that are particular to their status as trainees. Expressing one's discomfort with a clinical situation is considered appropriate now. The inner struggle between the feeling that one should be able to handle the situation and desiring to seek help will never go away. But hopefully, it will be made easier as educational institutions recognize their responsibility to assure that no physicians are expected to perform without appropriate support for their level of training and knowledge, and students are made aware of their ethical responsibility not to bend to such coercion.

COMMENTARY

Gregory L. Larkin

The above cases center around the drama of doctoring in the face of ineptitude. The discomfort and self-doubt shared by the collective conscience of the clinicians involved reminds us that patients should not be treated as a means but as ends in themselves. Issues of pride, embarrassment, and peer pressure are tertiary; their subjugation presents little, if any, moral challenge. After all, the patient is never the appropriate battleground upon which the ego should wage war. These anecdotes of trial by fire in which young, unskilled professionals expand the scope of their practice, in the absence of patient consent, underlines our need to honor basic ethical principles of beneficence and nonmaleficence.

At once, professionals attempt to do good (beneficence) for patients while avoiding harm (nonmaleficence). Of these two principles, nonmaleficence has arguably formed the bedrock of Western medical ethics since the Code of Hammurabi. From the Hippocratic writings up until the modern day, the imperative to provide quality in the care of patients is one of the few constants in medical practice. *Primum non nocere* is a mantra of nonmaleficence that has withstood the test of time. Today, in fact, "first, no harm" has assumed increasing relevance in our modern era of cost-consciousness and changing health care priorities and goals. Attempts to trade quality for other values (such as cost-containment) in health care systems have met with considerable resistance, particularly in the West. While gatekeeping practices and resource scarcity has often made it more difficult for health care professionals to act in their patients' best interests, the expectation and need for safe, competent, high-quality care has never been more important to the consumer.

The American Medical Association defines quality of care as "the degree to which care services influence the probability of optimal patient outcomes." (1) As health care providers have expected this of themselves, so have their patients come to expect high quality care. While conflict-laden interactions with other health care practitioners, nurses, administrators, and third-party payers can obfuscate our true clinical goals, cases such as the above demand an honesty and integrity that is strong enough to transcend such peripheral concerns. It is when professionals are most distracted by the chaos of an Emergency Department or during their early training periods that they are most likely to overlook their allegiance to a *patient-centered ethic*. This may be contrasted with a more utilitarian or society-centered ethic, wherein the physician fulfills duties to patients up to the limit imposed by scarcity of resources or the needs of others in society. By contrast, the patient-centered ethic compels the physician to do whatever is best for the patient without regard for the interest of society, other individuals, and most importantly the physician, him or herself.

For example, the Emergency Department saga of the surgical intern treating a young Latin male with a pneumothorax is illustrative. The intern enmeshed in this scenario was uncomfortable putting in a chest tube without supervision, and was also uncomfortable sharing with the Emergency physician his feelings of incompetence. However, a society-centered ethic may compel him to realize Stage Two of the "see one, do one, teach one" paradigm. He has certainly seen these procedures before, and society has a need for him to learn this procedure. One may argue that the societal need to have excellently trained physicians provides a warrant for using patients as training material. On the other hand, this same principle may be used to argue that complications at the hands of this intern could scar the reputation of all physicians in the eyes of not only this patient, but all other patients who hear of this case.

The more patient-centered ethic compels the intern to ignore his discomfort and his fear that he is not meeting the expectations of other professionals by doing what is optimal for the patient. This intern's relative inexperience at chest tube thoracostomy and his reluctance to acknowledge this inexperience suggests that a bewildering array of obstacles must be overcome in order to ensure that patient safety, and hence the

principle of nonmaleficence is upheld. One obstacle is hubris. Some interns may feel confident that doing such a procedure themselves is safe and will yield outcomes as good as those of physicians who have not done one in a while. They may even argue that it is better for the patient to have it done expediently, allegedly decreasing the risk of tension pneumothorax and other time-dependent complications instead of awaiting supervision. Note however, that these reasons are patient-centered and are legitimate, depending on the given context.

On the other hand, an overinflated sense of competence is tantamount to fool-hardy arrogance and has no place in the practice of medicine. Patient safety would be severely compromised if, for example, the patient needed only a needle decompression and not a large-bore chest tube placed into the thoracic cavity. While it is important for interns to learn by doing such a procedure, practice can usually be obtained on cadavers or swine, so that in the case of a real life patient, a more well-trained resident will be able to respond. Given sufficient time and repetition, the "training wheels" of supervision may ultimately be removed. The wings of competence must be allowed to unfold slowly however lest our impatience threaten the integrity of both our patients and our profession.

It is important not to get into the habit of ignoring the patient-centered ethic. Habits such as trustworthiness and honesty are important virtues in the Aristotelian sense; such virtues can buttress professionalism when well practiced. Failure to practice such virtues can lead to an erosion of values and a cavalier disregard of the patient-centered ethic, leading one to "fly by the seat of one's pants" as seen in the case "Operating without experience." This case of a trainee surgeon in the United Kingdom reveals that an initially conscientious and appropriately frightened new surgeon has trepidation borne of inexperience. As he succumbs to peer pressure from the operating room staff, it gradually becomes easier and easier for him to embark upon procedures (sigmoidoscopy, hemorrhoid treatment, circumcision, etc.) for which he has little or no experience. He goes on to suggest that "In a short space of time, I came to accept this lack of supervision as almost normal." The slippery slope implication of this value erosion is perhaps obvious. A disregard for professional habit and virtue in daily practice can quickly lead to a loss of the patient-centered ethic. This abdication of values and virtues can lead one to ignore personal ineptitude and displace principles of beneficence and nonmaleficence under the weight of an ever-enlarging ego. While "operating with no experience" may be acceptable or even *required* under austere conditions, a cavalier attitude toward patient safety may generate a modern incarnation of the Nuremberg slippery slope.

It would certainly be better for the profession not to have to have a tribunal set up every time the patient-centered ethic is forgotten. There is no question that we think less of our interns and students when they do not call for help, e.g., if they harm patients, resulting in damage to their own self-esteem as well as the integrity of the profession. It would be better if we did not rely on the National Practitioner Data Bank or medical malpractice claims as the "black marks on our soul" that motivate change to the patient-centered ethic. (2) A more pro-active and less reactive approach is to write down and adhere to personal codes of conduct in professional life. (3) The first principle in the *Code of Conduct for Academic Emergency Medicine* is that of "competence . . . that before all else benefits patients and society." Competence forms the core of the patient-centered ethic and is invoked in the first principle of the American Medical Association (AMA) Principles of Medical Ethics: "A physician shall be dedicated to providing competent medical service with compassion and respect for human dignity." This first principle trumps all others. Similarly, Principle V also speaks of the need to render competent care, asking assistance whenever needed: "A physician shall continue to study, apply and advance scientific knowledge,

make relevant information available to patients, colleagues, and the public; obtain consultation, and use the talents of other health professionals when indicated." Perhaps the Declaration of Geneva says it best: "The health of my patient will be my first consideration." This captures the spirit of beneficence, in which the physician's commitment to her patients generally supersedes other obligations. This idea of patients at the center of concern is best realized when there are compassionate, inner-directed, self-motivated, and ethically principled physicians taking their patients' best interests to heart. (4)

Codes of ethics may be only one small way in which issues of competence and integrity may be addressed. In this modern era in which the doctor–patient relationship has been replaced by the provider–patient relationship, it is clear that mid-level providers and alternative providers are often practicing medicine without a license. It is in the spirit of patients' best interests that we should maintain our core competencies and strive to improve professional integrity. It was medical charlatanism that inspired the foundling AMA to write its first code of ethics in 1847 and we must continue to maintain our quality in this "Snake Oil Sellers" market of today. We must maintain rigorous peer review and appropriate whistle-blowing beyond hospital-based credentialing "arms races." We must learn to become better teachers, leaving behind the pedagogical orientation that pervades medical education today. We must not reduce teaching to a show and tell, wherein magnificent scholars proclaim and exhibit their erudition. We must truly study the science and art of teaching in order to avoid what Sean Stitham has called "educational malpractice." (5)

The widespread lack of quality, supervised postgraduate education will continue to erode a patient-centered ethic. Such improvement in medical education can lead to enhanced professional accountability, credibility, trustworthiness, and a reinstatement of the patient-centered ethic. Doing a lack-luster, half-hearted job of educating

students and residents as if to create more wid-
gets serves neither the profession nor society.
Similarly granting privileges to unqualified physicians is penny-wise and pound foolish. For too
long, the ivory tower has ignored the need to
foster ultra-high quality clinicians. We do not
need more doctors. We do need a few highly
talented, committed, and conscientious professionals.

In all of the above cases my view is that any
argument for the young physicians doing these
procedures themselves must be based on whether
or not it is in the patient's best interests. In austere scarcity, wilderness, or rural settings, it is
possible that a lesser qualified physician may
need to expand the scope of his or her practice,
but as Samuel Papper once said, "Not to recognize one's limitations is a serious matter, but to
recognize them and not to act accordingly is an
unforgivable testimony to personal vanity. Vanity
has no place in medicine." In any of these scen-
arios, if the physician were to treat this patient
personally, he or she must do so with the patient's expressed informed consent, including an
admission of the physician's inexperience. Any
attempt to hide this information would be deceptive, dishonest, and unethical.

Substandard or marginal care is defensible only
when there is an advantage to the patient to receive such care, and not because it benefits the
consultant or the resident. If there is any compromise it should not be at the patient's expense,
since the physician–patient relationship implicitly assures the patient that the physician is looking
out for his best interests. All physicians and
trainees should remain vigilant against practices
that endanger patient safety or fall below accepted standards of care.

In closing, these cases of treating despite discomfort and self-doubt, underscore the wisdom
of a professor who early in my medical training
asked us to start intravenous lines on one another. The wisdom of this exercise made the principle clear that we should not be practicing on
our patients. More importantly, it gave us a sense
of respect for the pain experienced by patients
and the realization that ultimately we are all patients. Hence, the Golden Rule reigns: Do unto
others as that which you would have done unto
you. This rule, however overused, is not out of
date and reminds us that physicians' self-concern
must never be in competition with respecting a
patient as a person. Ultimately, medical care is
about patient care. Without patients, there would
be no need for doctors. Physicians are not expected to be God-like creatures and paragons of
perfection, but they are expected to provide acceptable, compassionate, and reasonable care
which does more good than harm. The patient-
centered ethic is in need of reinstatement into the
medical conscience.

Notes

1 American Medical Association. *Policy Compendium.*
   AMA, Chicago, 1992, p. 315.
2 Cullen DB, Cullan SK. Black marks on your soul. *The
   National Practitioner Data Bank, Missouri Medicine,*
   1991;88(5): 285–8.
3 Larkin GLL. A Code of Conduct for Academic Emergency Medicine. *Emerg Acad Med* 1999;6(1):45.
4 Larkin GLL. In *Ethics in Emergency Medicine*, ed. KV
   Iserson, AM Sanders & D Mathiew. Second Edition.
   Galen Press Ltd., Tucson, AZ, 1995, pp.362–6.
5 Stitham S. Educational malpractice. *JAMA*
   1991;266:905–6.

Blaming the patient

CASE

"If you weren't so fat"

After undergoing a Cesarean section, a very fat woman developed a wound infection that was not healing. The chief resident, who had also performed the surgery, became very frustrated over the fact that this untoward event had occurred on his watch. He rebuked the patient in front of a room full of students and house staff by telling her, "If you weren't so fat this simply wouldn't be a problem."

The patient happened to be Tongan and, consequently, she did not understand most of what the chief resident was saying. He continued to rail away at her in front of the assembled group, punctuated by an occasional, "You understand what I'm talking about don't you!" The patient would simply smile and nod, clearly uncomprehending.

I believed the patient was being used for the chief resident to absolve himself of any responsibility for the infection. As on-lookers, and underlings, what should we have done?

CASE

"The patient removed the traction"

When my friend and I were students on the ward, he was assigned the responsibility of arranging for traction to be set up for a patient. From subsequent events, I believe that he mistakenly ordered the wrong traction and then blamed the patient.

It started when the attending came into the patient's room and was told she was still having pain. The attending took one look and said "This patient isn't getting better because you have the wrong weight." Immediately, the chief resident demanded "Who rigged this traction?" My friend was accused of writing down the wrong weight and was ordered by the resident to "Get me the chart." By the time he retrieved the chart and handed it to the chief resident there was a critical smudge in the chart making an exact reading impossible. The original order could have read the required 15 pounds, or the erroneous 5 pounds that were actually rigged.

My friend maintained that he had ordered the proper weight and offered that "the patient changed the weight," since unused weights were stored at the bottom of her bed. When asked in Spanish, the patient, a native of Latin America, vehemently denied taking off any weight. The nurse, when questioned, said she did not remember altering the weights.

I think this was a case of succumbing to the temptation to try to preserve a rotation evaluation. I didn't want my friend to suffer, but at the same time I didn't want to see the patient accused falsely. What, if anything, was my responsibility?

COMMENTARY

Alan Steinbach

You've seen the chart notes:

"The patient did not take the medication as prescribed."

"The patient failed to follow instructions, and did not improve."

"The patient was lost to follow-up."

Whose fault is it when medical treatment does not succeed? Are some patients to blame when your treatment fails? Is it *ever* all right to blame a patient? Is there a constructive kind of blame? Is blame simply a song of guilt, or could it be helpful in making things right? This section is about a very human action: laying blame.

Blaming the patient is not a terribly toxic medical treatment. Compared to many of the actions (or non-actions) outlined in this book, blaming the patient is often more of a kind of "pop off" mechanism. It damages feelings, not tissue. And yet the slippery slope that begins with blaming the patient can, with time, and the encrustation of many slimy little blames, lead to a toxic professional practice.

As the two cases indicate, blame is often associated with a failure to communicate. If the Tongan patient ("If you weren't so fat") understood the ranting resident, she might protest the blame, or more likely just laugh and defuse the whole situation. When the Latina woman ("The patient removed the traction") received a translation of her blame, she did protest. Preliterate children are safe targets for blame; e.g., "He was wiggling around so much I couldn't see the vein," and the demented elderly as well, "If she took better care of herself this wouldn't have happened." A barrier such as language, gender, or age can become a channel for blame, creating the habit of using such channels, and leading to a culturally insensitive practice.

In one of the case examples provided, the patient is blamed for being fat, thus for having a wound infection, thus a prolonged stay in the hospital, with attendant costs to the hospital, to society (who paid the bills via Medicaid) and thus the continued embarrassing reminder of a treatment complication for the resident (something his fellow residents certainly remind him of often). In the other case, a student blames the patient to avoid admitting an error in writing down an order for a traction weight. The cases illustrate that blame knows no station, as well as the important fact that both leaders and beginners may seek to assign blame. Does blame hurt the patients? Not really. The primary damage of blame is to the blamer.

The temptation to shift just a little part of the blame for a bad outcome to the patient is almost irresistible. This is accentuated by being part of a team. In a solo practice, without witnesses, there is no opportunity for a practitioner to express blame, and perhaps less to even think of it. But in teaching hospitals where everyone is looking over your shoulder, surely something about the patient must explain part of why things did not work out as well as desired! Those things that make us obviously different, such as race, gender, obesity, language, are all easy targets.

Blame spelled backwards is acceptance. Accepting that a mistake has been made is the beginning of a blameless practice. Of course, team leaders can make it easy or hard to accept mistakes. Beginning rounds with a story illustrating the possibility of mistakes in practice can be a good educational tool. When a problem is encountered (such as the wrong weight on the traction bar), the superior team leader does not hold a kangaroo court to lay blame. What are the facts? Who was involved? Was a mistake made? If the resident or attending is skilled in team function, they will not rub the student's nose in the mistake. Take note, learn what you can, and move on. Knowing that admission of a mistake will be heard and not become the basis of ridicule may make it possible for team members to admit mistakes, and not try to blame someone else.

In "If you weren't so fat," should the resident lay the blame for his surgical outcome on the patient's fat? No, he should not. Most particularly, he should not lay such blame in a relatively public setting (on rounds), repetitively, and in a language the patient cannot understand. Clearly, the resident is chagrined that his intervention produced a wound complication. He is certainly entitled to think, "If the patient were thin and fit, it would have taken me less time to complete the procedure, and I would have been able to close more easily, and healing might have been better." But that is only a part of recognition of limitation, and the beginning of an atonement process.

The next entitled thought might be, "I wish I had better skills in surgery, so that even in difficult cases I would be able to proceed faster. I wish I knew more techniques for closure so that fat would not be so daunting." Such recognition might lead to the resident asking his attending for tips on working with fat; a very complex problem that requires advanced skills. I believe that blaming the patient derails the travel from, "This surgery did not produce an optimal outcome," to "This is what I need to learn to improve my outcomes." Blaming deflects the resident's attention from self-improvement. Even worse, it may lead to a permanent defect in his surgical techniques. Suppose the resident becomes a doctor who is anxious about fat? Will he objectively assess fat patients' surgical needs, or will he tend to triage the fat patient to nonsurgical status because of his own fears? When he does have to operate, will he be confident and cool in his approach, or anxious and flustered?

As an onlooker what can be done? As always, calling a Code E is the last resort (example follows below). Perhaps asking for time to talk privately, and expressing your feelings, couched in terms of professional behavior, might work. If it is too risky, creating a caucus of junior team members and having a slightly more confrontational meeting with the resident might work. As a last resort, tattling to the attending or chief is a possibility. In a bad team situation, any of these will be very risky; in a good situation, any will be effective. I would argue against a confrontation at the time

of the first blame; rather, intervention can prevent subsequent displays, and avoid the "channeling" that leads to toxic practice.

What about the situation in "The patient removed the traction"? Here a junior team member who does not feel it is safe to admit a mistake uses blame. This case illustrates the slippery slope phenomenon of blame, since it seems the student may have altered the medical record to help cover the mistake. This is clearly a high-stake situation; a mistake found by the attending, and laid on the chief resident might, if admitted by the student, change his career.

Occasionally, situations like this lead to blame-taking where someone with "wide shoulders" takes the blame to avoid damage to a less-strong person. We are all familiar with these schoolyard heroics. Remember, Tom takes a beating to protect Becky from the schoolmaster; what a hero, how adoring she is! The resident might accept some responsibility for the mistake, and then later privately discuss the matter thoroughly with the student, since some serious stuff is involved here. Just remember, if you take on blame, do not turn it into resentment and later penalize the person you have protected.

As a fellow student, your responsibility is, I believe, to the student. Without blame, you can have a conversation about the incident, and talk through feelings and help to sort out whether the record was changed, how the mistake was made, and so forth until the student has a better grasp of what happened.

So, blaming the patient comes easily in team situations, where the social pressures create embarrassment. However, blame is laid even in one-on-one situations. The traces of it are found throughout medical practice.

My favorite example is pretty benign. Assigned to draw blood on a patient, I applied a tourniquet, prepped the antecubital fossa, inserted the needle, drew the blood, removed the needle, applied compression and a bandaid, thanked the patient and prepared to leave.

"Aren't you going to do the other side?" asked the patient.

"No," I said, "I got the blood I need from that draw."

"Oh," said she, "but they always do both sides. They said I have bad veins."

It seems that on more than one occasion, the patient had been a "hard draw." Presumably the first try always failed, and a second was needed. The patient was then informed, at least once, that her "bad veins" made drawing blood from both sides *necessary*. She was not told (or at least did not remember), "Oh, I am sorry but I failed to get the sample I need from this arm, and will have to try again on the other side." Instead of knowing that it might be technically difficult to draw blood from her veins, and thus being able to warn future phlebotomists, the patient kept quiet about her "bad veins" because she was somewhat guilty about being so "difficult."

Suppose that a Code E situation really does exist? A Big Blame has just been laid, and you know it; maybe all the students know it. Maybe it is not the first time. What to do? Well, as always, Basic Ethical Resuscitation begins with E(xcuse me). Here are some examples of possible verbal actions, ranked in order of deepening doo-doo.

"Excuse me, I am not sure I heard what you said correctly; could you repeat it?" At which point the colleague mutters, *"I said 'if the patient's skin was lighter it would not be so hard to see the sutures'"* and you can either propose a solution without blame, *"Perhaps using a prolene suture might make it more visible,"* or reframe the statement, *"I hear your frustration; I guess you mean that the patient's dark skin color requires using a different technique; perhaps another color of suture would work?"*

If the blamer continues to blame, ask for specific clarification. *"I hear you saying it is somehow the patient's fault her skin is not the right color for the suture you are using. Is that what you mean to say?"* At which point, the colleague may say, *"Oh, I get it. You think I am blaming the patient? No, not really. I guess I should switch to blue suture material."*

Of course the blame may escalate, *"Dammit, I am sick of having to work with these people, I am sick of their color, and their fat, and the way they do not eat right or even bathe enough to stop from stinking!"* In such escalation, the blamer is making a cry for help. She or he is clearly having trouble with the pressures and workload, and is conveniently blaming that on attributes of the client population. As a colleague, you might want to get involved yourself, *"You sound really angry and stressed. Is that something you would want to talk about with me after this shift?"* or you might want to mention the matter to a team leader.

In a situation of blame, if you can at least detect the problem, you may save the colleague from the more toxic complication that a simple little blaming the patient may bring at the bottom of the slippery slope. How to detect that there is a problem? Well, a good place to start is the Rule of M. If the patient was your Mom, would you be acting this way?

COMMENTARY

Francis Kane

"It is hard to be good." So said Aristotle. Today, we veer more to a Platonic view and sometimes imagine that understanding the good is sufficient for virtue. Cases in medical ethics tend to focus on complex and exotic issues, like stem cell transplantation, in an effort to achieve some sort of conceptual clarity about what exactly is involved. Action follows from that understanding, quite literally, as an afterthought. The two cases presented here, however, are neither extraordinary nor difficult to understand. What makes them hard is both the determination of what to do and the actual doing of it. They are disturbing in part because they are so ordinary; they have the grime and grimace of reality about them. What they require of us is not brilliance but virtue.

Before we speculate on what ought to be done

in each of these cases, however, we need to depict the moral atmosphere in which the characters in these mini-dramas must frame their actions.

In each case we are confronted with an individual (the chief resident in "If you weren't so fat" and the medical student in "The patient removed the traction") attempting to cover-up a potential liability or error by blaming the patient. The chief resident blusters his way through the embarrassment of the infection by displaying incredible insensitivity toward his patient; while the lowly medical student seemingly resorts to an old-fashioned smudging of his mistake with an accusatory charge hurled, for good measure, at his patient. In both cases the patient becomes the convenient scapegoat in rather obvious and crude attempts to "cover your ass." While the moral scotosis of the two culprits is rather painfully visible, we might notice how their obvious faults, which they might argue are mere peccadilloes, morally contaminate, in a serious way, the whole therapeutic and educational environment.

First of all, no meaningful communication takes place with the patients, other than to blame them. Particularly disturbing in this culture of blame is the way in which the female patients' cultural and linguistic backgrounds make them even more vulnerable to the scapegoating tactics. The insensitivity to the Tongan and Latino women (and is it just accidental that both are women?) is not only inexcusable but also forestalls any opportunity to respond adequately to the needs of these women of color.

Secondly, while the image of the physician as teacher and role model is a powerful one in medicine, in both of these cases the educational value of the encounters has been almost completely nullified. The chief resident in the infection case has compromised whatever moral authority he may have had with his students. Furthermore, no one inquires about how much cultural expectations might play in the weight gained by the Tongan mother; nor does anyone point out how the language barrier obviates any involvement of either of the patients in her own care. The attend-

ing physician and the chief resident in the traction case seem totally focused on who is responsible for the wrong weights and thereby miss an opportunity to let students learn by their mistakes. By lying about his mistake, the medical student has violated the bottom line in any learning situation: academic honesty. Even the nurse, in the latter case, may have entered into collusion, however unwittingly, with the medical staff's finger pointing. While she deftly avoids the blame game by a convenient memory lapse (aimed perhaps at covering for the student), she would surely know how unlikely it was that the patient would have altered the weights.

Punctuated in the one case with embarrassment over an unexplained infection and, in the other, with the cut-throat pressure to pass a rotation, the moral atmosphere is rife with fault finding and finger pointing. A culture of blame is created wherein the accusations fly down the line until they stop at the lowliest player in the drama, the final scapegoat, the patient. The scenes play themselves out in an eerie and ironic mockery of the Hippocratic Oath:

I swear . . . to hold him who has taught me this art as equal to my parents and to live my life in partnership with him . . . I will come for the benefit of the sick, remaining free from all intentional injustice, of all mischief . . . In purity and holiness I will guard my life and my art.

Now, for the hard part. What is to be done in each of the cases? In the face of the boorish, insensitive chief resident and the mean-spirited, lying medical student, what do the bystanders do? It would not be easy for medical students, themselves vulnerable to a hierarchical and authoritative system, to cast the first stone. A prudent admonition of "Don't rock the boat" seems appropriate in such situations. And prudence, ironically, is called for here; but not its modern connotation of a cagey diffidence and hesitancy to act. Rather, what is required is the Aristotelian virtue of practical wisdom: the right person does the right thing at the right time and place, in the right way for the right reason. That sense of prudence may place too much expectation on callow medical students; yet when and where else would they learn it?

The temptation *not* to act would certainly be strong in light of the intimidating atmosphere and could be supported by the rationalization that no big harm has been done. "After all," the students could argue, "the infection is being treated in the one case and the right traction set in the other. Better to leave well enough alone." I suspect, however, that for them and for us such excuses would leave us with a sense of unease. As I have pointed out, the therapeutic and educational purposes in both cases have already been seriously compromised. To let the evil stand is to become an accomplice in it.

To decide, on the other hand, what ought to be done is problematic (in both cases) and I doubt that there is a clear-cut answer to the students' questions about what is the right thing to do; excepting, of course, the obvious wrong of participating in and exacerbating the scapegoating of the patients. Furthermore, one cannot replace or override the role of practical wisdom to decide on the spot and that requires the prudent actor to have a developed sense of the uniqueness of the situation and of the characters involved. There are no handbooks for moral action. There are, however, some moral guidelines for cases like these and we can use our moral imagination to think through and evaluate possible courses of action. Some fairly obvious principles operative here would be: (1) whatever action is taken, its purpose ought to further the patients' good; (2) correct, to the extent that is possible, whatever injustice has occurred; and (3) promote the educative values in the situations, particularly by putting an end to the blame game. In hindsight, had the chief residents acted more circumspectly, all the above principles could have been followed. They could have dealt with the medical situations in the patients' rooms and, then, out of earshot, discussed the problems – thus avoiding the charged atmosphere of fixing blame. Here, the

causes and intractability of some infections and the appropriate traction weights could have been dealt with in an atmosphere that would be more supportive and allow for whatever clinical assessments and judgments that needed to be made. The participants, however, do not have the benefit of hindsight and, so, we need the foresight to imagine some possible responses that could have been made in the immediacy of the situations.

One possible strategy – which would seem to carry minimal risk to the students – would be to return later to the patients, express concern about what happened, apologize perhaps for the insensitivity of colleagues, make efforts to communicate about their respective conditions, and promise to follow up on their progress. Empathy demonstrated in this way would at least counter the lack of compassion displayed to the patients. The mere mentioning of this option, however, suggests the obvious rejoinder: "Is that enough?" Probably not, since this after-the-fact response leaves the moral behavior of the participants unchallenged.

Another course of action, again after the fact, would be to go to one's superiors and register a complaint. That would probably create resentment and, unfortunately, just ratchet up the blame game one more notch. In the Tongan woman's case there is no obvious malpractice and the altered chart, in the traction case, would be impossible to prove. Certainly, such an appeal to higher authority would be more warranted if these individual situations represented patterns that left unattended could compromise the educational purposes of rounds.

Prior to taking that route, prudence would most likely counsel that the chief resident and the medical student in each case be confronted. I surmise that the right time and right place, along with the right way (the when, where, and how) would prescribe that the encounter take place later and in a less threatening environment. It still would be difficult to cut through the chief resident's pedantry but perhaps the indirection of suggesting that cultural views may have played a part in the Tongan woman's weight problem and offering to study the issue and report back to the rotation might open the door to a more frank discussion of the initial cause of the infection. Not to confront the friend in the traction case seems inexcusable, if only for the sake of the friendship. A private chat that raised the issues of his deception and his false accusations against the patient might even shame him into an admission of wrongdoing or at least force him to feel the sting of a friend's rebuke.

The question tendered at the end of the Tongan case is evocative: what should *we* have done? The solidarity of the students would make a more powerful and potentially less risky approach than the individual complainant. The students, along with the faculty, do form a moral community; they have to be up to some good, some common purpose. To transform the *de jure* moral community into a *de facto* community of character, again to invoke Aristotle, is hard. If, however, there is any hope of redeeming these two cases from the degeneracy of the very purpose of medicine, a communal effort is called for. By addressing, honestly and courageously, the issues together there is certainly the possibility of re-forming a learning community. In the first case, by jointly discussing with the chief resident their concerns, pointing out the obvious but (for him) overlooked fact, that the Tongan woman did not understand what he was saying, the students would not only better protect themselves from retaliation but could transform the whole learning environment. In the second case, together they might confront their fellow student and express their understanding of how much pressure they are all under in these rotations but also point out that all of them have to have a bottom line: honesty with

teachers and respect for the patient. What a powerful example could be set if the whole rotation then went to the attending and chief resident and discussed what happened and what could be done to create a more nurturing environment. A subsequent apology to the Latin American woman might in some measure redeem the situation.

The above suggestions are meant to be illustrative rather than proscriptive. Both cases are meant to be opportunities for foresight rather than to provide solutions in hindsight. Situations that demand quick thinking on the spot and on one's feet in a threatening environment can have an enervating effect on the actor. In the immediate moment, the participants are often caught unawares, struck with an element of surprise and, before they have a chance to react, the group has moved on to the next case, leaving them in startled silence and with a sense of unease and guilt. We have all been in those situations. The only hedge against the paralysis the unexpected brings is a certain preparedness that comes from a reflective mind and a disposition to act wisely, justly, and courageously. The "actual" situation is a bounded one for the participants; for those of us who think, discuss, and judge a deeper awareness is possible. In the distancing artifice that constitutes a case study, we can not only imagine what we as students would do but we can also put ourselves in the position of the patients and even recognize ourselves, however ruefully, in the chief resident's blustery cover-up and in the panicked medical student's fudging of the chart. If the culturally dysfunctional blame game is to be halted, such discussions could serve as important antidotes. These cases are good medicine.

4

Breaking the code: is a promise always a promise?

CASE

"How 'confidential' is confidential?"

The patient was a 13-year-old African–American male who presented to the pediatric clinic with his acting guardian from the boys' home for an entry physical examination. The clinic is staffed by a group of physicians who rotate through on different days of the week, as do the residents and medical students like myself. Providers at the clinic see children from underserved populations and frequently have patients from the local boys' home for physical exams and minor treatment. This young man was like most other children his age, basically healthy and active. He had been sent to the boys' home after driving a stolen car under the influence of alcohol, in addition to a previous history of other legal infractions.

His only health complaint was that he suffered from significant allergies that were causing him congestion and discomfort. He worried this problem might affect his trying out for the freshman football team. As the resident proceeded with the history, I examined the patient and listened. He appeared to be having trouble understanding the resident's accent and clearly did not appreciate how she was phrasing some of the questions, particularly the one implying drug use.

When she left, I remained with the patient, who had denied any drug use. We had a relaxed conversation about the importance of confidentiality in the doctor–patient relationship and how greater accuracy of the history will lead to greater efficacy of treatment. We talked some more, and the patient disclosed that in addition to still drinking alcohol, he was also smoking marijuana and thought this fact might be contributing to his allergies/congestion. I reassured him that his disclosure was the correct thing to do and confirmed with the "attending of the day" that the patient's records were confidential and could not be accessed by the boys' home.

The patient returned one week later irate that when he had returned to the boys' home, several counselors approached him in a public hallway about his drug and alcohol use. As it turns out, my resident had told the patient's guardian about his health issues, which included his substance abuse. Apparently, the clinic usually shares all medical treatment issues with the guardians from the boys' home and does not necessarily delineate sensitive issues from this policy.

As a result of what he views as a breach of confidence, the patient no longer trusts health providers and is now less amenable to treatment for his problem. What, if anything, could be done to ameliorate this situation? In the future, what should I say to patients about what "confidentiality" means?

COMMENTARY

Robyn Shapiro

This case study is a poignant illustration of the reasons for and significance of patients' privacy rights. The ethical principle of respect for autonomy has long been recognized as one important justification for respecting patient privacy. Privacy promotes individual autonomy in two important respects. First, by respecting patients' privacy we respect their autonomous wishes not to have information about them made available to others. At a more fundamental level, respect for privacy is instrumental in individuals' development of a sense of self and a capacity to be self-governing.

Respect for privacy also enhances the development and maintenance of intimate human relationships – including the physician–patient relationship. In fact, one defining characteristic of all intimate relationships is that they involve the sharing of private information and acts. As described by Charles Fried, "[P]rivacy is . . . necessarily related to ends and relations of the most fundamental sort: respect, love, friendship and trust. Privacy is not merely a good technique for furthering these fundamental relations; rather, without privacy they are simply inconceivable." (1)

Respect for patients' privacy is also critical for safeguarding patients' well-being and the good of society. Health care information relates to profoundly personal aspects of an individual's life. Typically, medical records include not only objective observations, diagnoses, and test results, but also health care providers' subjective impressions about the patient, and information or suppositions about the patient's life style, dietary habits, and recreational activities. Because of the highly sensitive nature of this information, improper disclosure can result in lost business opportunities, compromised financial status, damage to reputation, or personal humiliation. Yet, at the same time, in order for the health care giver to establish an accurate diagnosis and provide optimal medical treatment, he or she must be fully informed about these issues. An environment that facilitates full and open communication between doctor and patient must be maintained; yet without the assurance of confidentiality, patients are reluctant to share medically relevant information with their providers.

These ethical and policy justifications for health information privacy protections are reflected in statutes and court decisions that establish the legal duty to maintain patients' rights to privacy and confidentiality. Many states have statutes, regulations, or case law recognizing medical records as confidential and limiting access to them. At the U.S. federal level, the Alcohol, Drug Abuse and Mental Health Administration Reorganization Act, and implementing regulations, (2) prohibit disclosure of any information about patients who receive substance abuse treatment from federally assisted health care facilities, except in specified, limited instances.

The case study involves a 13-year-old whose guardian is an employee of the boys' home where he lives. As a general matter, children's rights must be exercised on their behalf by their parents or guardians. However, with respect to certain types of medical problems – including drug and alcohol abuse – almost all states have statutes permitting minors to receive treatment confidentially without the involvement of their parents or guardians. In Illinois, for example, any minor who is 12 or older may consent to substance abuse treatment (410 Ill. Compiled Stat. Ann. §210/4, 210/5); and in Michigan, a minor who abuses or is dependent upon drugs or narcotics may consent to care by a hospital, clinic, physician, or registered nurse, and the provider may, but need not, inform the minor's parents or guardian (Mich. Comp. Laws §333.6121). Moreover, federal law governing substance abuse treatment states that if a minor acting alone has the legal capacity under applicable state law to apply for and obtain substance abuse treatment, only the minor patient may give consent for disclosure of related health information to his/her parent or guardian. The intent behind these laws is to facilitate substance abuse treatment of minors who might be reluctant to seek such treatment if they thought their parents or guardians would be informed.

The home state of the 13-year-old patient in the case study is not specified, so exact legal requirements and prohibitions regarding health information disclosure cannot be ascertained.

Nonetheless, the case clearly illustrates the rationale underlying laws that facilitate minors' ability to confidentially access substance abuse treatment. It was only *after* the medical student explained the importance of and reasons for confidentiality in the doctor–patient relationship that the patient disclosed that he was still drinking alcohol and smoking marijuana and expressed concern that these activities might be contributing to his allergies and congestion. Moreover, when the patient later learned that, despite assurances of confidentiality, this information had been disclosed to his guardian and counselors at the boys' home, he retracted the trust he had placed in the health care system.

It is critical to avoid the situation posed in the case study by assuring that (1) the health care team has a clear, common understanding about confidentiality parameters of the doctor–patient relationship; (2) the health care team clearly communicates these parameters to the patient at the outset; and that (3) these parameters are followed. Since the pediatric clinic providers in this case often treated children from the local boys' home who had histories of legal infractions, the clinic should have been acutely aware of the need to develop guidelines, grounded in ethics and applicable law, about disclosure of patient information. These confidentiality ground rules should have been well understood by and agreed and adhered to by all of the clinic's providers, and communicated to the patient and his guardian at the outset of the clinic visit so that care could have been sought elsewhere if the patient or the guardian objected. In the case at hand, it appears that while the medical student and the attending physician believed that the confidentiality of the patient's health care information should and would be protected, the resident believed otherwise and followed the alleged common clinic practice of sharing all health care information with guardians from the boys' home. The resulting damage to the trust between this patient and his health care providers may permanently hinder his health care and damage his health. His

story illustrates the dangers of failure to take confidentiality seriously.

Notes

1 Fried C. *An Anatomy of Values: Problems of Personal and Social Choice.* Harvard University Press, Cambridge, MA, 1970, p.142.
2 42 U.S.C. §§290dd-290 dd-2, 42 C.F.R. §§2.11-2.12.

COMMENTARY

Pablo Rodriguez del Pozo

Modern medicine is the realm of the scientific and the technological, where day by day the borders of progress are expanded to allow people to enjoy longer healthier lives. So goes, at least, conventional wisdom, which turns today's doctors into something close to scientists – objective professionals, even a bit dehumanized. To a large degree, doctors share this notion about themselves and their profession.

It is obvious that medicine today is constructed on a scientific foundation. It is no less true that medicine today is loaded with considerations related more to cultural beliefs and taboos than to reason. These factors affect the essence and style of everything that goes on in the examining room and in hospital corridors, and have particular bearing on the crucial issue of doctor–patient confidentiality. The case under study, in which a troubled 13-year-old male undergoes a routine check-up complaining of allergies, and ends up receiving unwanted confrontations and counseling in drug and alcohol abuse, is very eloquent.

There are many particulars of this case which I find disturbing. Before seeing a single patient, a medical student should be familiar with the rules of confidentiality, rather than having to ask about them after he or she has received sensitive information. This would be the case in any clinic, but is particularly true at a clinic specializing in underserved populations and residents of a local boys' home, where patients are more likely to have a history of socially conflictive behavior and serious problems which their parents or guardians may or may not know about. It is doubly disturbing that, even after asking authorities at the clinic, the student is given inaccurate information on what will be told to the patient's guardians. Once the information is turned over to the guardians, "several" counselors approach the patient in a "public" place.

One can hardly blame the 13-year-old for his irateness afterwards, and we certainly will know who to blame if the young man, or others from the same center, never again confide in a doctor out of fear of being betrayed.

Moving beyond those considerations, which reflect a lack of organization at the clinic and a disregard for patient privacy, I would like to start by examining the meaning of confidentiality.

The efficacy of medical treatment depends on the doctor's own knowledge and the depth of the information obtained about the patient. Diagnosing and treating require exploring the physiology of patients, and also learning something about their family, their personal life, their lifestyle. Typically, however, only a fraction of the physiological and personal information is truly relevant. Patients cannot distinguish between what is and is not of medical interest; for that reason they are obliged to give the doctor access to all physical, psychological, and social details.

But patients aware of potential embarrassment among peers and possible problems within their family or social group can distinguish what information is socially problematic. This was already known to the ancient Greeks: because there are medically significant aspects that may carry social penalties, doctors must guarantee confidentiality over what they discover about their patients during a medical exam. Practicing medicine is possible after Hippocrates because doctors make the commitment that information will not be used for any other purpose than for treating the patient. Because there is professional confi-

dentiality, patients take the immensely intimate step of undressing physically, and to a degree, emotionally in front of the doctor.

With professional confidentiality it must be understood that (1) all information received by doctors is, in principle, absolutely confidential, even among colleagues; and (2) confidentiality will be breached only under exceptional circumstances, and must be duly justified. As a corollary, medical providers who reveal information must be ready to prove that without this revelation it would have been impossible to treat the sickness that motivated the visit to the doctor. (I will avoid entering into a discussion of the legal mandate to reveal information which is another complementary consideration – see preceding commentary by Shapiro).

After receiving all of the information from a patient, doctors should take into account only that which is relevant to diagnosis and treatment. This converts doctors into a warehouse for excess information that lacks genuine medical interest. When more than one doctor treats the same person, a common occurrence in today's practices, what part of the information must be passed on to colleagues and what must remain confidential? In my opinion, doctors should pass on only that information required for the concrete problem that prompted the appointment.

It could be said that the greater the potential embarrassment or social ramifications for the patient and the less medically relevant the information, the stricter confidentiality must be. Without any mathematical pretenses, this could be illustrated by the following formula:

$$\frac{\text{potential embarrassment} + \text{potential social penalties}}{\text{medical relevance}} = \frac{\text{confidentiality}}{\text{obligation}}$$

The problem is that medicine is not so scientific as to override values, and many times what is considered "medically significant" may be, rather than a scientific fact, a contingent social value, an expression of the beliefs of the dominant culture at that time. That may make it complicated for doctors to define what is and is not medical, and should or should not be passed on to colleagues.

Doctors, beyond their scientific knowledge of biological phenomena, are not removed from their cultural and social environments. On the contrary, they exercise their profession immersed in the coordinates of the culture to which they belong. While diagnosis and treatment may appear to doctors and patients alike to be scientific pronouncements, rarely are they exempt from moral, social, and religious considerations.

The concepts of health and sickness themselves, as evidenced by medical sociology and anthropology, have a cultural and historic character. The diagnosis is culturally constructed, and the designation of "illness" is a social act that chooses some human attribute, brands it undesirable and makes an effort to find its physical recipient, and then seeks to eradicate it. This means that what is considered health and what is considered illness can and do vary depending on time and place.

This is valid for some somatic conditions, although it is more evident in mental illness and, obviously, in syndromes related to cultures. (1)

The social construct of illness is what provokes its scientific study, and not the reverse. However, given the same physical constitution of all humans, and given that sickness almost always has a physiological basis, medicine tends to concentrate on the scientific study of these elements, and we end up viewing medical problems as independent of the social and cultural variables.

Returning to the specific case at hand, it is difficult to determine whether the young man's drug and alcohol use in any way aggravated his allergies; for that, I would have to know more about the nature of his allergies. On the surface, however, the two are unrelated. It is also impossible to determine the degree of his involvement with drugs and alcohol, whether it is occasional usage (anathema to most of us in a 13-year-old, but less medically important) or whether it is obvious and detrimental abuse. To better appreciate the cultural nuances that color the diagnosis, and the medical obsession related to the use of marijuana and other substances, I would offer examples from outside of the United States. In the predominantly Moslem countries of northern Africa, where cannabis is tolerated but alcohol prohibited, the latter may be the medical equivalent of our cannabis. And the amount of wine that a person drinks daily to be considered a health risk is not the same in the U.S. as it may be in France or even the Vatican.

In some countries and cultures, it would be socially unacceptable, not to mention illegal, for an unmarried woman to take birth-control pills. If this fact were to become known, she would suffer social exclusion and even legal penalties. Her life would be ruined in some ways. Would there be a strictly medical reason for another medical student to tell a resident that the patient was taking birth-control pills if the young woman consulted her doctor about allergies that were causing her discomfort and congestion?

Doctors should be able to evaluate the use of substances and drugs by their patients according to their physiological impact, and not according to whether they are socially unacceptable. By social consideration I also include the legal status of these substances. Again, the information shared with colleagues should be limited to the influence these substances might have on the pathology that originated the visit to the doctor. That is to say that the medical student should not have passed on the drug information to the resident. (And surely the clinic's policy of sharing all treatment issues with the boys' home regardless of how sensitive is a breach of patients' privacy.) In this case, the breach is particularly grave since the patient was given assurances by the medical student that all information would be kept private, and only divulged the drug and alcohol issue after receiving those guarantees.

Thus, we should take a critical look at the practice of our profession, to understand that medicine reflects values; that medicine is not simply applied biology but rather biology applied according to the dictates of the social interests and prejudices of each time. To the degree that current and future doctors are so preoccupied with educating themselves in the scientific aspects of medicine that they do not have time to study sociological and philosophical issues contained in them, they will run the risk of becoming ideological gendarmes to their patients.

And if doctors are incapable of guaranteeing confidentiality, patients will do it for them by hiding information and avoiding seeking medical attention. This is particularly true for the segments of the population that are most vulnerable medically and socially, who need models to follow and adults in whom to confide.

Note

1 These consist of a series of symptoms that: (1) cannot be understood outside a specific cultural or subcultural framework; (2) its etiology symbolizes certain beliefs and norms of conduct that are at the heart of said culture; (3) the diagnosis is based on technology specific to that culture and its ideology; (4) the successful treatment is done only by the participants in that culture.

5

The newly dead

CASE

"Patient or cadaver?"

One evening during my first year of medical school I was observing a preceptor in the Emergency Department. A paramedic-staffed ambulance brought in a man who had been in cardiac arrest for some time. In the Emergency Department it was clear from the start that the situation looked very grim. The doctor asked if I was CPR certified and if I wanted to do cardiopulmonary resuscitation on this patient. I told him that I was certified, but I wasn't ready to take on this situation. He brushed aside my reluctance and said, "Don't worry about it. Go ahead and try. I'll be here next to you." I administered effective CPR. Yet nothing worked, and eventually the patient was declared dead.

At that point, the curtain was pulled around the bed and the doctor told me he was going to practice intubation using the corpse that, only moments ago, had been his patient. He explained that since all the paramedics were now trained to intubate patients in the field, he seldom had the opportunity to practice this important skill. Since he didn't want to lose his proficiency, he felt this was a good way to maintain it. Later, I heard that there was also a group of training paramedic students who needed intubation experience and were invited to make use of this "practice opportunity."

* Portions of the following article were previously published as: Iserson KV. Life versus death: exposing a misapplication of ethical reasoning. *J Clin Ethics* 1994;5(3):261–4.

COMMENTARY*

Kenneth V. Iserson

Physicians do not learn in a vacuum, but rather amidst the blood, pain, and gore that medicine entails. The learning process is often not pretty, but it is effective, as the quality of American medicine demonstrates. This case raises questions about the educational methods surrounding the most consistently time-dependent physician specialty – emergency medicine. What part should medical students and paramedics play during their training? What should emergency physicians do to ensure their continued competency?

Current debates and future changes

Before concerning ourselves with this case, we should acknowledge that within not too many years, radical changes in educational technology will make most of these questions moot. Highly realistic computerized simulations will allow students and physicians to learn and remain proficient in nearly all medical procedures without involving either patients or their cadaveric remains. No one will do their first (or second or third) procedure on patients as they now must do. Rather, they will become proficient on models, only being allowed to perform procedures on people once they are technically proficient. While that won't guarantee success, it will greatly improve the novices' procedural skills

when they encounter patients. It may also mark-
edly shorten the timeline needed for medical
school and residency training. We live in the
present, though, and must deal with the educational and ethical problems our current environment presents.

Our first problem, however, exists in both our
current and future educational systems. The
medical student says that he learned CPR. He
would have used a common (but soon to be an-
tique) training manikin. Using these models, CPR
students get a rough approximation of what it is
like to perform cardiopulmonary resuscitation.
Depending upon the model used, they can get
various types of feedback on how well they do.
Yet there is a problem – the same problem that
will haunt future educators using more sophisticated models. Using models, students have none
of the fear, hesitancy, or personal involvement
that they have when confronted by real patients.
In this case the patient is dying, and the student
is suddenly being asked to take a "high-stakes
test" – transferring his classroom knowledge into
potentially lifesaving behavior. His hesitancy, not
uncommon among medical students, only demonstrates the rift between medical school class-
rooms and clinical settings, between theory and
practice. Yet does it demonstrate any ethical
problem?

No. CPR is a simple technique that, unlike a
surgical incision that once made cannot be eras-
ed, can be altered with each successive compression. Standard practice is for someone to feel the
femoral pulse during resuscitations to give people
doing CPR, whether novices or experts, feedback
so that they can alter the depth and rate of their
compressions. That the emergency physician
encouraged the student by standing at his side
and that he did not substitute someone more
experienced during the resuscitation attempt
showed both that the physician had excellent
educational skills and that the student must have
performed CPR well. Medical students and residents commonly need this encouragement during their training. This student was only lucky

that the attending physician had the patience and
experience during the hubbub of a cardiac resuscitation to provide this type of support. We will
continue to need this form of educational assistance – in transition from simulator to patients,
from classroom to clinic, and from nonthreatening to ego-threatening experiences – as long as we
train physicians.

The second problem, ethically sexier but with a
much shorter half-life, is that of using cadavers to
practice and teach noninvasive or minimally
invasive procedures such as intubation. As I have
previously argued, physicians not only can but
must remain proficient in lifesaving techniques.
In emergency medicine, the most practical, egali-
tarian, and effective way to do this is to use the
cadavers of recently deceased patients.

The knowledge base

Good ethics begins with good information – in
policy development as well as in clinical consultations. The necessary information to develop a
policy concerning practicing and teaching on the
newly dead comes in two parts: the setting in
which clinicians use lifesaving skills such as intubation, and what happens to corpses, both in
the hospital and elsewhere. Clinical ethicists can
easily obtain the former information from their
colleagues in emergency and intensive care medicine and from paramedics in their emergency
medical system. While they might not experience
first-hand the dread of not passing a tube into the
trachea of a dying child, or of having to reach for
the scalpel to cut a surgical airway when their
skills at intubation failed, they can certainly vi-
cariously feel these experiences. They can view
the patient's neck with a fresh cricothyrotomy
scar, or visit the morgue and see those in whom
the clinicians could not obtain any airway.

The latter information concerns what can and
does happen to corpses. While this information
has not been readily available, it is now. (While
developing this issue in another setting, this
question prompted me to do further investiga-

tion, resulting in the book, *Death to Dust: What Happens to Dead Bodies?*) (1) Yet even without this source, clinical ethicists can easily determine what happens to corpses in and just after they leave the Emergency Department, intensive care units, or wards.

As some misguided ethicists belatedly found out after promoting an intrusive policy requiring informed consent before practicing and teaching on cadavers could occur, cadavers do not idly lie around in busy hospital beds. Rather, nurses or in-house morticians quickly whisk them to the morgue, so valuable bed space can be opened. (2)

Despite what some would have us believe, no public outcry has demanded that clinicians stop using the newly dead in this manner; it is only misguided lawyers and ethicists. (3) One recent situation may be instructive in this matter. The U.S. media publicized an exposé in Germany that cadavers were being used as crash dummies, and then tried to create public outrage that the same practice was occurring in the United States. The public, once they were quickly told that the cadaver studies were saving lives through innovations in automobile safety, showed no concern at all, even though the source of many of the cadavers used is uncertain. (4)

The corpse as a symbol

Despite all this, societies should respect their dead; it remains the mark of a civilized society. Respect is due because the newly dead corpse symbolizes the recently deceased person, as well as all of humanity. Yet to what extent must we pay homage to the symbol? Respecting the symbol by denying physicians the skills to keep the living from joining the dead is, as Feinberg says, "a poor sort of 'respect' to show a sacred symbol." (5)

Another way of viewing this situation is to see postmortem practice as the ultimate respect for the corpse. The clinicians who worked to save the patient's life (and failed) now will use the per-

son's shell to hone skills with which they will try to save their next critical patient. Anyone who has seen this practice knows that it is done with respect, some would say awe. If respect means paying homage, showing deference, and bestowing honor, this procedure is more respectful than many of the after-death rites in our society such as embalming. (6)

The main question is whether the living, in the person of the next patient needing the health professional's critical lifesaving skills to survive, should be sacrificed to the memory of the dead. We must ask, on a utilitarian basis, which obligation weighs most heavily on both the physicians and society – paying homage to the symbol of a former patient (the cadaver) or being adequately prepared to help save the next life. Posed that way, few would have a doubt about the correct course of action. Human life always takes precedence over symbols of life; common sense always survives emotional and legal excess. As I understand it, human sacrifice was banned in Western religious practice in Biblical times (*Genesis: 22*). It would be a travesty to reverse this noble advance for civilization under the guise of "bioethics."

Skills and societal expectations

Imagine for a minute that you are traveling in a commercial airliner when the intercom comes on and the captain informs the passengers that unfortunately, both he and the copilot have neither flown nor been in a trainer for the past six months, having just returned from a wonderful prolonged vacation in Tahiti. "Don't worry," he says. "It's just like riding a bike." Think about how reassured you would be. Flying a commercial jet is not like "riding a bike," and neither is placing an endotracheal tube or a central venous catheter in a dying patient. In both circumstances, new and unexpected problems occur, variations from the norm exist, and the equipment changes over time. Unfortunately, unlike most commercial pilots, not all clinicians needing to perform these procedures have exhaustive training to make them even initially proficient. Yet their skill levels will be what saves (or loses) lives. Those who excel at these procedures need to teach others while remaining proficient themselves.

The question of keeping current in lifesaving skills is not hypothetical, but rather increasingly troublesome for many practicing physicians. It is obvious that experienced clinicians neither appear *de novo* nor remain experienced without practice. As the emergency physician in this case took pains to explain to the student, until recently, physicians who worked in emergency care areas had little need for added practice in endotracheal intubation or central line placement, because the mere frequency of these critical care procedures produced competence. Now however, highly trained ambulance personnel often perform procedures such as endotracheal intubations in the field; only the most difficult procedures are left for the Emergency Department staff, who consequently may lose proficiency in their lifesaving skills. (7) This expertise is a genuine value both to society in general and to all patients needing emergency care. Therefore, it is society's responsibility to encourage practitioners to develop lifesaving skills in a manner that will help patients, rather than harm them.

Requiring clinicians to formally request permission before practicing these lifesaving skills guarantees that many of them will simply either not ask and not practice (putting many lives in jeopardy) or practice without asking (placing other bioethics policies and any respect for bioethicists in harm's way). Putting any barriers in the way of maintaining these skills does a disservice to all patients relying on these clinicians to save or maintain their lives. (7–9)

A prescription for clinicians needing lifesaving skills

All of the above leads me to the conclusion that those clinicians who need to learn or keep current in lifesaving medical skills to decrease their patient's morbidity and mortality not only may, but *must* use the newly dead to practice and teach. Artificial barriers must not preclude this. Beneficence, doing good for the (next living) patient, must be the clinician's guiding principle. If physicians (and paramedics and medical students) continue to use this readily available and realistic model to develop and maintain their lifesaving skills, I will never again have to hear a colleague say, "If I had just been a little better at intubation, she would still be alive."

Conclusion

While societies should respect their dead, the living should never be sacrificed to their memory. Difficult, lifesaving skills in medicine, as in other fields, must not only be taught, but also be constantly practiced and refined. Putting any barriers in the way of physicians practicing and upgrading their skills in performing endotracheal intubation threatens the lives of their future patients. The guise of patient (surrogate) autonomy is stretched thin when ethicists use it to cover postmortem practice and teaching, especially that which is rapid, nondisfiguring, and potentially lifesaving for others. (Perhaps we should first concern ourselves with ensuring patient autonomy for the living, who can still be affected by decisions.) The common alternatives, practicing and teaching on animals (a poor model) or on unsuspecting patients under general anesthesia can only be considered abhorrent, given the availability of bodies who can no longer be harmed.

While pedants, far removed from the tumult of emergency care, worry over unusual permutations of solid ethical issues, I will encourage my colleagues to continue practicing and teaching, *ad lib*, on the newly dead. I submit that doing this is not only permissible, it is required. For health professionals to lack needed lifesaving skills even once because one has not done so violates the most basic ethical principles.

Little Red Riding Hood unmasked the deception, discovered her peril and avoided harm. Would that our society will do likewise.

Notes

1 Iserson KV. *Death to Dust: What Happens to Dead Bodies?* Galen Press, Tucson, AZ, 1994.

2 Perkins HS, Gordon AM. Should hospital policy require consent for practicing invasive procedures on cadavers? The arguments, conclusions, and lessons from one ethics committee's deliberations. *J Clin Ethics* 1994;5(3):204–10.

3 Goldblatt AD. Don't ask, don't tell: practicing minimally invasive resuscitation techniques on the newly dead. *Ann Emerg Med* 1995;25(1):86–90.

4 Iserson KV. *Death to Dust: What Happens to Dead Bodies?* Galen Press, Tucson, AZ, 1994, p.99.

5 Feinberg J. The mistreatment of dead bodies. *Hastings Cent Rep* 1985; 31–7.

6 Iserson KV. *Death to Dust: What Happens to Dead Bodies?* Galen Press, Tucson, AZ, 1994, pp.182–215.

7 Iserson KV. Using a cadaver to practice and teach. *Hastings Cent Rep* 1986;16:28–9.

8 Iserson KV. Requiring consent to practice and teach using the recently dead. *J Emerg Med* 1991; 9:509–10.

9 Iserson KV. Postmortem procedures in the emergency department: using the recently dead to practise (sic) and teach. *J Med Ethics* 1993;19:92–8.

COMMENTARY

Michael L. Gross

News item:

"Unjustifiable Paternalism"
It took a bereaved father, himself a doctor, to reveal a long-standing practice of surreptitiously using the fallen bodies of soldiers in training for emergency surgery. An embarrassed IDF (Israel Defense Forces) first defended the practice, citing the need to save lives, but yesterday announced that it had been stopped. (Jerusalem Post, 6 April 1999)

The Israeli case, like the one under consideration in "Patient or cadaver?" raises a number of issues that are not easily sorted out. It is a classic moral dilemma that pits firmly entrenched ethical principles of dignity, individual autonomy, and the common good against one another. Like any dilemma, there are at least two possible outcomes, either to permit or to ban the practice of surgery on the newly dead. The task is to decide which outcome is better.

By most accounts the practice of operating on the newly dead is extraordinarily beneficial and the benefits are easy to enumerate. First, the most commonly practiced surgeries, tracheotomy and similar resuscitation techniques, are the staple of emergency room medicine. Performing it well will undoubtedly allow paramedics and emergency room physicians to save lives. Second, operating on the newly dead allows medical personnel to perfect their skill in a way not available if a manikin or cadavers are used. Third, the dead are not harmed. Under these conditions – substantial benefits, dearth of alternative teaching methods, and no possibility of harm to others – resolution should be easy. Yet, the practice often meets with considerable resistance. Why? What considerations, if any, outweigh these considerable benefits?

The importance of informed consent

The most obvious objection to operating on the newly dead is the lack of respect shown the now-dead patient and his family. The objection hinges on the principle of informed consent, the overriding imperative that a patient's body may not be violated without his permission. But is the newly dead a patient? What rights to his body does he and his family have?

To answer this question, it might be useful to

look at the analogous case of organ transplants. Harvesting organs generally requires explicit consent from the patient or his family. Shouldn't similar consent be obtained for surgery? One answer is yes, without consent surgery cannot be performed. Another answer, not common in the U.S., is more qualified. Many European nations recognize the principle of *presumed consent*: patients are presumed to allow physicians to harvest their organs at death unless they specifically refuse their consent. This is based on a communitarian model of citizen–society relationships that see individuals' rights subordinate to the common good. Rights are not abrogated by any means, rather they are formulated in such a way as to further the common good. Unfortunately, presumed consent works better on paper than in practice. Many countries which have presumed consent laws on the books, Israel and France for example, still demand explicit consent before they will harvest organs. If practice surgery is akin to organ transplant then it, too, would require informed consent. Perhaps another analogy is more applicable.

Although consent is required for organ harvest, it is not, one might argue, always required for autopsies. This analogy would help were it true that practice surgery is more like an autopsy than organ retrieval. However, this is clearly not the case. Organ retrieval and practice surgery have only a localized benefit. If not performed only a limited number of individuals will benefit or suffer. This limited benefit is balanced against a patient's right to control what happens to his own body, and in most cases, the patient's wishes take precedent. Autopsies are different. Because they may reveal a communicable disease or heinous crime, the failure to conduct an autopsy may threaten the public good. In the case of operating on the newly deceased, as in the case of organ transplants, there are no far-reaching social benefits to override the need to obtain consent.

The social costs of non-disclosure

Additionally, one may weigh the social cost of not obtaining consent from the patient or his family. As the Israeli case shows the costs can be considerable. Not only is the family outraged when finally informed, but the public nature of the disclosure severely damages the trust that the public places in the medical profession, the military, and the government. This is not because the public believes that the practice of operating on the dead is unnecessary or not beneficial but because they assume that the bodies they are getting back have not been tampered with. They had sufficient faith in the authorities to assume that if there was a need to use their son's body they will be informed as such. This trust was violated in the most flagrant way imaginable.

As the cost of nondisclosure grows it might only be offset by other costs associated with trying to obtain informed consent. As a result, some observers argue that the need for informed consent creates unnecessary delays (that damage the lax neck tissue required for practicing intubation techniques), or causes stress to families. While this might be true, these costs are localized and only affect a limited number of patients. They are insufficient to override the need for informed consent for the potential damage to the public trust caused by nondisclosure gone astray.

Similarly, some physicians fear that the need for informed consent will forever preclude the possibility of practicing on patients. As one senior Israeli physician put it:

After death the issue of consent is irrelevant. No one is going to give consent to an operative procedure which won't benefit anyone. Look how difficult it is to get people to consent to donating organs and that can save the lives of several people. It's not an issue that can be discussed, it should just be done and everyone should keep their mouths shut about it.

Fear that the public will look askance at physicians is, however, misplaced. The public, it appears, is not entirely unreasonable and will, in fact, often assent to the surgical procedures once they are explained to them. (1–3) Not only is informed consent necessary, it is also available for the asking.

Emerging guidelines for the profession and the public

On balance, informed consent can be respected while preserving many of the benefits of practicing on the newly dead. For this reason, some medical centers have outlined a set of guidelines that not only stipulate informed consent but also limit practice on the newly dead to procedures that are not terribly mutilating (in an effort to respect the dead and increase the chance of gaining consent) and to those medical personnel who can truly benefit from the experience. Using newly deceased patients for teaching resuscitation techniques is thus carefully monitored rather than a spontaneous, sporadic event. (4)

Informed consent, however, can be a two-edged sword. In response to the Israeli case, the Jerusalem Post pointed out that if citizens want to be drawn into the process, they must contribute as well:

The public is correct to demand its right to be consulted, but the public also has a responsibility to give consent for life-saving medical procedures . . . Some parents interviewed . . . said publicly that they would not have given permission to doctors to practice an emergency operation on their son's body. One wonders, however, how such people would feel if such training could have saved their son's life (ibid.).

The newspaper is right to chastise the public, but it also needs to recognize that informed consent also means the possibility of informed refusal. Only experience will tell if consent will be forthcoming. If not, one can easily imagine the army backsliding and slipping into its old ways.

Alternative policies: banning the use of deceased patients for teaching intubation

The problem of backsliding might not have been far from the thoughts of British and Norwegian policy makers for the practice of operating on the newly dead is largely banned in those countries as it was in the Israeli military following public disclosure. (3) The difference between the proposed policy for some American hospitals and the decisions taken in Norway, Israel, and the U.K. rests on the way moral principles are ordered and the weight attached to respective principles. In these countries social utility is calculated differently than in the U.S. First, the utility of practice surgery is discounted. According to the Royal College of Nursing and the British Medical Association, intubation training on the newly deceased:

. . . is justified only in the most exceptional circumstances where the deceased patients has suffered severe head, neck or facial injuries. It may then be acceptable for learners *already skilled* in intubation techniques to extend their knowledge . . . (5)

In other words, practice surgery on the newly dead is not necessary to acquire basic intubation skills. Not only is the utility of practice surgery discounted but it is offset by two additional calculations: the possibility of backsliding and subsequent stress this may place on the health care system if revealed, and the distress caused to family members if asked for consent. If the possibility of backsliding is high, the probability of distress great and utility questionable, then it makes sense simply to ban the practice and let surgeons practice on cadavers and manikins.

Ethics can and should avoid the sobriquet that it can "justify anything." Disparate policies are possible but not all are justifiable. Justification policies are not just those that pay homage to respect for autonomy but those that give moral weight to competing principles in a way that is deliberative and public. Those emphasizing the need for informed consent will reformulate policy to obtain permission from next of kin (or from the patient himself by advance directive) before undertaking surgery on a newly deceased patient. Yet many commentators recognize the difficulties that this may bring. Faced with the prospect of not obtaining consent there exists the real possibility of backsliding. The English and others have thought it best to ban the practice. Either approach is acceptable because it gives careful consideration of respect for autonomy, the benefit of practicing the procedure, and the cost of operating without consent. The choice of policy hinges on an empirical question, namely the efficacy of practice surgery on the newly deceased, and on local assessment about the distress caused by consent requests, the cost of public disclosure, and the likelihood of backsliding.

These assessments will vary from nation to nation and the resulting calculation of expected social utility may tip the decision one way or another. But each is a legitimate decision. The old Israeli approach, one that still occurs in hospitals around the world, is ethically flawed because it fails to give weight to all those bioethical principles – dignity, autonomy, and the common good – that underpin life in modern democracies. No single principle is ever sacrosanct but each always deserves careful consideration. Ethics, more than anything else, demands deliberation. Dilemmas are solved as we try to accommodate conflicting principles and avoid dogmas.

Notes

1 McNamara RM, Monti S, Kelly JJ. Requesting consent for an invasive procedure in newly deceased adults. *JAMA* 1995;273:310–12.
2 Benfield DG, Flaksman RJ, Lin T-H, Kantak AD, Kokomoor FW, Vollman JH. Teaching intubation skills using newly deceased infants. *JAMA* 1991;265: 2360–3.
3 Brattebo G, Wisborg T, Solheim K, Oyen N. Ethical dilemmas when teaching intubation techniques – what does the public think? *Tidsskr Nor Laegeforen* 1994;114(13):1534–7.
4 Burns JP, Reardon FE, Troug RD. Using newly deceased patients to teach resuscitation procedures. *N Engl J Med* 331(24):1652–5.
5 Intubation training: an ethical practice? *Nurs Stand* 1993;7(44):38–9.

COMMENTARY

Jonathan Wyatt

This case description raises several interesting and difficult issues. One of these issues is the extent to which it is reasonable to allow medical students to learn practical procedures by contact with patients. This issue, which is covered in other chapters and commentaries in this book, is perhaps overshadowed by a separate one: whether or not it is acceptable to permit tracheal intubation practice on the recently deceased. Although this practice is generally frowned upon, it appears to be in widespread use.

Certainly, in the United Kingdom, for example, the British Medical Association, the British Nursing Association, and the Royal College of Anaesthetists all believe that the practice should not be performed. (1) They strongly argue that intubation practice on the newly dead is not only unethical (chiefly because consent is lacking), but also that it is unnecessary, because there are plenty of opportunities for doctors and other health professionals to learn how to intubate elsewhere. However, a recent survey of 200 junior doctors from the same country suggests that the practice is fairly common and that lack of other realistic opportunities are cited as the justification. (2)

Tracheal intubation involves the insertion of a tube (usually through the mouth, sometimes through the nose) down into the trachea. This is, and has been for many years, part of the standard management of patients who suffer cardiac arrest. (3) Becoming proficient in intubation is acknowledged to be difficult and to require practice. The procedure involves coordinating several different skills: using suction and a laryngoscope, positioning and handling human tissues, manipulating a tracheal tube.

It should be acknowledged at the outset that there are situations where practising is clearly unacceptable for other than ethical reasons – this includes cases where there is suspicion of homicide or suicide. In these cases, the coroner is likely to be involved and to require an investigation and autopsy. Obviously here, minimum disruption of the body and the evidence is required.

Despite the aforementioned concerns about disrupting evidence, it must be conceded that tracheal intubation does not usually result in detectable injury to dead tissues. (4) In this respect, practising intubation is very different from other practical procedures, such as central venous cannulation and chest drain insertion, which leave a definite wound in the skin and disruption of underlying tissues. Indeed, the fact that there is likely to be no trace of intubation having been performed may be partly responsible for the way that the practice on the newly dead goes relatively unchallenged. This, however, is no excuse for not considering the rights of the patient and the issue of consent. Clearly, if the patient was alive and conscious, they would be asked before any "practising."

The natural extension of this argument is that informed consent should always be obtained from the patient. This does, of course, present an obvious practical problem – having suffered cardiac arrest, the patient is not in a position to give consent. In the mid-1990s, this argument brought human cardiac arrest research in the United States to a virtual standstill. (5) It could be argued (using the parallel with organ donor cards) that it would be possible for the patient to give consent prior to sustaining cardiac arrest. In reality, however, this would be extremely difficult.

As an alternative to obtaining prior patient consent, it is more feasible to try to obtain consent immediately after death from the next of kin. Although this presents certain difficulties, this approach is actually followed in some hospitals when there is a stillbirth. There are, again, parallels with organ donation. It must also be noted that technically, in some countries, the person legally responsible for the body after death may be the coroner or other legal equivalent (e.g., in

Scotland it is the Procurator Fiscal).

Having established that ideally, intubation practice on the recently deceased should not proceed without consent, is it unethical to proceed without? Those who advocate the practice would argue that consent is not necessarily essential, that no damage results and that, in any case, the benefits for future patients justify "bending the rules." In order to see the strength of these arguments, it is worth examining the evidence for possible benefits of future patients. For a variety of reasons (which include fewer elective intubations in the operating theater and more competition amongst health care professionals for intubation), there are decreasing opportunities to practice. Manikins are clearly not the same, although some would argue that the latest models offer realistic alternatives. In some countries, animals may offer an alternative, although many find this concept equally distasteful. As already explained, intubation has for many years been considered to be the "gold standard" method for securing the airway in cardiac arrest. (3)

The consensus of opinion is that individuals who sustain cardiac arrest will do better if they are intubated early. It is therefore argued that the chances of a patient receiving the best treatment may depend upon the last patient having been practised upon. However, the evidence to support this viewpoint is distinctly lacking: studies of out of hospital cardiac arrests in Scotland have shown no difference in survival between those patients treated by paramedics capable of tracheal intubation and those treated by ambulance technicians who do not possess this skill. (6) Indeed, the evidence suggests that as far as the vast majority of adults with cardiac arrest are concerned, the overriding concern is to provide them with early defibrillation. It is for this reason that Advanced Life Support courses around the world concentrate so heavily on teaching safe and rapid defibrillation. Similarly, as the emphasis on intubation has diminished, laryngeal masks are increasingly being advocated for use in adult cardiac arrest by those who lack the skills to intubate. (7) The situation is perhaps different in the resuscitation of young children, especially in the newborn, where securing the airway at an early stage with a tracheal tube may, theoretically at least, provide the best chance of survival.

Given that there are ethical concerns, it must be acknowledged that there are ways of "dressing the process up" to make it less distasteful for everyone present. This includes allowing only those actively present during resuscitation to practice intubation, asking all staff present if there are any objections and not proceeding if anyone has an objection.

In conclusion, the practice of intubation of the recently deceased raises difficult ethical issues. Certainly, if acquiring the skills of intubation could be shown to be important, then it would be important to maximise ethical opportunities for real practice on real live patients. However, considering that intubation remains of unproven value in cardiac arrest, practice on the newly dead appears particularly hard to justify.

Notes

1 Tonks A. Intubation practice on cadavers should stop. *BMJ* 1992;305:332.

2 Campbell-Heweson et al. unpublished data.

3 Kloeck W, Cummins R, Chamberlain D, et al. The Universal ALS Algorithm – an advisory statement by the Advanced Life Support Working Group of the International Liaison Committee on Resuscitation. *Resuscitation* 1997;34:109–11.

4 Benfield DG, Flaksman RJ, et al. Teaching of intubation skills using newly deceased infants. *JAMA* 1993;265(18):2360–3.

5 Levine RJ. Research in emergency situations – the role of deferred consent. *JAMA* 1995;273(16):1300–20.

6 Guly UM, Mitchell RG, Cook R, Steedman DJ, Robertson CE. Paramedics and technicians are equally successful at managing cardiac arrest outside hospital. *BMJ* 1995;310:1091–4.

7 Baskett PJF. The use of the laryngeal mask airway by nurses during cardiopulmonary resuscitation. *Anaesthesia* 1994;49:3–7.

6

Asking for help: who's listening?

CASE

"I fled from the room"

As a female medical student I was conducting my first physical exam on a male patient, in the presence of classmates and supervising faculty, when it became quite apparent to all that the patient had an erection. I was taken by surprise, flustered and embarrassed, and not knowing how to deal with the situation, I fled from the room. Later, my male colleagues couldn't understand my response. I know my unprofessional behavior added to the discomfort of the patient, a young man not very much older than myself. For that I am profoundly sorry. I was not prepared for such a situation and still have received no instruction as to how best to manage a similar future occurrence – for the patient's sake as well as my own.

CASE

"I still don't know what I did wrong"

I was a third year medical student when one of our patients needed to have a nasogastric tube put in. The team turned to me and told me to see to it that this was done – and then they all disappeared. Before, in similar situations, a resident would say "Let's get the stuff and do it" but this time I found myself entirely alone.

A day or two earlier, a resident had showed me the procedure; so, I went to find him. However, this time he just said "I've already shown you how to do that, just get it down. Call me if you have any problems."

I returned to the patient and tried, as the resident said, to "just get it down." The patient was pretty demented, was only semi-conscious, and couldn't consent to the procedure, which is very uncomfortable under the best of conditions. When the tube is inserted, it is usual for patients to gag; but if they gag and cough excessively, the tube may be starting to go to the lungs. My patient was really gagging a lot and I just couldn't continue. I left him again and went to find the intern on our team who was on another floor. I told her the problems I was having. She went through the procedure and said when I finished the patient should get a chest X-ray to make sure the tube was inserted properly.

I finally got the tube in on my own. The X-ray showed that everything was correct. Later the intern approached me and said that what I did was improper and I shouldn't have tried the procedure on my own. I couldn't understand why, when I sought her out and told her of my concerns, she didn't just say "Wait, I'll be there to supervise." She let me go and do it without saying anything, but later reprimanded me. How could I have handled this confusing situation differently? I still don't know what I did wrong.

COMMENTARY

Barbara Supanich

"I fled from the room"

Why did the female medical student run from the

room? And, why did she conclude that she behaved in an unprofessional manner?

The scenario gives us a partial answer – she was embarrassed, flustered, and felt unprepared for such an event. I think that there are more profound issues hidden within this story and I think that we as medical educators have a moral obligation to our students, residents, and patients to properly address them, as we engage our students in the process of becoming professional persons and physicians. (1)

The aspects of professional education in medical schools are somewhat variable across the country and are often referred to as the "hidden curriculum." (2, 3) It is probably more accurate to say that the hidden curriculum describes elements of medical "professionalization," rather than "professional education." The hidden curriculum includes such areas as learning how to work with interns and residents, how to work with various staff within the hospital, understanding the medical "pecking order," an assumption that the student will be competent and comfortable in any medical or surgical setting starting with their first experience, and the proverbial "see one, do one, teach one."

The female medical student in this scenario was performing her first physical exam on a male patient, which will create enough anxiety on its own for most students. However, she had the additional pressures of also performing the examination in the presence of peers and faculty. The actions and reactions of the students and the teaching faculty in this scenario are quite common and highlight the need for improving the style and environment for learning both clinical skills and personal interaction skills between students, residents, faculty, and patients.

An important aspect of human development is the integration of our sexuality into the fullness of our personhood. In U.S. society, sex acts are very often equated with sexuality and this narrow understanding is what is exemplified in this scenario. The male colleagues in the scenario express their discomfort in a stereotypical, yet not un-

common manner – with the false pretense that they were "o.k." with what happened and could not "understand" why she was flustered – or male "bravado." This male "bravado" is all the more significant in medicine, where the pressure is on for the student or resident to "always" be able to perform in any setting "perfectly." And so, the student in this scenario, according to this culture, was expected to live up to the "criteria" of never becoming flustered or embarrassed.

Another key aspect of this case is the poor responses that the faculty member, her classmates, and she had concerning the patient's erection. Every encounter with a patient is an opportunity for our own personal and professional growth and learning. It is often a rude awakening for many students when they have their first encounter with a patient closer to their own age, social background or of the opposite sex, who is ill in the hospital or in the office setting. They often come to the clinical setting thinking that most of the patients that they will provide care for will be much older. Rarely do they think about the reality that many of these patients will be similar to them in some manner, i.e., ethnic or racial background, socioeconomic status, religious affiliation, etc. It is a challenging moment for many students when they first provide care for a person of the opposite sex, especially if that person is close to their own age. For the most part, up to this point, they have related to persons in this age group as peers, friends, or potential lovers. Now, they need to develop another skill, that of a professional relationship with the person as a patient.

How easily this occurs will depend upon many factors, including the student's family upbringing, personality development, and current professional development in her or his medical school. Given this student's experience, I would say that her current medical school's curriculum is sorely lacking in the areas of sexuality for men and women and how our sexuality impacts and influences who we are as professional persons. I think that medical schools have a significant obligation to provide solid educational experiences preclinically for students to help them develop a healthy understanding of sexuality in human growth. These experiences should include teaching students strategies for how to handle a variety of encounters that they will have with patients, including the one described in this scenario.

As educators we need to remember that our students and we come to any encounter with a patient with all of who we are – including our sexuality, as do our patients! We also need to remind ourselves that many cultures within U.S. society are at best neutral and at worst relatively repressed when it comes to sexual issues. The dominant cultures in America have not dealt with sex in a healthy manner and so we observe extreme behaviors related to sex – adolescent "acting out" and promiscuity, idealizing women or men or exploiting them, inaccurate stereotypes of men and women, etc. Given this cultural context, it is not surprising that when something like this happens, the student can run the whole spectrum of guilt, immature humor, embarrassment, and a misunderstanding or lack of understanding of what is proper professional behavior.

I think that it is a failure of our medical education system that we have not adequately prepared students and residents and helped them to develop an appropriate knowledge base concerning sexuality of men and women and how to use this information to cope with these types of situations. (4) I would not blame the student's colleagues. I would challenge the faculty member to create a learning setting that allows for safe discussions of such events within a supportive and nonjudgmental setting. I think that we have a moral obligation as teachers to respect the integrity of patients and students. This respect for personal integrity requires that we understand and honor the person for who they are, understand and honor the person's values and fulfill our obligation of helping in the development of the person professionally.

Specifically in this case, I would suggest the following strategies:

The faculty member should create an atmosphere and expectations at the beginning of the rotation that is open, responsive to student questions, and supportive of learning and not one that sets the bar at "perfection."

In the setting of this case discussion, the faculty member should have readily observed the student's discomfort and the patient's erection. In this case, it would seem that it would be helpful for the faculty member to discreetly make a supportive comment to the student, such as, "It's nothing that you've said or done. Let him know that you are here to do a professional examination." If the student is still too flustered, then the faculty should take the lead in making a comment like: "I know this can be a startling or embarrassing situation. It's all right, you are human, these things can happen. Would you like us to step out for a moment and give you some privacy?"

If the patient agrees that he needs a moment – the faculty member can take the opportunity then to let the student know that this did not happen because of anything that she did – it was most likely an unintentional physiologic response of the patient. It would also be important for the faculty member to stress the importance of taking an opportunity later to process this experience so that it will be a positive growth experience and not an emotional scar for this student.

In returning to the room, if it is evident that the patient is being inappropriate with the student then that has to be confronted; if there is no indication of provocative behavior, then the exam can be resumed.

During the debriefing session with the students, the faculty member should lead a nonjudgmental discussion about how to handle such encounters in the future. The faculty member (or one who is skilled in such issues), should assure the student that she did not act in a manner that "brought on" the erection, and that the fact that he had an erection did not mean that this was a come-on by the patient. There should be an opportunity for the student to discuss her feelings and future approaches and strategies.

"I still don't know what I did wrong"

What are the "real" issues here? Why does this student find herself alone this time and I think literally abandoned by the resident on her service? What are the expectations of the student for learning and patient care obligations and those of the resident and intern?

The situation presented in this scenario is very common in most of our teaching hospitals. Residents and interns are given increasing responsibilities for patient care and often feel overworked and underappreciated. Many residents have not received adequate training in how to teach students or residents. In this type of work environment – high stress to get the work done, an atmosphere which demands that students and residents be competent and efficient "immediately," and a very low tolerance for mistakes, it is all too predictable that the resident in this situation can choose to "kick the dog." In other words, when you are stressed and overworked and someone makes a request, even a legitimate request, you blame them for their "incompetence" rather than owning up to your own frustration or tiredness. Misdirected feelings in this scenario are harmful to both the student and the resident.

From the student's perspective, I think that there were at least two significant issues – needing assistance with a procedure in a more complex type of patient and having "unresponsive" residents; and the patient was unable to give informed consent and this was not resolved with the resident or attending. Let's turn our attention to discussing these troubling ethical concerns.

Students come to their clinical rotations both with a set of learning goals and expectations. They want to learn at least a basic set of skills and knowledge base for that particular speciality. They want to feel as if they are a part of the health care team. They want their experiences and observations of patients heard and respected by the other members of the team. They also learn relatively quickly that they are on the lower end of the medical hierarchy and as such their contributions are not always well received or appreciated. When this is the experience of students, they also are concerned about how and with whom to discuss these concerns.

From the residents' perspective, they are often all-consumed with "getting the work done," and often find it frustrating when students approach them with a question or request for what the resident understands as a very minor concern. In this scenario, the resident is viewing the placement of a nasogastric tube as a very routine and minor procedure and is not at all attuned to the student's learning needs. The apparent concern of the resident is "simply" to get the "tube down." It is probably one of many procedures and tests to be completed on a very long list for this resident, just for today! If they are also stressed by overwork and attendings that are making other multiple demands upon their time, this student's request could be the proverbial "straw that breaks the camel's back." It does not excuse the behavior, but it might help to explain the work atmosphere in which the resident finds himself.

And, as was mentioned in the previous case, there is the ever present milieu of "see one, do one, teach one." The student in this case unfortunately is living out this experience. Two days prior to this experience, she had a resident show her how to place a nasogastric tube. So, the assumption has been made by her residents that she now "knows" how to properly insert this tube under all circumstances! For the student, this sets up a tremendous amount of pressure to perform and unnecessary guilt when she doesn't accomplish this procedure.

I also am wondering about the dynamic of male resident and female student as a factor in this scenario. It is becoming better understood that there are male/female dynamics present in the classroom – male children are called upon more frequently than female children are. I think that there can be a similar dynamic that comes into play between male residents and female students. Residents with a more traditional understanding of female roles may have less tolerance for female students making "demands" on their time, which takes them away from other important duties.

So, how should we approach this scenario's issues? Why did the resident and intern give the student such confusing responses? What should have been done for the student?

First, I think that the student made a very reasonable request of the resident. The student had a patient with significant complications, which increased the risk for a complication from placement of the nasogastric tube. Any procedure performed by a student *must* be supervised by a person with the competency and skills to perform the procedure. There are no exceptions to this rule! The resident really can't say, "just do it, call me if you need me or have questions." It is mandatory for the resident or another supervising physician with the privilege, to be present for the entire procedure. There are two basic reasons for this – to assure that the procedure is being properly and safely performed and to assure a good learning environment for the student.

Secondly, I would like to briefly address the issue of informed consent. The patient in this case had a diagnosis of dementia and was semiconscious. The resident or attending physician needed to model for the student how to properly obtain informed consent in this case. Briefly, the physician needs to document an examination, which verifies that the patient does or does not have the capacity to make decisions regarding this treatment. If they do not have capacity, then the physician needs to identify who is making decisions for the patient and obtain consent from them for the treatment. Again, it is the obligation of the attending physician to obtain this consent or appropriately delegate this to another physician with the necessary skills to obtain the consent.

I would posit that we have an obligation to assure proper and competent teaching and supervision of residents and students. A part of that obligation is to assure that the learning environment for both residents and students is not oppressive, but truly conducive to learning and caring for patients. We need to abolish the acceptance of the philosophy of "see one, do one, teach one." It is a dangerous philosophy; it breeds arrogance and fear, and does not assure that patients receive high quality care.

We have an obligation to our residents and students to create teaching and learning environments that allow for asking questions and seeking help. (5, 6) If the student in this scenario was in this type of environment, she would have been able to ask for help and she and the resident would have worked out a time to meet to obtain proper consent and place in the nasogastric tube.

Since the world is not perfect, students will not always find themselves in such a supportive learning environment! So, what then? I would suggest identifying supportive faculty and residents with whom the students can discuss cases and situations. Another option would be to have an ethics course or a Balint group for third and fourth year students in which they could discuss cases and situations like this with a skilled facilitator or faculty member. (5, 7) There are several medical schools which have created such opportunities for students, including Michigan State University's College of Human Medicine.

And so, residents have an obligation to teach students in a supportive learning environment. They need to learn how to prioritize and organize the work of the day, including time for student case issues. Students need to learn and use appropriate assertiveness techniques with residents and attendings. They need to understand that residents and attendings will be inconsistent at times in their responses. For example in this scenario, the resident at first said, "just get it down," and later admonished her for doing the procedure on her own. There are some definite communication problems here on this service! This is an opportunity for both the resident and the student to have a clarifying conversation about these issues. As medical professionals, we are ethically obliged to provide care in a safe and caring manner. We can no longer tolerate medical teaching environments which do not allow for questioning and asking for help without undue repercussions to students.

Notes

1 Andre J. Learning to see: moral growth during medical training. *J Med Ethics* 1992;18(3):148–52.
2 Hafferty FW, Franks R. The hidden curriculum, ethics teaching, and the structure of medical education. *Acad Med* 1994;69(11):861–71.
3 Sanders M. The forgotten curriculum: an argument for medical ethics education. *JAMA* 1995;274(9):768–9.
4 Zoppi K. Sexuality in the patient–physician relationship. [Pulse column]. *JAMA* 1992;268(21):3142, 3146.
5 Osborne LW, Martin CM. The importance of listening to medical students' experiences when teaching them medical ethics. *J Med Ethics* 1989;15(1):35–8.
6 Dwyer J. Primum non tacere: an ethics of speaking up. *Hastings Cent Rep* 1994;24(1):13–18.
7 Feudtner C, Christakis DA. Making the rounds: the ethical development of medical students in the context of clinical rotations. *Hastings Cent Rep* 1994;24(1):6–12.

COMMENTARY

David N. Weisstub

Witnessing withdrawal and abandonment

Images that cause embarrassment are normally responded to by avoidance and emotional withdrawal. In extreme cases, it is an understandably personal reaction when persons abandon or even deny exposure to situations, which have led to deep embarrassment. In well-established cultures, images are important, if not central to the creation, maintenance, and perpetuation of what is deemed normal in a given social context. In male-dominated cultures in the West, which have had defining norms and mores as part of long-standing examples of guild identity, matters which could bring social embarrassment to an ordinary bystander such as witnessing a sexual reaction to a medical intervention are something which the group has often prepared for by relating stories in the inner circle from past experiences, thereby explicating the range of normalcy that is permitted and recommended in the response options available. Female introduction into the medical guild is not uncomplex in this regard. To begin with, it has been part of the Victorian legacy that females who have entered the profession are prima facie desexualized beings. It is part of that particular mythology that women who join a professional fraternity either are male-like or should become male-like because any form of sensitivity should be interpreted as forms of overreaction, something akin to hysteria. Therefore females caught off-guard with any form of perceived female-like behavior are regarded as having been unprofessional.

It is important to distinguish appropriate sensitivity and respect from examples of hypersensitive reaction, which could lead to the unfortunate diminution of the interacting party, in this instance the subject as patient. In order to exercise appropriate control as a professional where the social relationship has distinct parameters and by necessity an overlay of formality, it is critical in the early stages of education to find one's moral footing, such that one begins the process of coping with predictable incidents which could lead to undignified or embarrassing responses on the part of either the professional or the recipient of care. Because in the modern world of medicine there is a baseline respect for the principle of maximizing patient autonomy in decision making, there is an overwhelming professional obligation to put patients at ease so that they can behave naturally as partners in accumulating information upon which to make informed decisions affecting their welfare. Putting a patient ill at ease and even worse in situations of being flustered or disoriented detracts from the professional ideal at hand. Part of a professional's early obligation is to find the balance between being normal and social, that is, not denying one's human and indeed bodily presence, while at the same time ensuring that any sexual nuance or even opening for stimulating or directing one's attention to a sexual nuance should be downplayed, in order to maintain a clear line of professional vision. It is equally wrong to ignore the variable of one's sexuality in the professional context. This is well known from the extensive treatment of the transference and countertransference dimension in any psychotherapeutic encounter. Because of the built-in power imbalance in any form of medical diagnosis and treatment, and given that healing is connected to a weighty psychological component, there is a challenge to every professional to mature into and attain roles which define the right boundary conditions for professional interaction. This should include avoiding unreflective apologies or admitting defeat or acquiescence to the novice mores of the profession which are a euphemism for peer revelry or camaraderie.

The introduction of females and ethnic and racial minorities into modern-day professions is an opportunity for finding new and more respectful avenues of greeting, interacting with, and responding to a wide range of patient populations in potentially embarrassing surroundings. In ideal terms, embarrassing or awkward incidents should motivate a sharing of reactions such that there could be new peer pressures evolved to relocate embarrassment signals so that some decades from now responses will have shifted orientation in other directions. Above all, the model of instruction and experience should be to dictate to professionals in training the need for a group to

"hold strong" in minimizing embarrassment to patients even where uncomfortable moments could give rise to group humor.

Persons often leave the scenes of accidents because it is wounding to the observer to see a person in a state of destruction or great pain. Unable to initiate help or in fear of doing so inadequately, even well-meaning individuals can find themselves fleeing or abandoning persons left in great distress. Panic ensues and people are left frequently with feelings of guilt in having contributed to a further loss. An example of a student in training leaving a hospital room where there has been a group peer presence is a soft form of abandonment behavior. As a weak form of panic, it suggests the unresolvable dynamic of the sexual reality having presented itself in a depersonalized environment, which in some instances could understandably catalyze anxiety, fear, and even panic leading to an abrupt withdrawal reaction. However it should be observed that such withdrawal may tell us more about the universe of peer pressure and social expectations than the morally grounded intentionality of the actor. Therefore emphasis should be placed on peer assessment and the articulation of "boundary conditions" so that emotions do not run aground and get buried, leading to more disturbing examples of either repression or group bravado that could be morally damaging to the relevant professional interaction. Where medical consultations involve sexually transmittable diseases, the sexual organs themselves, and where differences of age present subtle interactions, students should be trained early on to come prepared for emotional reflection among themselves and should not be allowed to abandon the moral high ground in reacting to perceived examples of hypersensitivity.

Being witness in a wide variety of circumstances can carry with it a moral burden, as Elie Wiesel has so insightfully documented in his work on the Holocaust. Whenever we see even the mildest version of human degradation, it is incumbent upon us to speak and reflect but not abandon. Avoidance or withdrawal is not a good course of action for morally responsible behavior. Equally, to remain standing as a witness and either to do nothing or worse to seize the occasion for humor and then derision can be highly violative of the person found in a diminished light. To remain as a witness or to participate in a recuperating dialogue where one contributes to the autonomy and self-respect of the individual is not only restorative of the individual but also constitutive of a mature and moral group solidarity. This should be the professional ideal that governs the education of persons entering the healing profession.

One of the realities surrounding medical diagnosis and treatment is that, as a fundamental value in our society, privacy is by definition compromised in order to achieve the higher stated goal of health care. When in possession of good health as observers or practitioners, there is a well instantiated sentiment in Western societies that our body should be absolutely protected from the unwanted surveillance of others. In teaching hospitals, we may wish to question the extent to which illness creates the conditions for unnecessary and exaggerated communal surveillance of disease including regions of the body that may be particularly sensitive among vulnerable populations. It may be that as our sensitivity increases in this area to patient responses, we may achieve much more than presently in meeting educational objectives through the use of computers, videos, and other advancements in communication techniques. This may be conducive to reducing the number of privacy intrusions that occur in the everyday life of hospitals and clinics. On the one hand it is important that we do not mystify the body such that patients and practitioners alike contribute to a sense of hiddenness thereby associating disease with uncleanness or evil. On the other, it is consistent with our contemporary expressed ideals of respect for the personhood of patients that through dialogue and attitude the subjects of our healing be approached in such a fashion that cues and sentiments are acknowl-

edged that are enhancing to patient wishes to the maximum extent possible.

Standards in training

Torts Law is packed full of introductory cases where the issue at hand is to locate the relevant standard for persons in the course of training. Learning to ride a bicycle, drive a car, or fly an airplane, there are always moments where the trainee is let go, released from the shared control of a mechanical act or to perform solo or to do an intervention which requires dexterity and/or finesse. This represents a threshold whereby the individual begins to execute professional acts at a reasonable, if not highly experienced, level of performance. In teaching persons how to be professional, there are sometimes ambiguous zones of communication where at least according to some theories of how-to-do-its, persons are thrown into cold water, sometimes to the point of being traumatized or at least put at high risk. Such shock theories of pedagogy are now regarded as crude and ineffective although there are persons found in most systems that still swear by the old school. The more dominant theory is that we should give careful instructions and then allow for cautious ventures in the direction of conducting unfamiliar tasks. Most medical schools would prefer not to rely on instinct and do not wish to suffer allegations against them for premature release of their offspring. In this sense, the birds and the battlefield are distinguishable from institutions of higher learning.

Moral transgressions in public institutions would seem to occur when there is an unfair reliance on either instinct or pressure. It is assumed that there is a positive obligation in order to avoid professional liability that serious attention be given to adequate supervision for professional debuts. Having placed medical students in situations where there has been an undertaking to train, withdrawal of such supervision where there has been reliance on the part of the supervisee could give rise to a demand for tortious damages on the part of patients if not equally on the part of students in training where damage to reputation could be an issue. These of course would be extreme examples. However, there remain many nonlitigious occurrences where persons in supervisory roles give mixed messages about who should be responsible for what in which circumstances. That is, there are troubling cases of inadequate supervision and withdrawal, such that untrained or partially trained individuals are pressured to perform at a level of skill for which they have been inadequately prepared. Unfortunately, there is a preponderance of such cases in large urban environments where there is a disproportionate representation of the chronically ill, the elderly, and demented populations. In the cut and thrust of large urban hospitals where novices have been put in jeopardy by ambiguous signals from their supervisors, there can be frivolous reprimands, even for nonnegligent behavior. The depersonalized flow of traffic in environments of fatigue and harassment can predictably produce a high level of tension and acting-out behaviors even on the part of experienced beleaguered staff. In addition, there are cases which routinely arise of outright meanness. The reality is reconstituted, such that the overseeing professional creates the impression that they were at all times standing by if the real need had occurred. That is, with the benefit of hindsight had something untoward occurred, the trainee would have been held to the standard of a reasonable practitioner. The message being, behave as a professional, or do not do it at all. This presumes a tight standard, one that begins with a notion of reasonableness or prudence and seems to end with a nonnegligent standard so airtight that it borders on the unrealizable objective standard of something akin to absolute liability.

Because of ambiguity in the torts system, many jurisdictions remain unclear about the level to which an intern can be held liable. There is a tension between legal and moral standards stretching from among the professionals themselves, both within the legal and medical communities through the patient population and throughout the general public. The assumption is made that in order to perform at an exacting professional standard, institutions of higher learning practice-oriented clinics and even research laboratories all have a moral–legal obligation to "get it right" for the recipients. However, the reality exists that even before recent cutbacks in health care funding trainees found themselves with surprises and unpredictable variables such that it became a necessity to act with imperfect training. From a moral point of view it would appear to be unfair to judge individuals or institutions that have acted with best intentions by forms of absolute liability standards. Rather as is the case with constructive common-law reasoning we should develop an internal professional jurisprudence based on reasonable ethical guidelines such that professionals should hold themselves to reasonable standards of supervision and avoid cases where patients can be put in jeopardy.

The rule that students in training, interns and residents should uniformly identify their inadequacies to the patients for whom they are administering treatments is a textbook ideal but in practice one that can put terror into the hearts of patients whose dependency can in any event frequently lead them into cases of acquiescence even when they are aware of the fact that they would have insisted on better treatment and a higher standard if conditions had been otherwise. Knowing that patients in many cases have no choice and that institutional training is inadequate, we are left with moral dilemmas of a very pressing nature. What are the reasonable demands on institutions and each other that can be made by supervisors, trainees, patients, and indeed administrators and government officials?

COMMENTARY

David Bennahum

Listening is so very difficult, especially for men.

One can listen and not hear. To "hear" another person requires seeing as well as listening, sometimes even touching; perhaps smell and taste and certainly memory all play a part. It is not enough to listen to the patient, as one must also listen to the family, to nurses, ward clerks, students, and colleagues, to all who are entrusted with a patient's care. I have had a difficult time learning to listen and learning to hear. I so envy those with a wondrous capacity to listen. These gifted people seem to anticipate what they must listen for, a Delphic quality of foresight. Helping by listening can be a silent task, ascultating without a stethoscope, having the courage to step forward to cover an exposed patient on rounds or to sit with a patient while the crowd of white coats hurry in and out of rooms. Even the simple act of knocking and listening for permission to enter rather than barging in as most physicians do, expresses an awareness of the patient as a person.

A student embarrassed by a patient's sexual response needs a house officer or attending courageous enough to cover the patient and steady the student with a reassuring touch, shielding both patient and student from shame. Freud tells us that shame is the most primitive emotion, learned very early in life so that we will do as the group does. Thus we make private the essential acts of urination, defecation, and certainly tumescence and erection. Of course she felt shame, haven't we all, stumbling over words, embarrassed to be out of sync with those about us, wanting to sink into a hole or float away, depersonalized. Shame sets off the *fright–flight* response causing us to want to flee. Not so guilt, which is learned, internalized and drives our lives of life-long study and obsessive preparation. Physicians, especially in training are too often subject to the agonies of shame and the stress of guilt. The system of training creates these tensions which the establishment does little to resolve.

I empathize with this hard-working young woman medical student feeling surprised, taken aback and embarrassed by her patient's frank sexual response. Flustered and incapable of handling the situation she fled. No one warned her that this could happen and no one intervened to help her. She asks how she can cope? I too have stood silently on rounds with a dozen medical students watching a professor pull down a middle-aged woman's dressing gown so as to demonstrate her heart sounds. There she lay, breasts exposed yet no one moved until after what seemed an interminable hour a young, female intern stepped forward and covered her right breast. She was *listening* to the patient, and to the group and to herself.

In my student days in the late 50s and early 60s it was routine for the medical students to come in early and draw all the bloods, place nasogastric tubes and collect body fluids from patients. Having collected samples of blood, urine, stool, sputum, and gastric fluid it was the students who went to the tiny laboratory, a walled-off corner of the ward, where we dutifully prepared the specimens for staining and analysis. counted and described red cells and white cells, checked for urinary sugar and protein and stained sputum and gastric fluid for the delicate tuberculosis bacillus. It astonishes me to think of the responsibilities we carried, for no one that I can recall ever checked up on us. I do remember how slithery the nasogastric tubes felt, greasy with vaseline and then frothy with sputum as one would pass the tube down the unfortunate patient's nose and into his stomach in order to suck out with a huge syringe any tubercle bacilli that might be hiding there. One felt awkward, diffident perhaps, coming over to someone's bed, these were 25-bed wards, the beds extending out from the four walls of a very large room and sometimes not even protected by curtains. I can recall an elderly Black man who accepted my ministrations without protest, but he may be a composite of many faces. I was probably polite, perhaps kind, but certainly not gentle. It was hard to pass the thick tube up one nostril and down the throat as the patient would gag and you would have to stiffen your spine and push and probe and force, sometimes there would be a little blood from the nose. I hated passing those tubes each morning, hunting for microbes. Of course that was why we were set at the task, to find the fragile but deadly tubercle bacillus that infected the patient's lungs and were coughed up and swallowed during the night. And we never wore masks, nor did the patients! Curiously it is now thought that such practices were almost useless; but medicine is so certain of itself. At any one period everything that we do has an aura of infallibility.

I can't say that I did anything "wrong" in this exercise; but so much seemed wrong in those days. The vague sense of fear that we would make a mistake or would not know a pertinent fact when asked by our attending. The helplessness of the patients in the county hospital. The unstated power of race. All but one of the students in my class were White, mostly male and very young. It was so easy to assume the mantle of medicine, to ignore vulnerability and power imbalance. What was wrong was the abuse of power that was and still is too often part of medicine.

On the obstetrics service there was a long tradition of 3-hour professor's rounds on Saturday morning. All 20 or so students, interns, residents, and nurses would follow the chairman of the department from bed to bed. The chief resident would present each patient's case while some of us, exhausted from having been up for 24 hours would try to maneuver ourselves behind someone else so that we could close our eyes, actually sleeping standing up for a few seconds at a time. On one of these mornings a pregnant, Black woman was presented. She was at great risk of losing her baby and even death as she was an achondroplastic dwarf. This lady was expected to have a difficult delivery, perhaps one that would result in a cesarean. Without a word to the patient who was standing before us, the professor pulled down her gown to reveal a deformed spine and pelvis and her swollen abdomen. I watched in horror, but said nothing. Apparently the unfortunate chief resident had failed to measure her pelvis accurately. The professor said viciously "you'll be packing your bags if this happens again." As we passed to the next patient I could see that the chief resident was crying and sweating. It is supposed to be better today and it certainly is in my department and school. Still there are stories that students tell and one sees residents who seem so beaten down. Perhaps the power, the authority of medicine is intrinsic and is so easily wielded to the detriment of patients and the men and women in training.

DISCUSSION QUESTIONS

Section 1. Performing procedures

1 Is a medical trainee's lack of experience with a procedure sufficiently relevant to warrant informing the patient of that fact before the procedure is performed?
2 If a patient is being used for training purposes must this fact be disclosed?
3 What should you do when you do not feel competent to manage a procedure?
4 How hard should health professionals try to change their patient's mind?
5 When do medical personnel have the right to discuss their patient with others? (e.g., professionals? family? legal authorities?)
6 Under what conditions is it better to violate a patient's confidentiality than to preserve it? Are there any valid conditions that would justify breaching confidentiality?
7 What are the moral limits on keeping commitments once they are made?
8 What do we owe the dead? (e.g., cadavers? recently deceased patients? even families of the deceased?)
9 Is practicing on the newly dead without consent morally wrong?

Problems in truth-telling

Truth-telling is a major feature of physician–patient interactions. On the one hand, professionals must tell the truth so that patients can adequately make decisions about their health care. On the other, patients must have sufficient trust in the relationship to give accurate and forthright responses to their doctors. In this section some of the complexities of truth-telling are raised. Questions about the appropriateness of disclosing information only arise when there is some sort of psychological resistance to disclosing a particular kind of information. What are the limits of disclosure? Is misleading through dissembling and obfuscation justifiable?

7

Omissions: failing to come forward

CASE

"Omit the mistake"

When I was a third year medical student, I observed that a patient was suffering an adverse drug reaction because he had been given an overdose of the medication. The patient was informed that his discomfort was due to an allergic reaction to the medication. He was not told that an order had been written improperly. I was then instructed to write a note documenting the incident, but omitting the "mistake."

CASE

"Was I acting under false pretenses?"

I was a resident in internal medicine when a patient, to whom I was not assigned, was admitted to our service with pulmonary emboli in both lungs. I happened to meet a fellow intern outside the patient's room who said "If you want to hear some really clear rubs, check this guy out." When I entered the room, the patient obviously assumed I was another of his physicians coming to do an exam. He lifted his gown so I could listen with my stethoscope. I was aware that the patient was under the impression he was receiving medical care, while in reality he was serving as an educational experience for me. I said nothing to enlighten him, but I wondered, was I acting under false pretenses?

CASE

"White lies and omissions"

I am often torn by how much information to give a patient. For example, often when giving a differential diagnosis some low probability diagnosis, such as cancer, would have to be included to give full disclosure. But a cancer diagnosis has high emotional impact for a patient and I wonder about the wisdom of exposing the patient to such a possibility, particularly if there are only minimal supporting data. I find myself relying on white lies and omissions. How much should the patient be told in this kind of situation?

CASE

"I hated disappointing them"

Mr. G was a 60-year-old man with chronic obstructive pulmonary disease who was transferred to the medical intensive care unit after he "coded" on the floor. I was the intern on call accepting the transfer. My job was to keep him alive. Immediately I placed a central line, an arterial line, two intravenous lines, and a tube through every body orifice. Mr. G was in a coma. He had minimal brainsteam reflex and an electroencephalogram showing little activity. Despite the poor prognosis and hoping against hope, his family wanted everything done to keep him "alive." One day I was writing my notes while Mr. G's daughter was visiting. She held his swollen hand. "Daddy," she whispered in his ear. "Daddy, if you can hear me, do nothing." Mr. G just lay there.

Mr. G's organ systems were all going into failure. I just could not do enough to keep up with their deterioration. I knew it was futile. I was not sure whether I was prolonging his life or prolonging his suffering. But the family kept pressing me for good news, any bit of good news to hang their hopes on. I hated disappointing them. I would sometimes take the back entrance to avoid walking through the family waiting area, if I had nothing new or good to report to the family. Mr. G died one week later, after the family finally agreed to withdraw life support.

I am still uncomfortable with my role in this case. I was at a loss with sufferings that I could not fix; and since I could not "fix" Mr. G, I felt I had little to offer if I did not have any good news. What was my job here? If the family needed compassion and some TLC was it enough to order social work's help, a psyche consult or a meeting with clergy?

CASE

"Sin of silence"

During my internship in a Dutch Catholic hospital there was an elderly woman on the ward who was dying. When the nursing staff contacted the family to tell them she might not last much longer the family's first thought was whether there would be enough time to have the last rites performed. The family was assured that the hospital priest would be contacted immediately. He was told of the family's request and asked to come with some speed. When the priest arrived I saw him stopping to speak with some colleagues that he had not seen for some time. After 20 minutes he inquired as to the patient's room number. He was informed he was too late, the patient had died. The priest told the nursing staff that instead of the last rites he would go and bless the deceased. He was in her room less than one minute before he left to attend to other business. When the family arrived they were relieved to hear that the priest had just gone. They clearly believed that the last rites had been administered. Later, the priest phoned the family

and said that if they had any more requests they should call him. Should the family be told the truth? Is not telling in such circumstances participating in a sin or conspiracy of silence?

COMMENTARY

Lawrence J. Schneiderman

"Omit the mistake"

When I was a medical resident I prescribed an overdose of an anticoagulant for an elderly man who was in the hospital to be treated at bedrest for deep vein thrombosis. Just at that time, the drug Dicumarol was being replaced by Coumadin, which was 10 times more powerful. In writing the prescription I used the more up-to-date medication but inadvertently put the decimal point in the old-fashioned location. Within a few hours the patient was producing beet-juice urine. I was horrified. I had just turned the patient's illness from one that was potentially life-threatening to one that was imminently life-threatening.

I told the patient what had happened but cannot take credit for lofty virtue in doing so. I had no choice. We were in this together. I spent the rest of the day and the entire night by his bedside following his heart rate and blood pressure, and after giving him vitamin K, checking his urine and stools, and sticking the poor man's fingers to draw hematocrits – all this after I had typed and cross-matched his blood, and indeed ended up transfusing him with three units of blood. It seemed he was bleeding everywhere I looked.

Throughout this adventure the patient kept trying to console me as much as I was trying to administer to him. Every time I had to do a painful pinprick of his finger to get blood, I must have conveyed my own pain so vividly that the patient kept reassuring me that it wasn't so bad. In the early hours of morning he began to produce a more elegant vin rose, and we both took the occasion to offer it to each other in celebration.

I was struck by how much the patient continued to trust me even after I had given him good reason not to. Somehow, the fact that I promptly confessed my error, promptly tried to correct it, kept close watch and thereby made clear that I would do my best to protect him – all this reassured him. He could see we were in this together.

The outcome made it easier, of course. We both were lucky. He came away intact. And I came away wiser.

This, in fact, is how most physicians absorb their most powerful and unforgettable lessons: from their mistakes. So that today, when I hear on rounds about a student's or resident's mishap, I'm quick to confess my own failings. "If it's true you learn from your mistakes," I say to the miserable soul, "someday I'll know everything."

"Was I acting under false pretenses?"

I cannot get too upset by this person's self-doubt, although that is not to say things could not have been done better. But I wonder what the man's expectation was. If he was a patient in a teaching hospital, almost certainly he was aware that the hallways are filled with eager learners. He readily raised his gown and exposed his chest, not exactly a big deal in a male patient.

The sensitive resident was "aware" that the patient was "under the impression" he was receiving medical care, while "in reality" he was serving as an educational experience. The resident draws a bit much, I think, on his own categories of subjective and objective reality. All things considered, I submit that as long as the medical resident (a qualified doctor) was in the room, the patient was medically better off than when he was alone, hence he *was* receiving medical care.

That said, I still think things could (and should) have been done better. Did the patient even know he had a pulmonary friction rub? The patient's intern could have explained the physical finding

to him and then said: Oh by the way, this is the kind of physical finding doctors have to learn to recognize. Would he mind if some of his colleagues dropped by and listened? In my experience, patients invariably welcome the attention. Also, when they are informed they are less puzzled and disturbed when they receive the attention.

My own bad experience in the category of Physician Seeking Physical Finding in Uninformed Patient is a distressing example. I was a resident supervising a medical student who was scheduled to present a patient to the attending physician – a Young Turk infectious disease specialist. The patient had been admitted for pyelonephritis – right up the attending physician's alley. The patient also had a large spleen, which we discovered incidentally, and at the time had no explanation for. As we wanted to wait until we had obtained some more information, we hadn't told the patient about his large spleen.

The student nervously began his presentation and the more he stumbled and hesitated the more impatient the great man became. When the student got to the part in the physical exam where he described palpating a large spleen the attending got fed up. "Pyelonephritis doesn't give you splenomegaly," he expertly pronounced. When I confirmed the student's finding, he demanded to see the patient right away. Before I could say anything more, he strode to the bedside, threw off the sheets, pressed his hand into the man's left upper quadrant, widened his eyes and whistled. Then left it to me to hastily and shamefacedly fill the patient in on this "incidental finding."

There too, things could have been done better.

"White lies and omissions"

The physician admits that when faced with disclosing the possibility of cancer, which has "high emotional impact for a patient," he or she resorts to "white lies and omissions."

Part of this avoidance behavior may reflect the

physician's own discomfort more than the patient's discomfort. And why not? Is the emotional impact not also experienced by the physician, who fears that the patient may have a condition over which the physician has no control?

However, if we stipulate that the physician is capable of dealing with the situation personally and has a well-founded concern about the patient's own emotional state, then I think several issues ought to be considered in presenting bad news:

(1) Context: If cancer is at most a remote possibility, then there is no need to force the issue into the patient's consciousness. If, on the other hand, the patient is worried about the symptoms, then it is quite possible he or she is already wondering about the possibility of cancer. Telling the patient that cancer is only a remote possibility could in fact be reassuring. In short, if the physician thinks the patient is thinking about it, then it's best to talk about it.

(2) Preparation: We all know we're going to die, yet most of us spend most of our time not thinking about that. Except when we go to the doctor. That's when we look at ourselves, all our body parts and laboratory tests, with one deep question in the back of our mind: How much longer do I have? The physician who makes use of routine visits to include advance care planning in the discussions gradually prepares the patient for what is inevitable. By initiating discussion on that deep question, the physician sets the tone and builds trust. The patient gets to know that this physician will not be afraid to talk about anything. Also the patient gains confidence that his or her wishes are understood and will be honored.

(3) The whole truth: Giving the patient the diagnosis of cancer provides only part of the truth. The whole truth is much larger. It consists of saying: You have cancer and here is what we can do. If there's a chance to cure it, let's go for it. Here's what you can expect. Many patients like you have recovered from your kind

of cancer. On the other hand, if the physician is forced by the facts to say that there's no realistic chance to cure the cancer, the physician still says: Here's what we can do for you. We can make sure you have the best quality of life for your remaining days. You've probably heard a lot of horror stories about cancer. What are you afraid of? Pain? We can keep you pain-free if that's what you want. It may require sedating you in the end, but I guarantee I'll do that if that's what you want. You'll die in your sleep, which is what everybody wants. So don't worry about pain. Think about what you do want and in so far as it's possible we'll work together to make it happen. We all die, as you know, and as your physician I'll stick with you all the way. When your time comes I'll do my best to make sure it comes as peacefully, comfortably, and with as much dignity as possible. And so forth.

That comes closer to the whole truth.

"I hated disappointing them"

The intern feels at a loss because she could not "fix" Mr. G and could not do her job which she thought was "to keep him alive." The family added to the impossibility of the situation by whispering in the nearly dead man's ear, "Daddy, if you can hear me, do nothing."

Not surprisingly, the intern was so uncomfortable she found herself hiding from the family. Indeed, empirical studies have shown that medical providers don't like bad news any more than their patients do. Right after a diagnosis of a terminal illness is made, the number of visits to a hospitalized patient plummets.

The intern made her life more miserable by accepting the unrealistic expectations put on her by the family and by her own sense of what her job was. She "knew it was futile," yet she hated disappointing the family who "kept pressing me for good news."

I submit the intern missed an opportunity to get the family to reconfigure the good news. The good news is how much the patient was loved, what a wonderful man he must have been, and for which he will be remembered. The good news is that everyone cared about him, his family, even the intern, and wanted to do what was best. All the people were dedicated to do just that. Which meant that this man was luckier than most people in the world. Most people don't have such love and caring at any time in their life, much less when they are helpless and dying. And most people won't leave such good memories.

I believe in getting all the help you can, so indeed, the intern should call upon social service, psychiatry, and the clergy. In short, the job of Mr. G's physician was not to "keep him alive," but to provide optimal end-of-life care.

"Sin of silence"

The priest performs a ritual of blessing the dead rather than the ritual of blessing the dying. He missed out by less than 20 minutes. Does that spoil the patient's chances to gain his just reward? If there is a God, and He takes such distinctions seriously, I would not want to affiliate with such a Supreme Being, much less take Him seriously. Besides, in such matters who are we, mere mortals, to make judgments? The priest performed a ceremony designed to comfort the living as much as it honors the dead. Apparently someone doesn't like this priest – who in my opinion is already worthy of respect for working in a hospital – because he was observed to speak with colleagues he had not seen in a long time and then to spend less than one minute with the deceased before hurrying on to other business. People who make such observations should be willing to consider how fallible they are. Not only their observations. They might also consider how they themselves measure up to this imperfect man. In my opinion, the family's relief should not be poisoned by someone who is so insensitive as to regard the tact and discretion of those who do not tell the family "the truth" to be a "conspiracy of silence."

COMMENTARY

Ben Rich

"Omit the mistake"

Both medical ethics and medical jurisprudence are implicated in this case. Because our primary focus in this volume is "ward ethics," I shall briefly allude to the legal concerns and then discuss the ethical implications at greater length.

A patient's medical record is sacrosanct in the sense that it must be consistently maintained with scrupulous attention to completeness and accuracy. Under no circumstances, and certainly not for purposes of disguising someone's mistake, should any misleading information be placed in the record. Writing a note that suggests that a patient experienced an allergic reaction to a particular medication when that is not in fact the case cannot be justified on any grounds. To do so would deprive the patient of that medication in the future when it may be critical to his or her health.

If the treatment of the patient during this hospitalization became an issue in subsequent litigation, and the person who entered that note in the record were called to testify about the incident, that individual would be put to the choice of acknowledging the inaccuracy of the note or committing perjury by standing by the accuracy of the note as a factual representation of what happened to the patient.

Medicine is practiced by fallible human beings. Mistakes are made, and when they are discovered and have adversely affected a patient, they must be forthrightly acknowledged. The place of truth-telling in medical ethics has been encumbered by what might be referred to as "the therapeutic privilege." Technically, that phrase refers to one of only two recognized exceptions to the general rule that the patient's informed consent must be obtained to a procedure with any risk that is not *de minimus.* If, in the physician's judgment, disclosure of certain details about the patient's condition are likely to create an unreasonable risk of serious harm to the patient, the physician may invoke the therapeutic privilege and withhold that information. Except in these (presumably) exceedingly rare circumstances, the general rule (of medical ethics and medical law) is that a physician has a duty to disclose to the patient all information that is necessary for an informed decision to be made about treatment options.

Historically, something like the therapeutic privilege was exercised by many physicians when they withheld the diagnosis of a terminal or life-threatening condition from patients. Unlike the confidentiality of information pertaining to the patient, which has roots that run deep into the Hippocratic medical corpus, truthtelling as a general principle of medical ethics was not recognized until late in the twentieth century. This strikes me as a curious artifact of the history of medicine if we are to think of the physician–patient relationship as fiduciary in nature. A fiduciary is one who owes another the duties of good faith, trust, confidence, and candor. It is by definition, therefore, inconceivable that one can discharge the responsibilities of a fiduciary while at the same time withholding from the person to whom those responsibilities run information that bears directly and substantially upon that person.

"Was I acting under false pretenses?"

It is an assumption, but in all likelihood a safe one, that the patient believed the student to be a physician who is examining him for some therapeutic, as opposed to educational purpose. In raising his gown to facilitate the examination, the patient is impliedly consenting to it, but presumably because he believes it to be part of the therapeutic undertaking. There appears to be, without much, if any, foundation in fact, an assumption that many, perhaps even most patients would decline to be examined by a medical student if they were informed in advance that it was merely for the purpose of educating the student. In this

respect, patients are given insufficient credit for being sensitive to the educational needs of students.

There is another common perception, also without sufficient factual support and which is actually in conflict with the previous one, that patients in hospitals that are affiliated medical schools or health professional training programs do, or at least should assume that any young person in a white coat whom they encounter is a trainee of some sort. Hence, there is no need to belabor that fact by identifying each and every student whom they encounter during the course of their treatment.

Treating patients in this way deprives them of the respect to which they are entitled by those who stand in a professional relationship to them. Most patients, if dealt with honestly and courteously, will consent to an examination by a student or other trainee. The few who decline are exercising their right to do so. Receipt of appropriate medical care cannot be conditioned upon some presumed consent to be examined or otherwise touched by those who stand outside the patient–professional relationship.

"White lies and omissions"

There is more than a difference of degree between the impropriety of withholding of a confirmed diagnosis from a patient and the nondisclosure of a remote possibility of grave illness that is part of a differential diagnosis. The former is categorically wrong unless the patient has made it clear that he or she does not wish to know. The latter raises questions of relative benefit and burden. Subjecting a patient to days or weeks of doubt and distress while additional examinations and tests are undertaken out of a meticulous adherence to the principle of full disclosure may not confer a benefit to the patient that is not outweighed by the burdens.

One approach to consider would be to identify those conditions which most plausibly account for the patient's symptoms, and merely allude to the remote possibility of others which might have to be considered further if each of the more likely candidates is ruled out. Unless the patient presses for more detailed information about those remote possibilities, there is no need to do other than allude to them at that time. However, if a definitive diagnosis remains elusive, so that a more remote and more serious possibility has not been ruled out, then the need for candor and adherence to a shared-decision making model of the patient–physician relationship militates toward broaching the subject.

An exception to this approach would be if the physician has concerns that there is a risk that the patient may be lost to follow-up or not be diligent in pursuing the additional diagnostic procedures that are indicated. If that were the case, it may be both necessary and appropriate to admonish the patient that at this point there remains a possibility of a much more serious cause for the symptoms, in order to impress upon the patient the importance of continuing to work cooperatively toward an accurate diagnosis and the appropriate treatment.

"I hated disappointing them"

What immediately strikes any reader who is familiar with intensive care units that participate in graduate medical education programs is the question: Where is the attending physician who must be ultimately responsible for the care of the patient? No resident, and certainly no intern, should be left with the impression that his or her "job" is to keep a dying patient alive and to be the individual primarily responsible for dealing with the patient's family. If an intern is actually abandoned as this one seems to have been, they should proceed without delay through the chain of command until they have secured the appropriate level of supervision in dealing with this most difficult of all cases. If that process does not produce appropriate responses, then they should request an immediate consultation from the hospital's ethics committee, for their abandon-

ment alone raises significant ethical issues.

Actually, this case raises many more ethical issues than can be adequately considered within the scope of this analysis, so I will address only the most troublesome. Beyond the plight of the intern, the next major issue is why there is no care/treatment plan that has been discussed and agreed to by all of the team members and the family. Blind adherence to a vague admonition to preserve life is unacceptable when a patient, as this one does, clearly demonstrates that he is actively dying. Mr. G has multi-organ system failure; he has suffered a cardiac arrest and received CPR; he is comatose with virtually no brain function; and he is showing no positive response to any interventions. Hence, Mr. G can only be described as actively dying. Further treatment, including continuing life-sustaining interventions, can confer no benefit on this patient, but only prolong the suffering and delay the inception of the appropriate grieving and bereavement process of the family.

This case characterizes the deplorable care of dying patients documented in SUPPORT and decried by a host of recent reports by major medical organizations, including the Institute of Medicine and the American Board of Internal Medicine. Such care suggests that many intensivists are unable or unwilling to identify patients who are actively dying and effectively make the transition from therapeutic to palliative interventions. There is absolutely no reason to conclude that with the proper guidance and counsel from senior physicians, this family could not have been helped to realize that what is in Mr. G's best interests at this time is that he be made comfortable and that his loved ones gather near him while the dying process is completed with respect and dignity. While most teaching hospitals certainly have social workers and pastoral counselors available to help families come to terms with the fact that a loved one is dying, physicians, particularly attending physicians with the responsibility for both patient care and the mentoring of residents and interns, cannot ethically delegate these matters to others. To do so sends precisely the wrong message, which is that when therapeutic interventions cease, so too does the responsibility of the physician.

The intern was uncomfortable in this case because much was wrong about the care and treatment provided. The ultimate responsibility for that lies with the attending physician. But that is not to say that in the default position in which the intern found him or herself, more could not have been done to help the family understand and appreciate that Mr. G was dying and that good care for dying patients does not include a tube through every orifice. When interns and medical students are actively involved in patient care, as in this situation, they have an increased obligation to articulate questions and concerns about troubling situations that involve patients in whose care they are participating.

"Sin of silence"

As this case is described, the medical personnel are less implicated in the family's erroneous conclusion about the administration of last rites to the patient than the priest. Whether it is morally imperative for the family to know the truth of the matter – that the priest only blessed the deceased but did not perform last rites – may depend in part on church doctrines which are beyond the scope of this commentary. At this point the focus of concern has moved from the patient to the family. From a purely ethical perspective, there are competing considerations. Revealing the facts of the matter when nothing can any longer be done will be likely to increase their emotional distress. Failing to reveal the facts of the matter to the family does, to a certain extent, render the treatment team complicit in deception, however well-intentioned. A middle course might be to express concern to the priest that the family is laboring under this misapprehension, and request that he make clear to them, as sensitively as possible, what he was and was not able to do for the patient with regard to the rites of the Church. Only when he has apprised them of all of the relevant (religious/spiritual) circumstances will they actually be in a position to avail themselves of his offer to respond to any further requests they may have.

8

Commissions: deliberate deception

CASE

"The chief resident 'lied'"

In rounds I began to notice that the chief resident occasionally misstated information in order to avoid criticism from the attending. On one occasion I believed patient care and safety were possibly jeopardized when the chief resident "lied" by saying he was unaware of a serious abnormality, even though I knew personally that he had had the knowledge for more than 6 hours. Should I have corrected my superior in rounds? Talked to my superior separately? Talked to other staff? Let it go?

CASE

"A false report"

It was in the morning and my good friend and I were in our third-year clerkship. He very much wanted an honors grade in surgery. He had been busy xeroxing articles related to his preceptor's research project so, as he explained to me, he had not yet checked on his patients. The chief resident arrived and asked my friend if a patient whose temperature had spiked the previous evening was still febrile.

He responded, "No, 99.2." – a false report and I knew it.

COMMENTARY

Lawrence J. Schneiderman

"The chief resident 'lied'"

When I was a medical student, a resident achieved a much-admired reputation for one-upmanship. He simply carried a test tube of blood around in the breast pocket of his white jacket. The hospital was world-renowned for research that made nearly every issue of the *New England Journal of Medicine*. The researchers themselves were international celebrities from whose ranks were drawn the attending physicians. Daily rounds were more likely to be devoted to seminars on biochemistry than to more mundane patient care matters. To maintain status, the attending physician would feel obligated to suggest an esoteric diagnosis that no one else had thought of – which often happened to coincide with the attending's own area of research. The fact that the patient's problems were far more likely to have common garden-variety causes would not be considered worthy of the great man's time and brain power. Inevitably, during the course of rounds, the attending physician would say, somewhat smugly, "I think you should get a serum suchandsuch," naming an obscure substance most of us had never heard of; whereupon this crafty resident would raise the test tube in his pocket and intone, "It's just been drawn, sir."

We all regarded such a lie as amusing and harmless, a sly rebellion against pedantry. But his motive probably was not much different from that of the chief resident in this case scenario who occasionally "misstated information in order to avoid criticism from the attending."

Medicine is a harsh taskmaster, demanding inhuman perfection. That is because the stakes can be huge; the difference between life and death. However, this striving for perfection can so dominate the medical culture that it leads to its inevitable consequence. Physicians cannot be perfect, so they fake perfection. Then, like the legendary blue wall put up by the police, they put up a white wall in order to guard their own.

Years later in my career I took care of a lawyer who specialized in medical malpractice cases – a risk-taking on my part some might regard as flagrantly pathological. Falling under the category of Some of My Best Friends are Lawyers, he actually was a very decent fellow. And very honorable. Whenever he was not certain, and when a case was particularly complicated, he asked me to review the medical record to see whether in my medical judgment the doctor had performed negligently. Even though he knew I might be inclined to give undue weight to the uncertainties and complexities of medical care, he always turned down cases that I said did not strike me as being caused by physician malpractice.

One case, however, aroused my ire. A physician, who had no business doing surgery, ligated the ureters of a woman who had come to him to have her fallopian tubes tied. The physician's training was abysmal, his past history appalling, his record-keeping sketchy and incomprehensible, and on top of that when the woman went into renal failure, he proceeded to rewrite her medical record to cover his mistake.

Here, I told the lawyer, was a doctor he should go after and, if possible, put into involuntary retirement. The lawyer was forced to accept a meager settlement (the woman was Hispanic and poor) because he could not find a single specialist from the community willing to testify against the offending physician.

The reader will recognize that this happened several decades ago. Fortunately (or some would say unfortunately, since the tables have turned and now the law courts resound with the expert testimony of hired mercenaries), physicians are less likely today to get away with such egregious behavior.

I must say I am concerned about the behavior of this chief resident. Not only are patients threatened by his behavior, but he should know: so is his career. If his colleagues decide he is not trustworthy, he will not get referrals, not be consulted. In fact, he will be avoided as much as possible. A fundamental basis for good medical care, the ground on which just about every action depends, is truthfulness. Between patient and physician. Between physician and physician. Indeed, among all health professionals.

I do not know the exact relationship of the narrator in this scenario to the chief resident, although the power relationship of the chief resident is described as being superior. If the narrator feels secure enough to take the chief resident out for a beer and tell him his concerns, that would be the gentlest way to begin. If the narrator is a student or nurse, and is reasonably concerned about retaliation, however, then I would go up one step at a time, discreetly, the nurse to her supervisor who can take it to the next appropriate step, the student to someone like the clerkship director who can take it from there.

For everyone's sake I do not think the narrator should just "let it go."

"A false report"

The issues in this case are very similar to those noted above. Why couldn't the medical student simply admit he had not checked the patient's temperature? Because that would make him look imperfect. Because he was supposed to know it. That's all there is to it. No excuses. And why didn't he know it? Because he was too busy doing things in order to make an impression on his preceptor that had nothing to do with the patient. He got sidetracked by the drive to look perfect.

And ended up faking it.

Since the narrator is the student's good friend, he is, in my opinion, honor-bound both as a friend and colleague to discuss the problem with him. This can be done empathically. ("We're all under tremendous pressure. We're all tempted to take shortcuts. We all think we can do more than we really can. We all want so desperately to succeed we find ourselves doing things we shouldn't do, things that can get us into trouble" etc.)

If the narrator cannot bring himself or herself to do this task – which by the way is excellent preparation for some of the really difficult discussions involving patients and families that lie ahead for this doctor in training – then I would suggest calling the chief resident for a private session. During this session, the student can again quite empathically express a desire to help the friend who is "anxious about doing well."

In any event, intervention in this student's attitude and behavior now will be far more beneficial than intervention by the courts later in his career.

COMMENTARY

Jeffrey H. Burack

These cases are not about whether to lie, but about whether to "blow the whistle" on someone else who has lied. Whistle-blowing presents an ethical problem unlike many in medicine, because the individual patient may be only peripherally involved, whereas concerns about interprofessional relations and self-preservation are paramount. As a member of the treating team, the medical student has an obligation to seek the patient's best interest and to protect her from harm. If incorrect information is likely to cause inappropriate care, the student's obligation of beneficence requires that she come forward to correct that information. Furthermore, a colleague's lying may be an indication of impair-

ment, an overwhelming workload, or a misplaced belief in the importance of appearing to know everything. Intervening may help correct these underlying problems. Doing so sooner rather than later may mitigate the consequences to that colleague, who might otherwise tangle himself progressively deeper in a web of deceit, and may prevent harm to this and future patients. Other arguments favoring whistle-blowing include the obligations to preserve one's own integrity, and that of the team, the institution, and the profession.

On the other hand, whistle-blowing raises the possibility of doing harm, to one's colleague and to oneself. What if the colleague's belief in the importance of knowing everything is not misplaced after all: what if, in this teaching setting, admitting to not knowing information about a patient is considered inexcusable, while small lies are likely to pass unnoticed? What if being revealed to have lied damages the colleague's career prospects? What about the humiliation such accusations will cause? And what of the potential repercussions for the whistle-blower herself? Certainly, a relationship with a colleague may be damaged. In the case of the chief resident, that colleague may have the ability to retaliate in more substantial ways, perhaps making the student's life miserable, smearing her in informal conversation, or writing a damning evaluation. In either case, the student may face being labeled as "not a team player," and subsequently treated as a pariah. It is unclear to what extent such fears are borne out in reality. What is undeniable, however, is that they become important motivations, and that the impetus to stand by team members is a powerful one. (1)

Sometimes, what seems at first blush to be a lie in fact reflects the speaker's own misunderstanding, misinformation, or ignorance. A student who passes on incorrect information, derived from a source which she has no reason to doubt, is not lying. One must therefore be circumspect in judging that a colleague has intended to lie, and must often begin by seeking more information. Unfortunately, in these cases, we are led clearly to believe that both the chief resident and the third year clerk lied deliberately. Furthermore, it is plainly implied that both acted for reasons of self-preservation, or self-advancement, offering false information rather than admitting that they do not know answers which are expected of them.

Should the students in these cases speak up? To cut to the chase: yes, but in different ways. By committing themselves to the study and practice of medicine, the students have inescapably taken on membership in a moral community, which brings with it responsibilities for patient welfare, for their own conduct, and for that of their colleagues. What they ought to do does not take long to describe. But the details of the cases suggest different pragmatic strategies, and at the same time go far toward explaining why many of us hesitate to try them. What demands more comment than *what* to do is the set of conditions which place medical students in such positions to begin with, and which make it so hard to get out of them.

There are several morally significant differences between the cases, which suggest different responses. In "A false report," the student who lies is a peer, indeed described as a "good friend." A personal relationship pre-exists between perpetrator and putative whistle-blower. The student's motives are made clear: he wants an honors grade so badly that he uses the time in which he is expected to check on his patients to instead propitiate his preceptor, who presumably is able to ensure that grade. There is no suggestion that the patient's health is meaningfully endangered by the student's lie, particularly as third-year clerks generally have little authority over significant clinical decision making. Further, there is no suggestion that this type of behavior has happened before – it appears, in the eyes of the narrator, to be a "first offense." The offending student may, in a sense, be trying on a new mode of behavior for the first time; he most likely feels guilty and anxious, and has lied in panic. Nevertheless, there is a real risk that if the lie passes

unchallenged, this unthinking response in a moment of terror may become a conscious, adaptive strategy.

Intervention should therefore come promptly but gently, respectfully, and in a spirit of offering the benefit of the doubt. The narrator would be best advised to take her friend aside, privately, at some later time, and discuss her concerns about what she observed. Perhaps she can adopt a stance of understanding and compassion, indicating that she shares her friend's anxieties about not knowing enough, and about how to behave on the wards. Together, they can adopt strategies for dealing with similar situations in the future, or if unsure about how to do so, can seek help from their clerkship director or other faculty. Is it utopian to imagine that the student who lied would respond so positively? No; rather, it is unfair and incorrect to presume that such lies are typically born of uncaring or poor moral character. Respect dictates interpreting the behavior as an error and helping create opportunities to avoid its repetition. Many students, though deeply embarrassed, are relieved to be able to share their guilt and to take constructive action. It is, of course, possible that the student will angrily reject his friend's overture. In this case, she ought to put off taking any further steps (such as speaking confidentially with the clerkship director) unless and until the behavior is repeated, in order to give her friend a chance to demonstrate that he has nevertheless taken her concerns to heart.

In "The chief resident 'lied'", the chief resident, far from being a peer, sits high above the concerned student in the medical hierarchy – high enough both to wield considerable power over the student, and to make (or to negligently avoid making) decisions of grave consequence to patients. Indeed, the student has noted at least one occasion on which she believed that a patient was actually endangered. The chief resident's motive is as clear as was the student's in the previous case: his dominant concern in reporting information to the attending physician is to avoid criticism, rather than to communicate the truth about their patients' conditions. Most disturbingly, lying has evidently become a regular pattern for this chief resident: the student "began to notice" that it "occasionally" occurred. This is no one-time, unthinking response, made spontaneously in response to panic – though I have little doubt that a deeper, enduring, and desperate panic indeed underlies the chief resident's behavior. This is instead an established pattern of dishonest and clinically dangerous behavior.

The chief resident must also be responded to from a stance of compassion, and urgently, as patients may be at risk. But the behavior at issue is more worrisome, the accusation more serious, and the student's position much weaker. The student on this team has become as much a victim of the imposed culture of deceit and conspiracy as are the patients, the other trainees, and the chief resident himself. Speaking truth from a position of oppression demands great courage; speaking it to the oppressor's face may demand superhuman courage, and is sometimes reckless and ill advised. In my opinion, it is unrealistic and even irresponsible to counsel this student to personally approach the chief resident as she would have her peer. Too much is at risk for the student, and a counterproductive, punitive response too readily available to the chief resident, who is likely, to put it mildly, to be highly defensive.

The response to the chief resident must come from others higher in the hierarchy, and the student's responsibility is to alert them. The student should approach a trusted faculty member, perhaps the team's attending physician but more often a clerkship director, faculty adviser, or dean, and request that her concerns about this resident be relayed in strict confidence to his immediate supervisors. There is no reason that the student's identity need be revealed, as the intervention presumably would be to alert faculty to watch for future behaviors, rather than to call the resident to task for past ones. The student should feel reassured that others have almost certainly had concerns about the chief resident's behavior; her report is unlikely to take his supervisors by surprise. Finally, this highlights the point that the student should never feel that she has to take such risks alone. There will always be faculty who will respond positively and helpfully to the student's dilemma; her task, often with the help of fellow students, is to identify those faculty.

One of the truths revealed by these cases is that moral judgment under dilemma conditions involves weighing various priorities to decide not only what one must do, but also how to do it. These priorities may include the indisputably "moral," such as the obligation to protect patients or the commitment to truth, but also what are more commonly thought of as nonmoral concerns, such as self-preservation, professional self-advancement, social acceptance, and reticence. Active intervention in these cases may indeed seem supererogatory for these students – that is, it is morally desirable, but may go beyond what ethics can demand of them. But it seems supererogatory precisely because we admit that these values of self-concern can and should legitimately be weighed against moral ones. It is a counterproductive moralism which claims that concerns about harming oneself or one's teammates have no place in deliberating about one's response. Furthermore, the student may find it overwhelmingly unfair to be offered a choice between finding the tremendous moral courage to undertake such a supererogatory act as directly confronting the chief resident, or the moral cowardice of "letting it go." But this dichotomous choice is illusory: once one acknowledges the duty to do *something*, and the moral question becomes *what* to do, there is almost always a range of more creative options than the stark dilemma would suggest. The student can take seriously both her obligation to speak out, and the pragmatic need to protect herself and others.

The most important interventions for which these cases call out, however, are not individual acts of courage or moral decision making, but institutional responses to the conditions which permit, encourage, and conceal dishonesty. The cases speak eloquently about the role of *power* in determining the behavior of members of a medical team. (2) Most evident is the distorting effect of the team's own hierarchical power structure. Power is most tyrannical when it is wielded, or believed to be wielded, arbitrarily. It is the power of senior team members to capriciously influence career paths that drives junior members to deceptive behaviors in the first place. Insecurity about one's knowledge and one's "place," and explicit fear of unrestricted retaliation from above, further silence students. The cases also speak to the power of team members to control information about patients, and thereby quite literally to control those patients' lives. That this power can be misused to the patient's detriment is a reminder of the responsibility vested in even the most "junior" team members. While similar hierarchies exist, and likely have comparable chilling effects, in other occupations, the particular vulnerability of the patient creates an obligation to respond to medical hierarchy in at least two ways. First, all team members, however powerless they may feel, must be mindful of their personal responsibility for honestly sharing even apparently trivial information about patients. And second, all must work in whatever ways are available to them toward creating systems that both encourage sharing true information, and permit safe reporting of lapses.

That lying about test results or vital signs is more acceptable than admitting to not knowing them may be transmitted as part of the "hidden curriculum" of medical education. (3) This is the set of shared values, attitudes, and beliefs conveyed to students and residents, not as explicitly taught content, but through the behaviors of their superiors and the institutional structures in which they work. Medical schools must question seriously what encourages such lying. Do students perceive that faculty and residents are rewarded for apparent knowledgeability, comprehensiveness, and confidence, but not for humility, integrity, and attention to patients? Are these perceptions accurate? Are students berated

or humiliated for not knowing data? Is the radically honest act of saying "I don't know" modeled by faculty, up to the highest echelons, or is the predominant culture instead one of appearing to "out-know" one another? Perhaps the most important way in which educators can encourage trainees to treat patients with honesty and respect is to treat the trainees the same way. (4) Do we respect students as persons, altruistic learners eager to expand their knowledge base, or do we use them as means – as convenient and vulnerable foils for our own insecurities? Building up one's own ego by showing up a student's lack of knowledge may be temporarily satisfying to a teacher, but ultimately undermines the integrity and confidence of both.

A disturbing element of both cases is that the onus of responding seems to fall to the most junior members of the team. Where is the attending physician? Tellingly, the answer most of the time is: somewhere else. Students and residents generally spend only a minuscule fraction of their long hours under the eye of the attending physician, who is consequently ill-positioned to notice, let alone assess, their ethical comportment. Attendings see only the faces designed for presentation to them during brief, stylized encounters, and are not privy to learners' interactions with each other and with patients. Because of this detachment, their own insecurity within the hierarchy, and a variety of well-intentioned but misguided reasons, attending physicians are very reluctant to respond to evidence of unethical behavior. When they do respond, they do so in oblique ways that risk failing to clearly communicate a standard of acceptable or ideal behavior. (5) If we are to take seriously the encouragement of honesty, we must create a teaching environment in which attending physicians spend enough time with learners to get to know them, and are more willing to intervene, both to commend moral courage and to correct lies and like failures. Teachers can only be expected to promote these as the ideals of the educational culture if they in fact *are* the ideals of the culture, and if they feel supported in doing so.

Finally, it is striking that in a chapter on acts of "commission," the protagonists of both cases are not those who lie, but those who observe *others* lying. The real "commissions" at issue are in fact the commissions of others, acts that have already taken place as the drama begins. The central dilemmas as presented now concern whether and how to blow the whistle, not whether or not one ought to commit a deception oneself. Why not engage the prior question of whether, or under what circumstances, it may seem acceptable to lie in clinical teaching settings? Or even more, why not ask why students, trainees, and even senior physicians feel driven to lie in such settings? I believe that we in medicine cannot or simply do not face these questions because we assume one or more of three flawed premises. We believe: (i) that anyone seriously interested in ethical concerns would in the first place not even entertain such an action; or (ii) that the answer to such a dilemma is obvious; or (iii) that it is not properly cast as an *ethical* dilemma at all, since it pits ethical concerns against those of self-interest.

I will not dwell on these premises except insofar as to state that all are problematic, not simply logically or empirically, but also in that they sustain a conception of ethics that keeps it irrelevant to the exigencies of everyday life in medicine. When ethics cannot address the real dilemmas of practice, and the things we actually lie awake feeling badly for having done, it degenerates into the sterile moralism described above. As such, it risks being appropriately ignored as inconsequential or even damaging. I venture to claim that virtually every one of us has at some point lied or dissembled, in ways large or small, to protect ourselves from criticism, humiliation, or a poor evaluation, or simply to preserve others' esteem for us. Are we wrong to do so? Almost certainly. Is doing so understandable under the conditions prevalent in medical education? Quite often. A rigid ethical deductivism that has little to say beyond ruling on the wrongness of these acts

gets us nowhere in addressing their determinants. A more sociological approach, one that concerns itself with understanding the social structures within which medicine is taught and practiced, and ultimately with altering those structures so as to encourage more ethical behavior, would allow us to meaningfully ask about the root of the problem, the "commission" of the lie itself. But that would be another case.

Notes

1 Feudtner C, Christakis DA. Making the rounds: the ethical development of medical students in the context of clinical rotations. *Hastings Cent Rep* 1994;24:6–12.
2 Brody H. *The Healer's Power*. Yale University Press, New Haven, 1992.
3 Hafferty FW, Franks R. The hidden curriculum, ethics teaching, and the structure of medical education. *Acad Med* 1994;69:861–71.
4 Reiser SJ. The ethics of learning and teaching medicine. *Acad Med* 1994;69:872–6.
5 Burack JH, Irby DM, Carline JD, Root RK, Larson EB. Teaching compassion and respect: attending physicians' responses to problematic behavior. *J Gen Intern Med* 1999;14:49–55.

COMMENTARY

Ben Rich

"The chief resident 'lied'"

This case presents issues of both tact and truthfulness. From a strategic standpoint, challenging the chief resident in rounds, particularly with regard to his truth and veracity, would not be appropriate or necessary, even if patient care is implicated. The initial response to this clearly problematic situation is to promptly arrange a private conversation with the chief resident when you can, with candor and diplomacy, express your concerns. Assuming that patient health and safety are not at that moment in jeopardy, the goals for this conversation should be prospective rather than retrospective. First, of course, the chief resident's response to your concerns needs to be elicited. If you have in some way misunderstood or misinterpreted his statements, or if in fact you are wrong in any of your judgments of his credibility, this is the time to make that determination.

Both denial and hostility on the part of the chief resident must be anticipated. Consequently, a tactful presentation of your concerns, perhaps even acknowledging (though not conceding) the possibility of a misunderstanding might be considered. If your concerns cannot be satisfactorily allayed by the chief resident, then it is important to let him know that "letting it go" and saying nothing further about future instances is not an option. If the pattern of misrepresentations persists, and the chief resident will not take the initiative to address the problem, then you should make it clear that you see no reasonable alternative but to take the matter up directly with the attending.

The chief resident is placing his reputation at risk by such conduct, and seriously compromising the integrity of the health care team that participates in rounds. Furthermore, as this case illustrates, on occasion patient health and safety are also at times placed in jeopardy. Remaining silent in this situation tolerates, even tacitly approves the chief resident's unethical and inappropriate behavior, and renders the student complicit in the wrongdoing.

"A false report"

There are two distinctions between this case and the previous one. First, the misrepresentation of fact is made by a peer rather than someone higher up in the "chain of command." Second, the "false report" is presented as an isolated incident rather than an example of a pattern and practice. Neither of these distinctions, however, is sufficient to warrant a different approach to the problem or to make it any less difficult to confront.

As soon as the chief resident leaves, the student should confront his friend and insist that the record be set straight immediately. In the unlikely event that a prompt examination of the patient reveals that he or she is afebrile, the friend can merely be warned that you will not stand by silently in the event that there are any future instances of lying. If the patient remains febrile, then the medical record must be made to reflect that, and the patient's status relayed to the chief resident. The friend should be given the opportunity to do this, but you should make it clear that you will do so yourself if he or she does not.

Medical school, internship, and residency constitute the progressive development of professionalism. Intentionally misrepresenting important factual matters which bear directly on patient care constitutes unprofessional and unethical conduct. Any tendency to habitualize such behaviors must be resisted in oneself and confronted when they are manifested by others.

DISCUSSION QUESTIONS
Section 2. Problems in truth-telling

1 Are there any good arguments against telling the truth? Under what circumstances, if ever, should doctors keep secrets from the patient? From the family? From one another? From their own spouses or families?
2 Is there a morally relevant distinction between lying to the patient and merely being nonresponsive or evasive?
3 How should you deal with a request to lie from a superior? What if that superior evaluates your performance?
4 Much of medicine deals with uncertainties, is there a moral burden to acknowledge uncertainties? To what degree, if at all, should uncertainties be disclosed?
5 To what extent is it the physician's responsibility to educate patients about the state of their health?
6 What if you fear that telling the truth may cause more harm than good?
7 What if you witness an error being made or a falsehood being told to a patient? Do you have an obligation to set things straight? If you do, how would you go about carrying it out?
8 How far are you willing to jeopardize your own career in making sure those around you are being truthful and honest to patients? To peers? To their superiors?

Setting boundaries

Defining professional parameters can be especially complex and confusing for doctors in training. What counts as too close so that professionalism is lost? What counts as so removed as to lose the special connection that defines the physician–patient relationship? The blurry state of boundaries is underlined in our time by shifting role expectations and the importance of patient autonomy. Physicians owe patients clarity as to what they will or will not do, and patients must be clear with their physicians about their own values and limits.

In this section we stress three of the most difficult boundaries to establish in the physician–patient relationship. They define boundaries of professional parameters. Might sexual relations initiated by patients be justied? What are appropriate responses to sexual innuendoes? How to handle the common complaint about investing emotional energy in difficult patients? Is losing compassion inevitable?

9

From professional to personal

CASE

"Do you want to see me again?"

As a resident a very attractive woman came to see me with pityriasis rosea on her breasts. I examined her, made the diagnosis and told her that although it would take some time, her condition was benign and would heal spontaneously. I told her to come back in a couple of weeks and we'd see if her skin had cleared up. She came back and indeed I was able to tell her "That's fine, it's completely gone." Later, to my astonishment she made another appointment to come and see me. When I entered the room she had already removed her clothing and wanted me to check her. There was no indication she needed medical attention, and I began to suspect that something less professional was going on. She said, "Well, do you want to see me again?"

CASE

"I don't think I took advantage of her"

One night when I was a resident a female patient asked me to undress her. I did and, at her urging, got into bed with her and had sex. After that I went to her room for sex several times while she was in the hospital. We saw each other for some time after her discharge. I've never told anyone about this. She initiated the sex and it was entirely consensual, I don't think I took advantage of her.

COMMENTARY

Richard Martinez

Few experiences in the patient and health care professional relationship are more challenging than the introduction of sexual feelings. In my work as an educator and supervisor of psychiatry residents where sexual material is not uncommon in the context of the therapeutic relationship, I find it useful to utilize the concept of boundaries between health care professional and patient as the best means to understand these situations. This then allows us to consider the ethical issues involved in boundary situations where the professional and personal elements of relationships with patients become confused.

Boundaries in the patient–health professional relationship is a useful concept to define the limits and extensions of activity and behavior between patient and professional. The management of these boundaries reveals much about the individual professional as she negotiates the inevitable overlap between her personal and professional values. Broadly considered, boundary dilemmas in the patient–professional relationship have come to include sexual misconduct with patients at one end of a continuum, while discussions of how to respond to gifts or whether to attend the funeral of a former patient are included at the other end. Since most physicians, not just psychiatrists, are involved in intensely intimate relationships with their patients, understanding boundary dilemmas is essential for good patient care.

Ethically, issues of patient exploitation and coercion are the central concern. Boundary crossings and boundary violations are paradigms for understanding dynamic and complex behavior between patient and professional. The distinction between "boundary crossings" and "boundary violations" involves judgments about whether exploitation and/or coercion have occurred in the patient–professional relationship, and an assessment of the seriousness of the exploitation. That is, has harm occurred, and if so, how much harm to the patient has occurred because of the boundary crossing? If the crossing is judged to be of significant harm to the patient and involves exploitation on the part of the professional, then the "crossing" is then labeled a "violation." In psychiatry, where sexual misconduct has influenced discussions about boundaries, the "slippery slope" view of boundary crossings maintains that "crossings" often precede "violations," and thus the importance of vigilance and care in assessing and managing these interactions. That is, current recommendations discourage health care professionals from relationships with patients outside of the traditional patient–professional relationship. The American Psychiatric Association (APA) has declared all sexual encounters with current or former patients as unethical. The American Medical Association (AMA) through its Council on Ethical and Judicial Affairs declares that a sexual relationship with a current patient is unethical. The AMA also questions the appropriateness of a relationship with a former patient, but unlike the APA, the AMA leaves open the possibility that in certain cases, and after appropriate termination of the patient–professional relationship, a romantic relationship might be understandable.

Rules and guidelines from professional organizations are intended to protect patients, guide professionals, and support public trust in professionals. In most cases, this does happen. However, the "slippery slope" approach can have the unintended impact of simplifying the complex behavior and underlying processes by which professionals balance professional and personal values. While we do talk about our personal self as distinct and separate from our professional self, as if the two never touch, this is an obvious oversimplification. In real life, it is often difficult to separate the two, and perhaps, at times, it isn't necessarily desirable to have such a distinct separation. Cultural, racial, gender, religious, and ethnic considerations can be ignored when rules and guidelines alone define what is ethical in the domain of boundary dilemmas. While there is an emerging consensus around many boundary dilemmas that involve potential harm and exploitation of patients, there are many other types of boundary crossings that require further discussion and research.

To illustrate this point, some health care professionals provide discounted services to certain patients as a morally desirable choice. This violates the practice of treating all patients equally and avoiding "special" or "privileged" care. As an example, consider a patient, an unemployed artist, who barters with his health care professional by paying for his medical and dental services with sculptures and paintings. Is this an example of undesirable boundary crossing, or a legitimate moral choice by the health care professional and patient? In certain situations, professionals may choose to be friends with current or former patients, perhaps they attend the same church, or live in communities where it is natural to socialize with individuals who are or have been patients. For some health care professionals, the value of forming complex and enduring relationships with patients is an important part of professional identity. Unfortunately, the tendency to look suspiciously on all boundary crossings as "risky" or as "dual-relationships" can discourage professionals in pursuing moral ideals in their practice and professional identity. Rules and guidelines in the area of boundary crossings are intended to reduce risk and prevent patient harm. However, there are no singular and absolute definitions of professionalism. Discernment and acting with good judgment are necessary for proper management of boundary dilemmas in the patient–professional relationship.

In these two cases, while similar in that both involve sexual feelings, there are important differences. In the first, the resident is faced with a "seductive" patient, one who invites the physician into a boundary dilemma. Importantly, the case ends before the reader is told the outcome. Several important issues can be considered. The nature of the relationship between patient and health care professional can be described as a relationship that is highly intimate. The health care professional, often a stranger to the patient, requires physical and emotional disclosure from the patient in order to provide medical care. A significant differential in vulnerability and power between professional and patient characterizes this relationship. Trust is essential if the relationship is to serve the ends of providing healing medical care. Quite naturally, the intimate nature of this unique relationship can and does arouse sexual feelings in both health care professionals and patients. The sexualizing of the relationship can have many meanings, though. As with other behaviors that are presented to the professional, the ethical responsibility of the professional is to understand those behaviors, not to act upon them in exploitative and harmful ways.

Codes of professional conduct require the physician to act in the best interests of her patients, including the duty to place self-interests aside in certain situations. Some argue that this is at the core of professionalism, and to abandon this core value would be to dramatically damage the essence of medical care and the patient–professional relationship. Lastly, the sexualizing of the patient–professional relationship can obscure other understandings of such "seductive" behavior. Is this an attempt to control or dominate in a situation in which a patient is feeling vulnerable, helpless, and afraid? Does this patient have mental health issues that have not been addressed or noted? Is this an attempt to aggrandize the physician, or express gratitude? Obviously, we can't know in this vignette, but to engage in a sexual relationship and ignore the

professional responsibilities toward the patient is an ethical and clinical failure. Likewise, to rebuke and abandon the patient in such a situation is no more acceptable than engaging in a sexual relationship. The part of medicine and professionalism require a compassionate approach, where both a clear boundary is established, while remaining responsive to other ways of understanding such patient behavior.

In the second situation, a resident engages in a sexual relationship with a patient, while responsible for her medical care. Furthermore, the patient is in the hospital! The boundary dilemma is no longer a dilemma in this latter situation, but a boundary violation as defined by current professional standards of medical practice. A sick or injured patient in a hospital is not likely to be their emotional, physical, and spiritual "best self." Such a request from a patient should be looked upon with compassion and appreciation of the patient's vulnerable situation, not acted upon. The argument that this was a mutually consensual affair is not persuasive. Even if we give some merit to the "mutually consensual" argument, the current societal position is clear. Health care professionals should not have sexual relationships with current patients. By definition, the patient is vulnerable, and the risk of harm and betrayal in this situation cannot be minimized. Trust is damaged. The health care professional is using very poor judgment, placing his own desires before the patient's best interests, and then rationalizes the situation after the incident. This health care professional is harming the patient, the profession, and himself. In many states, this is a clear violation of standards of medical professional behavior with possible sanctions from the state medical licensing board. Such behavior creates significant liability for the health care professional, while often doing significant psychological and emotional damage to the patient.

COMMENTARY

Rosamond Rhodes

It is well accepted in medicine that doctors are committed to acting for their patients' good. In a peculiar way, both of these cases raise the question of whether the doctor or the patient decides on what counts as the patient's good. In that respect, these cases seem to be about the limits of patient autonomy and the grounds for appropriate paternalism. They are especially interesting, however, because they also raise the question of how to delimit boundaries for physician behavior.

To answer these questions we can begin by imagining far more standard doctor–patient encounters. The patient comes to see the doctor about some physical complaint. The doctor is a stranger or a near-stranger. Yet, for the doctor to be able to act for this patient's good, the patient will have to share details of her personal life, discuss her habits, and disclose intimate facts that she reveals to very few or no one else (e.g., about her sexual behavior, her bowel and drug habits). She will have to disrobe and allow the doctor to touch her body, to examine sexually significant areas, and to palpate in ways that are likely to cause pain. On the doctor's recommendation she may change her life habits. And if the doctor prescribes them, she may take medicines that are likely to be poisons. If he says they are important, she will subject herself to procedures or diagnostic tests, have things done to her body that she never wanted and would never choose again without a doctor's recommendation. And if the doctor says that it is necessary, she will allow herself to be made unconscious so that strangers can cut into her body and remove vital organs. Albeit, all of this is done for the patient's good. But none of it could occur without the patient having a particular attitude toward the doctor. In sum, the patient must trust the doctor to be acting for her good. Without trust, the practice of medicine would not be possible.

Because trust is necessary for the practice of medicine, seeking trust and engendering trust must be central to the ethics of medicine. In molding themselves, doctors must work to make themselves trustworthy. In their interactions with patients, doctors must strive to gain their patients' trust. And in setting boundaries for their professional behavior, doctors must consider which standards are most likely to earn and retain patient trust.

It is precisely because doctors must regard their patients' nakedness, and because they must touch sexually sensitive areas, and because they must probe areas of patients' personal lives that they would not have access to without being their doctors, that it is crucial for doctors to assure their patients that their looking, touching, and delving is purely professional. If patients had to worry about the nature of their doctors' regard, examination, or questioning, patients are likely to be far less open and doctors would be less likely to be able to do good for them. Clearly, then, the professional standard for doctors must be to avoid sexual relations with patients. To do otherwise would abuse patient trust and seriously undermine the future of patient trust.

While avoiding sexual relations with patients is the rule for doctor–patient relations, these cases raise questions about how far the rule extends and whether the prohibition on sexual relations with patients can be overridden by other considerations. In the case of the patient who invites the resident to have sex with her, the resident does not believe that he "took advantage of her." There are two implicit arguments in his position. If neither he nor the patient ever disclose their sexual interaction, his behavior could not undermine the public's trust of doctors maintaining a sexually disinterested stance toward their patients. Furthermore, if the patient rather than the doctor initiates the sexual interaction, it could be seen as the patient explicitly waiving her right to have no sexual attention from her doctor and proclaiming an autonomy right to decide what is best for her.

Nevertheless, I do not find either of these arguments persuasive. First, secrets eventually come out. In fact, here we are discussing the case, so we know that this doctor's secret is out. Betting on the unlikely eventuality that their secret will never be known is, at best, imprudent. And because patient trust in the nonsexual regard of their doctors is so crucial to the practice of medicine, it seems as if this chance could not possibly be worth taking. The idea here is that what each doctor does can impact on the public's regard of the profession. No one can know which incident will capture the attention of the media. So, while a particular doctor might choose to rashly risk his personal reputation, if his imprudent act involves professional conduct, it also puts the trustworthiness of the profession in jeopardy. No individual physician has the moral right to do that, and especially not for such a frivolous gain.

Second, there are professional limitations on patient requests that doctors should honor. For the most part, respect for autonomy requires that physicians allow their patients to make their own choices and to live by their own values. Respect for autonomy gives competent patients the right to choose between alternative treatments and the right to refuse having any treatment at all. Respect for autonomy is certainly a negative right to be left alone, and, in the medical context, I believe that it is also a positive right to have a physician provide treatments that clearly fall within the domain of services that only medicine has the power to provide. Respect for autonomy never gives a patient a right to have something done to her that lies outside the bounds of what is allowed by the ethics of the profession. There may be debate about the profession's stance on some medical interventions, for example about whether genetic screening for breast cancer should be provided to a patient with no family history of the disease or whether physician-assisted suicide falls on the prohibited or the required side of the borderline. When it comes to sex with patients, however, there is no debate. The relationships are professionally forbidden. There may be some vagueness about how long a patient remains a patient, but clearly so long as the doctor–patient relationship persists, any sexual relationship is prohibited. The patient is not violating a professional standard by asking, because the patient is not bound by the professional standards of medicine. It is the doctor who does something wrong by accepting the invitation.

While some authors have discussed the doctor–patient relationship as a contract or as an exchange relationship between equals, cases like these make the inequality between doctor and patient apparent. (1, 2) In assuming the ethical responsibilities of the profession, the doctor accepts duties that are not binding on others. Doctors take on a fiduciary responsibility to patients to act for their good. Thus, when the vast majority of reasonable physicians acknowledge that a particular kind of treatment can be good for patients (e.g., restoring function, controlling pain, not prolonging the dying process), no physician is justified in withholding it unless there are some overriding features of the particular case that other reasonable physicians could also accept as justifying a departure from the norm. Similarly, when the vast majority of reasonable physicians acknowledge that a particular kind of behavior should be forbidden for physicians within the professional practice, no physician is justified in engaging in that behavior unless there are some overriding features of the particular case that other reasonable physicians could also accept as justifying a departure from the norm in such a situation. While individuals who are not bound by the professional responsibilities of physicians may be free to offer and accept sexual invitations, within the confines of their professional relationships with patients, physicians do not have that moral liberty. The opportunity for a brief experience of pleasure cannot conceivably count as an adequate justification for breaching the standard that protects physician trustworthiness.

The resident who is asked by his patient, "Well, do you want to see me again?" appears to recognize the bounds of professional responsibility. As attractive as the patient may be and as much as he may want to see more of her or see her again, the importance of medical practitioners maintaining a disinterested sexual stance toward patients makes crossing the line of sexual disinterest unacceptable. Regardless of the patient's pleasure in her doctor's regard or her genuine interest in developing a fuller relationship, it should be out of the question.

In the course of treatment, a physician learns a great deal about the patient, particularly in long-term relationships, in the treatment of chronic illness, and in psychiatry. It is easy to imagine how a physician's insight into an admirable patient, coupled with a physician's proper concern for the patient's good, could grow and develop into something more than the special fondness for a favorite patient. Yet, at the same time, very little about the physician is, or should be, revealed to the patient during the course of treatment. So, a patient's interest in her doctor is more likely to be a manifestation of projection and fantasy, an understandable reflection of the caring attention from a genuinely concerned paternal figure. To respond appropriately to sexual interest, a physician must first be alert to the possibility of such interest from either party so that he can identify what is happening. Physician interest in a patient must be addressed with an unclouded understanding of the importance of professional sexual disinterest. Patient interest in a physician must be addressed with empathic understanding and a clear vision of the importance of maintaining this professional boundary.

Notes

1 Emanuel EJ, Emanuel LL. Four models of the physician–patient relationship. *JAMA* 1992;267(16):2221–6.
2 Veatch R. Models for ethical medicine in a revolutionary age. *Hastings Cent Rep* 1972;2(2):5–7.

10

Losing empathy

CASE

"Patients I don't like"

Patients I don't like fall into two categories: those who are rude, offensive and I wouldn't like them under any circumstances, and those who behave in a way that makes it difficult for me to do my job – they are noncompliant, don't tell me when they are taking alternative therapies that may have a bearing on the treatment program, etc. I find that I give these patients less energy, less time and their care necessarily suffers. When I expressed these feelings to my chief he came down very hard on me and said that physicians owe all patients equally, but I find it is only human nature to make distinctions.

CASE

"Why should I invest in these patients?"

I have very strong feelings about patients who engage in self-destructive behaviors, e.g., obesity, smoking, drug abuse, etc. I tell them the risk factors; but for the most part they won't change their behavior. They respond with giggles or a look that says, "So what?" I keep my involvement with these patients to a minimum. I don't need to bang my head against a wall since they're not banging their heads. Just because I'm a resident why should I invest more in these patients than they are willing to invest in themselves?

CASE

"A nurse said I should be more empathetic"

I was an anesthesiology resident in a small rural hospital when a patient was admitted with a gun shot wound after engaging in a shoot-out with the local police. As a member of a violent militia group, he had come to town in a car filled with false identification and automatic weapons for the purpose of furthering antigovernment activities. Although personable and neat in appearance (contrary to what one might expect), I was fully aware while we talked that he was a man who would kill anyone who stood in his way. Accordingly, I asked him the questions I needed in order to treat him, but I did so without enthusiasm and in a monotone voice. Later, a nurse criticized me and said I should have been more empathetic. I told her "Just because an evil person is in the hospital, he does not deserve considerations he denies others." I wouldn't compromise such a patient's care, but at the same time I do not feel obligated to extend myself personally.

CASE

"Where were the third year students?"

I was a third year medical student and had just started surgery. It was during the first days and I didn't know anything. I was seeing patients with a surgical resident when he said, regarding a patient, "Change her IV fluids to D51/2 normal." I opened the book to charts and wrote the date and time followed by "Change her IV fluids to D51/2 normal." Later, after seeing the notation, that same surgical resident shouted a stream of insults and obscenities, ending with "You are worthless. This is English and we start with a subject." He scratched out my statement and wrote in its place, "IV Fluids: change to D51/2 normal." I was humiliated but thought to myself "Isn't IV Fluids a directed object, and isn't the subject understood as 'you'?" I was very confused as to what I was supposed to be learning, medicine or grammar?

On another occasion we were rounding on a patient and I was trying to figure out where to find her information. I went to the Cardex that records the medications that are to be delivered. The resident had written that the patient was to be given her first dose of digoxin. So, I said "I think the patient got her first dose of digoxin." He angrily demanded, "Show me where you got this!" I showed him the Cardex, and it turned out the patient had not in fact been given her prescribed dose. Again, he screamed out, "You make sure when you tell me something it is the truth or you keep your mouth shut!"

There were many more instances of this particular surgical resident verbally abusing my classmates, and he made our surgical rotation a nightmare. One night when he left the hospital and was walking to his car, he was mugged and brought into the Emergency Department. He was not so badly hurt that the attending couldn't joke, "Where were the third year students?" as if we might be responsible. But it made me think very seriously about how I would feel if I were faced with treating someone I actively disliked. Could I, in all honesty, be as good a physician to them as I would be to someone else? If not, what should I do?

CASE

"I hope this patient dies"

I was a sleep-deprived resident in the intensive care unit when I found myself thinking one night, "I hope this patient dies so I can get some sleep." I was shocked and very much ashamed at what had gone through my head. I always pictured myself as compassionate and someone who cared deeply about patients. That incident has caused me to seriously question whether I am the kind of person who should be a doctor.

COMMENTARY

Richard Martinez

For many health care professionals, some of the most difficult patients are those who are angry, abusive, "noncompliant," and/or self-destructive patients. In the vignettes above, we see dramatic clashes between the values of the health care professionals and the patients under their care. All of these clashes have important emotional elements, while each illustrates important ethical aspects about the patient–physician relationship. From this set of vignettes, we can observe how the determination of what is ethical is tightly joined to the emotional element for many health care professionals, especially when the health care professional has firm ideas about what are in the best interests of his or her patients. The angry or abusive patient presents a difficult challenge to many health care professionals. Few health care professionals are adequately trained in understanding or managing such behavior. Patients who participate in behaviors that are counterproductive to the pursuit of good health commonly frustrate health care professionals. All of these cases illustrate ethical dilemmas where empathy is lost or compromised. Each of these cases illustrates the dilemma for the health care professional when one's emotional responses toward patients precipitates estrangement from one's ethical and moral ideals. Often, such an experience is most disconcerting for many health care professionals. In each case, the health care professional is challenged to maintain the physician's duty to compassionate and concerned care for all patients, while presented with situations that arouse strong emotional reactions that undermine this responsibility.

In the first case, a health professional openly discloses his dislike of difficult, "noncompliant" and even dishonest patients. In the second vignette, a resident makes it clear that she distances herself from "self-destructive" patients, those patients who she judges are engaged in behaviors that are destructive to health, and undermining her medical care. In the third vignette, a resident is rebuffed by a nurse for not being "more empathetic" toward a patient engaged in criminal activity, a patient who the resident judges to be "evil." In the fourth vignette in this series, another layer of complexity is introduced to the theme of empathy, as we hear a medical student describe a resident who is abusive toward the medical student, causing the medical student to question his own capacity to be empathic when he will someday face a difficult patient. Lastly, a "sleep-deprived" resident describes his secret wish for a patient to die so he can sleep. He confesses this with shame.

When human beings are sick, injured, and frightened, they express their fear and vulnerability in many ways. For some, compliance with authority is a natural strategy in order to get needed help, and avoid further helplessness or injury. Such patients are often considered "compliant" by health care professionals. For some health care professionals, these are ideal patients since they present no challenge to professional authority. On the other end of the spectrum are some of the patients described in the above vignettes. Difficult or "noncompliant" patients can challenge our psychological and moral limits. In order to face this challenge, a few considerations about the struggle with difficult and abusive patients are in order.

First, it is not uncommon for the very professional who selected medicine as a profession for good and laudable reasons, to confront unfamiliar and even distasteful aspects of herself through the process of becoming a physician. As an educator for 15 years, I have been impressed with the many decent, smart, and compassionate individuals who choose medicine as a profession. Likewise, I've watched many students become angry, disillusioned, or emotionally distant and self-protective as they move through the medical education process. Certainly, the difficulty of the work and the constant exposure to other human beings in painful and at times tragic circumstances contribute to such developments. In addition, the medical education environment and the acculturation process by which professional identity is formed contribute to these problems. Acknowledging mistakes, discussing self-doubt and uncertainty with mentors and colleagues, sharing the sorrow and joy of what is witnessed in medical experience; such activities are not encouraged and in certain institutions, discouraged. The case of the abusive resident and medical student rings true for many. If we are to be consistent with our patients, then we must be consistent and fair with each other in the process of learning and caring for patients. However, even with changes in medical education and the professional acculturation process, the discrepancies between how one aspires to ideal professionalism with all patients and the reality of human limits – including the dislike and disdain for some patients – are unlikely to disappear.

The ethical issues raised by these cases can be divided into two main areas. First, central to the ethical tradition of Western medical practice is the belief and practice that all human beings possess intrinsic and equal value. This then creates obligations and responsibilities for all health care professionals to approach and engage all patients with respect for this intrinsic and equal value. In addition, professional codes and laws obligate health care professionals to resist discrimination and other forms of practice that compromise fair and respectful treatment of our patients. In the liberal philosophical tradition of Western society, this fundamental principle has been transformed into the language of "patient's rights." This does not mean that health care professionals are obligated to endure abuse, but that as health care professionals, we must move beyond the emotional obstacles that would have us behave in a disrespectful or abusive manner toward our patients. Does this mean that health care professionals must provide medical treatment in cases where one disagrees with the patient's judgment of what is best for him or her? Must a professional perform treatments that one is morally opposed to? Or treat people who engage in morally questionable behaviors? This then brings us to the second set of ethical issues.

The AMA, as well as certain state and federal laws, have created requirements so that patients are not abandoned. In certain situations, such as emergencies, health care professionals are obligated to provide care. In the nonemergency situation, the AMA, as well as other professional organizations and regulatory boards, have provided patient "nonabandonment" guidelines and requirements consistent with responsible professional behavior. In nonemergency situations, where moral conflict and other conflict interferes with the professional in providing proper care, health care professionals are required to transfer the patient's care. Such processes support health care professionals' rights to determine the nature of their practices, as long as discriminatory and prejudicial motives are not determining those decisions. Most of the patient "nonabandonment" guidelines are intended to guarantee that all patients will have options for treatment.

In the cases above, a piece of advice from one of my supervisors from 15 years ago comes to mind. "Act responsibly, not responsible for," this wise and older psychoanalyst told me when I was struggling with my own dilemma of evaluating intoxicated patients in the emergency room. In the cases of the abusive and "self-destructive" patients, this advice has value. As a health care

professional, we are responsible to act "responsibly," which means respectful of all patients, but we are not "responsible for" all of their life decisions and choices. Sometimes, the grand sense of responsibility interferes with the more realistic possibility of how we can and can't influence the lives of others. As professionals, we cannot and should not assume the responsibility of reforming and changing all the "bad" behaviors of our patients. Equally important, this judgment about what is "self-destructive behavior" is rooted in our own values and even biases of medical science, in selective concepts about health and illness that frame much of our training and medical practice. Some humility can go a long way in helping us see through the eyes of our patients, even when we are concerned about their behaviors. With the abusive patient and with the abusive resident, it is necessary to set firm limits. Health care professionals are not obligated to unconditionally absorb abuse from patients or supervisors. Dignified and appropriate confrontation with such abuse is in order. However, there are patients who can only ask for help by rejecting help. It takes an unusual professional to hang around and work with such individuals. Recognizing one's limits in this domain is important.

In the case of the resident who acknowledges his wish for his patient to die, it is important to recognize the huge difference between a fantasy and an act from a moral perspective. To have wishes for a patient's death is not the same as then translating this wish into action by neglecting a patient or providing substandard care. As a psychiatrist and psychotherapist, I hear often of the human longing to be free from burdens, even when those burdens are people and things usually cherished. Empathy, like compassion, involves the ability to see the world through the eyes of the other. Often, our work in medicine presents us with obstacles to such sight. The patient can become the obstacle, challenging our values and perspectives. The "evil" patient, as all patients, requires attention and fair treatment. A core value of professionalism is the obligation to transcend the personal and particular, and serve the needs of others. In law, the right to a vigorous defense, independent of guilt or innocence, and separate from the "feelings" of the lawyer about his or her client, is central to the ultimate moral integrity of the profession. Likewise, in medicine, if we allow our own views to influence each medical decision, determine who is deserving or not deserving of the best we have to offer, then we are on slippery and dangerous moral ground. Humility and empathy are practices, and like most practices that we wish to do well, they require hard work and discipline. Professional excellences in attitudes and behaviors must be worked toward, especially when the obstacles to such excellences are large.

COMMENTARY

Marli Huijer

The case vignettes present familiar situations. All interns or residents know patients to whom they are glad to say good-bye. It is difficult to feel empathy for patients who claim unnecessary interventions, whose manner is offensive, or who use the physician to "doctor up" or reverse the consequences of their unhealthy life styles without being prepared to make the necessary changes in their behavior. The basic ethical question raised by these cases is: As physicians, what do we owe patients in terms of empathy?

In the medical curriculum students are taught, as much as possible, to treat patients equally. Also, the law dictates that physicians must meet the standard of due care in all cases. The cases presented here demonstrate how these general rules about treating all patients alike are put under pressure when dealing with difficult patients.

Students know that ideally they should treat all

patients compassionately but sometimes their feelings intervene and they act differently. It is too simplistic to simply condemn the students' and residents' behavior. General laws, rules, and codes, although important moral guidelines, do not do justice to the particularity of each case. Making distinctions and connecting particularities to general knowledge and codes is an important medical skill. In both medicine and ethics, future physicians must learn to adjust to the specific patient, his or her diseases and behavior, and guard against allowing their own reactions to various types of individuals to interfer with the general rule that all patients should be treated alike.

The dilemmas in the presented cases can be perceived as conflicts involving:

1 The everyday reality in which students and trainees have many understandable reasons for losing empathy for some patients.
2 General medical, legal, and ethical codes stressing the patient's right to equal treatment.
3 A general agreement in medicine on the value of professional empathy as well as distance.

The dilemmas sketched by the cases in this section do come up rather frequently in discussions with Dutch students. Dealing with noncompliant, aggressive, neglectful, and denying patients are themes students regularly select to include in their clinical ethics education. They feel frustrated by these kinds of patients because they have learned to value both health and their relationship with patients. Having empathy for patients who move in the opposite direction on both counts is not easy to achieve.

Why do interns or residents lose their empathy?

In the cases presented, several reasons can be identified: (1) The first set of reasons is patient-centered: patients are rude, offensive, noncompliant, engage in self-destructive behaviors, are violent and dangerous, or have previously humiliated the trainee; (2) The second set of reasons is physician-centered: the intern or resident does not like certain patients, feels threatened, or is too tired to maintain empathy for patients.

The patients presented in these cases can be divided into subtypes: (a) patients who behave or behaved badly and/or dangerously, and (b) the noncompliant or self-destructive patients. The first group offend the expectations people have of normal social interaction. In public space, we expect people to behave according to etiquette. In business, people who act in an aggressive or offensive manner toward clients are fired; and similarly, clients who transgress expected standards can no longer count on the services of the provider. In medicine, patients are also expected to behave decently. Physicians set limits on aggression or rude behavior for their own and their patients' safety. Violent patients are usually not welcomed with open arms in the clinic hospital! Tolerance is limited by the serious tasks at hand.

Patients who engage in self-destructive behavior or who are noncompliant do not fall into the same category. They may not have bad manners. Students lose their empathy with these patients because they believe "that patient behavior makes it difficult for me to do my job." The aim of health care is to heal people and to prevent disease. Patients who are noncompliant, who do not provide the physician with the necessary information, who do not tell the physician when they are taking alternative therapies, or who are not at all inclined to change their unhealthy behaviors, thwart the physicians' policy. This often frustrates the intern's or resident's intentions. As in the case presented, a natural question arises: "Just because I am a resident, why should I invest more in those patients than they are willing to invest in themselves?"

The intern or resident, in turn, may have their own reasons for losing empathy. Some students do not have any empathy for patients who engage in self-destructive behaviors. The basis for their engagement of these patients is diminished when, as described in one of the cases, patients respond with giggles or a look that says "So

what?" when provided information on risk factors. Others might have a more balanced judgment about these patient reactions. The source of these different responses can be traced to the views, experiences, and characteristics of the different trainees. Core beliefs, personal philosophy, family influences, gender issues, and sociocultural influences clearly shape interns' and residents' behaviors when interacting with patients. (1)

Another physician-related reason for losing empathy is the interns' or residents' feeling of being threatened. In the case of the patient who was engaged in a shoot-out with the local police, the resident did not lose his or her empathy because the patient was aggressive – contrary to what the physician expected, he was personable and neat in appearance – but because the resident became aware as they talked that the patient was a man who would kill anyone who stood in his way. Although the resident did not want to compromise the patient's care, he or she lacked the ability or the inclination to treat the offender with enthusiasm. Feeling threatened can prompt a decision to keep some distance from patients, and not to "extend myself personally." This is to be expected and should not lead to opprobrium unless it affects the level of care.

The last reason illustrated in the cases is the physician's extreme fatigue. In this case, the resident's physical and mental limits were clearly exceeded. His or her capacity to care empathetically about patients was completely depleted. On the one hand, the circumstances under which the resident had to work are to blame. On the other, the mental and physical condition of the resident is a factor. It is hard to imagine a way to reform the workload that would realistically address this problem, but it surely needs attention.

Ethical, legal, and medical rules

Patients' behavior, circumstances and the condition of the student or resident are possible reasons for losing empathy. Identifying them as possible reasons does not mean that they therefore are good reasons. In general, ethical, legal, and medical guidelines contradict any idea that there could be good reasons to treat some patients less well than others. Assuming the responsibility of a physician requires resisting the inevitable temptations to lose patience and to forgo compassion and empathy.

In medical ethics, the rule of nondiscrimination is formulated as the ethical obligation of beneficence and nonmaleficence. The physician is obligated to contribute to the welfare of all patients and not to inflict harm on them intentionally. This ethical obligation is supported by law. In the Netherlands, for example, constitutional law as well as the law on informed consent dictates that all patients have an equal right to treatment and care.

Medical curricula often follow the same approach. The obligation to meet the standard of due care implies the double task of diagnosing and treating the disease, and of caring for the patients' experiences of illness. The rule of equality not only implies providing all patients equal access to diagnostic assessment and treatment, but also to create in all cases an optimal balance between empathy and professional distance, between emotional involvement and reasonable thinking. (2)

In medical practice, these general rules are passed on to medical students by way of example and correction. Whenever they trespass the limits of professional empathy or distance, that is, whenever they are too close or reserved in relating to the patient, the rest of the team corrects them, as noted in the cases: "When I expressed these feelings to my chief he came down very hard on me and said that physicians owe all patients equally." "A nurse criticized me and said I should have been more empathetic." After some time, the professional rules on empathy and distance, like the adequacy rules on diagnosis and treatment, become internalized. Students no longer need outsiders to correct their behavior, they become their own critic. Again an illustra-

tion from one of the cases: "I always pictured myself as compassionate and someone who cared deeply about patients. That incident has caused me to seriously question whether I am the kind of person who should be a doctor."

The general rules and codes about equal treatment do not permit treating patients differently, let alone losing empathy. When we stick to general rules, we have to conclude that losing empathy is never allowed. Reality forces us, however, to be aware of the fact that "it is only human nature to make some distinctions."

Emphasizing the general rule of equality, and forcing students to conform to this rule, bears the risk of smoothing over the fact that physicians actually do make distinctions among patients. Even if they are absolutely convinced that the general rule of equality has to receive the highest priority, students and physicians are not always able to put this idea into practice: controlling one's body language is a hard task, especially if caused by feelings of disgust or insurmountable fear.

Being aware of the distinctions one feels or makes, and discussing them with others, is a helpful means to find ways to deal with these patients. Instead of ignoring distinctions between patients, students should learn to value the patient's pleasant or difficult particularities and to connect them to the general rule of equality. The greater the variety of patients, the greater become the students' skills.

Discussing thoughts and feelings about specific patients can help physicians understand why they treat patients differently, and what they can do to change this situation. Expressing empathy and listening to patients are indeed thought of as "personality traits," but these traits can be changed through education. (3) As stated by De Monchy et al.:

While most physicians may find certain patients "difficult," some physicians, because of personal biases, may find some patients particularly difficult (e.g., alcoholics, obese people, dependent patients, hypochondriacs).

These biases may prevent some physicians from acquiring the skills to effectively treat these patients. By discussing their thoughts and feelings about specific patients, physicians can help each other understand their personal biases, relieve some of the emotional pain that may be associated with these biases, and help each other gain new perspectives . . . (4)

Empathy and compassion need to be taught, not by exclusively referring to general rules, but by discussing the reasons *why* one loses empathy and subsequently how this particular case can be adjusted under the general rule of equality. How can the student or trainee use the feelings, or lack thereof, to become a better doctor?

In this perspective the interns and residents who selected the cases are not rude and insensitive persons but rather sensitive persons who struggle with the fact that they do not measure up to the idea of a physician who treats all patients alike. By presenting their dilemmas they open up the possibility of talking about this important subject, and developing new maturity as professionals.

Notes

1 Novack DH, Suchman AL, Clark W, Epstein RM, Najberg E. Calibrating the physician: Personal awareness and effective patient care. *JAMA* 1997;278:502–9.
2 Suchman AL, Markakis K, Beckman HB, Frankel R. A model of empathic communication in the medical interview. *JAMA* 1997;277:678–82.
3 Smith RC, Lyles JS, Mettler J, Stofelmayr BE, Van Egeren LF, Marshall AA, et al. The effectiveness of intensive training for residents in interviewing: A randomized controlled study. *Ann Intern Med* 1998;128:118–26.
4 de Monchy C, Richardson R, Brown RA, Harden RM. Measuring attitudes of doctors: the doctor–patient (DP) rating. *Med Educ* 1988;22:231–9.

COMMENTARY

David Bennahum

The *suspension of judgment* is an ancient principle of medicine, honored more in the breach than in reality, yet it confronts physicians more often than they are likely to admit. There are patients that one doesn't like or who offend in one way or another. It can be difficult to be empathic with an agitated, disheveled, unwashed, ill-smelling street person who is roiling in delirium tremens on an emergency room gurney. There are also the endlessly demanding patients who come to the physician with lists of questions, with always another question just as the session seems over.

There is obviously a transition as physicians age. The young student is more likely to experience the offensive patient, but patients are less likely to offend an experienced physician whom they may trust. Overall, however, I think that what matters most is how a student or young physician presents herself. If the message is clear, that one is there to listen, to try to explain and to help, the vast majority of patients will entrust their care to you. Even the most difficult and untrusting patient will usually respond to competence and compassion and if they don't it is often due to the physician's failure to "hear" and communicate.

If a patient will not cooperate or agree with the physician's recommendation, more than a question of empathy may be at stake. Committed to a positivist philosophy, most physicians and many lay persons believe that science can improve their lives. The very idea of Progress, articulated by Sir Francis Bacon in the seventeenth century, has been the dominant philosophy of the Western world for almost four centuries. When a patient doesn't "go along" or is "noncompliant" he challenges the Cartesian logic and implicit meliorism of the idea that science, especially medical science, can make the world progressively better.

It is hard to like a patient who challenges not only us, but also our fundamental belief system.

Patients who reject a physician's instructions are labeled as noncompliant in current parlance, but we need to listen to that refusal. Empathy is not only an ability to feel another's pain and suffering, but an awareness as well of the whole person, her ideas, feelings, attributes, and prejudices and a belief that we can learn from our patients.

Physicians have a terrible fear of being in error. Training is rigorous and exhausting. Information is detailed and very technical. Not to have checked a patient before morning rounds or not to know the result of a specific laboratory test when asked or the mechanism of action of a particular medication or the pathophysiology of a rare disease is to experience shame and humiliation. I can recall when one of my residents called me over during my internship. Having been trained abroad it took me about a year to catch up to my more clinically trained peers. In the privacy of an empty wardroom she said, "Do you know what is wrong with you?" "No," I answered. "You are just no good. Just no good." I couldn't answer. In fact I think that I laughed. It was so preposterous, so cruel and egregious that I was taken aback, as I think, paradoxically, she was as well; but I had to live with that statement for ever after. It has, however, stood me in great good stead as I could never get worse, would only improve and had many an opportunity to laugh with troubled students when I would tell them what she had said to me. It was a gift. The gift of failure, of knowing what it feels like to be humiliated and shamed. Maimonides said that we can learn from everyone, teachers and patients and even unpleasant and officious caregivers. So especially can we learn from our failures.

11

The limits of compassion

CASE

"Does being a doctor include being a social worker?"

As a fourth year medical student I was assigned to care for an elderly Hispanic woman with frequent hospital admissions. As I got to know her it became clear that there were a number of nonstrictly medical issues that were having a decided impact on her health. She lived alone in a small unheated inner city apartment, accessible only by a long flight of steps. Because of her severe arthritis she seldom went outside. Her decreased mobility made it difficult for her to shop properly; she favored an ethnic grocery store at some distance from her neighborhood. The resulting poor nutrition contributed to her anemia. My patient was an extremely private woman who had few personal contacts and valued her solitary life. She confided in me that her greatest fear was losing her independence.

What are the boundaries of the doctor's professional responsibilities in such a situation? Does being a doctor also involve being a social worker? Was it part of my duties to be concerned about the separate, but not medically unrelated, issues of food and housing for this patient?

CASE

"I took a bus to his house on my day off"

I was a third year medical student and one of my patients was a frail, elderly Chinese man who lived alone at the other end of town from the hospital. At the time of discharge he was given an extensive regime of medications important to his recovery and health maintenance. What the medications were, how and when they were to be taken was explained. He asked no questions and I was very worried he did not fully understand the schedule. I grew up speaking Chinese and I called him on the phone several times to ask how he was doing with his medications but he seemed vague and unsure. Finally, when I had an afternoon off, I took a bus across town to where he lived. I spent time with him going over the medications in detail. I did this several times until I felt sure he understood and could continue on his own. When my supervisors heard of my personal concern for this patient they said my actions were unwarranted and inappropriate.

CASE

"How do I suffer with her?"

Ms. P was a 36-year-old woman with chronic pelvic pain. I have seen her for the past two-and-a-half years, and she is still having pain. She came to me with high hopes. She was referred to me by a graduating resident who had high praises for me. To prove myself worthy, I gave her my pager number and told her to "Page me if you need me." "We'll lick this pain," I assured her. After two laparoscopies, a colonoscopy, a cystoscopy, and multiple other tests and studies failed to turn up an apparent cause of her pain, I was at a loss. I had prescribed narcotic medications, muscle relaxants, antidepressants, physical therapy, and multiple other medications and therapeutic modalities, and nothing worked. Some of my colleagues thought that it was all in her head, and I told them that the head is connected to the body. I referred her for psychiatric counseling but she refused to go. I believe that her pain is real. Her life is ravaged and engulfed by her pain. She tries to work, but often misses work because she is laid up in bed with pain. She is not drug-seeking because nothing really works for her. She pages me every so often when her pain exacerbates, and there is little I can offer her. Sometimes I am afraid to answer her pages simply because I do not know what to tell her. Her pain has licked me.

Ask any resident which kind of patient is most difficult to show compassion, and the response is invariably the patient with chronic pain. The case of Ms. P exemplifies my difficulty. I am at my wits' end, and there is still no fix for her pain. Her life is being ravaged by pain, and I stand helpless. How do I suffer with her?

CASE

"You don't help your patients by crying with them"

I was a resident in pediatrics and followed the course of an infant born with multiple internal abnormalities. Throughout an unsuccessful course of surgeries the mother stayed by her daughter's bed. She even slept in the hospital to be near her child. From the beginning there was very little hope the infant would ever leave the hospital, but no matter how bleak the news, the mother continued to search for options that would save her child. We spent many hours together discussing her daughter's situation and the struggles of this mother and child affected me very deeply. When all attempts failed and the child finally died, I cried along with the mother. I didn't try to hide my feelings from her. My supervisor admonished me later and said that I would have to learn better control because, "You don't help your patients by crying with them."

COMMENTARY

Richard Martinez

In this series of vignettes, health care professionals describe personal and unique experiences of compassion toward their patients. Simultaneously, these health care professionals then pose questions about limits and obstacles that each individual professional confronts in the expression of compassion. Several of the vignettes illustrate the concept of health care professional as patient advocate, and what patient advocacy entails. In two of the cases, the hindrance to full expression of professional compassion appears in the form of critical supervisors. These supervisors challenge their trainees' concepts of advocacy and compassion, and create confusion and uncertainty. In one case, a medical student is criticized for visiting a patient on an afternoon off and at the patient's home. In another vignette, a supervisor criticizes a pediatric resident for crying with the mother of a deceased child. In the first vignette, a medical student is faced with aspects of patient care that are not directly "medical." She asks if being a doctor means being a social worker. In the fourth vignette, we read of a conscientious resident trying to take care of a patient with chronic pain, where many of the medical interventions have not relieved the patient's suffering. She asks, how does she suffer with her patient?

Compassion is a complex emotion. To understand the experience, the Latin derivation of "suffering with" another provides some help. Philosopher Lawrence Blum describes four conditions of the emotional attitude called compassion. (1) First, one must be able to "imaginatively dwell" on the situation of another. Second, the compassionate person takes an active regard for the good of another. Third, the person who is the recipient of compassion is seen and thought of as a fellow human being. Last, certain intense responses or actions are necessitated by the awareness of the first three conditions. In other words, in situations that are not hopeless, true compassion, unlike empathy or sympathy, requires that the compassionate person act or intervene in order to reduce or remedy suffering.

Unique to Blum's concept of compassion, in the case of the hopeless or irremediable situation, where some type of beneficent action is not possible, the attitude of compassion is a worthy good in and of itself. As an example of the latter condition, the resident who is caring for the patient with chronic pain has acted in every imaginable way to remedy the patient's suffering. She is no longer able to find beneficent acts that might remedy the patient's experience of pain. Now with no other obvious options, from Blum's perspective, there continues to be value in compassionately understanding the patient's continued suffering, acknowledging this suffering, and accepting the limitations of medical solutions. Many health care professionals feel useful and obtain meaning in their work through their ability to apply knowledge and skills that relieve suffering. Commonly, when faced with limitations in knowledge and skills, health care professionals feel they have nothing further to offer. For Blum, in such situations, the continued attitude of compassion has moral value. Likewise, the social and behavioral sciences argue that there is clinical value in such a stance as well. While limiting the patient's phone calls and expectations might be necessary and helpful, to avoid and abandon the patient would be clinically and morally unacceptable.

Similarly, in the other vignettes, we see evidence of Blum's criteria in the compassionate attitudes and actions of the medical students and residents. A resident understands, or "imaginatively dwells" on the experience of a mother who loses her child. A medical student worries about an elderly Chinese patient's understanding of his prescribed medications and makes the extraordinary effort of visiting the patient's home on several occasions until it is clear that the patient understands the proper dispensing of his medications. In this case, the understanding of the patient's condition is joined to an act that some might define as going beyond the call of

duty, a supererogatory act. In another vignette, a fourth year medical student is concerned about the "not medically unrelated" aspects of caring for an elderly Hispanic woman. The medical student asks whether these psychosocial concerns fall within the responsibilities of doctoring. Since compassion, by Blum's definition, requires a beneficent intervention when possible, the medical student articulates confusion over where to limit her patient advocacy. Compassion begins in empathy, which naturally leads to the desire to advocate for one's patient. But how do we define duties that arise from a compassionate ideal? When are professionals justified in setting limits? And when are health care professionals free to choose to act beyond the call of duty? If professional ideals are individually determined – that is, each health care professional must define his or her own aspiration toward excellence in attitudes and behaviors – then how do professionals justify limits, and distinguish between required professional duties and optional professional ideals? As with other service professions such as police and fire prevention work, health care professionals have obligations to certain self-effacement acts and even risk-taking while in the role of their profession. However, as with these other professions, there are limits, even if those limits on self-effacement and risk-taking behaviors are rarely clear.

Supererogation is a type of moral ideal that pertains to actions. In moral philosophy, supererogation defines those acts that are beyond what is owed, doing more than is required by the community morality. For example, in our society, to give money to a homeless panhandler is not a community moral requirement. However, for some members of our society, it is difficult to walk past such a person without giving support. To qualify as a supererogatory act, commonly, four conditions must be met. First, a supererogatory act is optional. It is not required by the values of a community or, in the case of medicine, required by the profession. Nor is it prohibited. Second, the supererogatory behavior exceeds standards of expectation. This means going beyond the call of duty. Third, supererogatory acts are undertaken specifically for the benefit of others. Lastly, these acts are intrinsically good and praiseworthy.

Of course, like any simple model, there are limitations in its usefulness in the real world of patient care and setting limits. For many, the first condition is never clear. What is morally optional for one person can be clearly obligatory for another. The medical student visits a patient's home to instruct the patient on his medications. For some, apparently the supervisor in this case, this is an optional and extraordinary act. However, the vignette implies that for this student, a failure to visit the elderly Chinese patient would be a failure of duty, a failure to fulfill a robust notion of professionalism and doctoring. Likewise, the resident who cries with the mother of the deceased child, is joining the mother's suffering. The sharing of tears becomes an act of compassion. Once again, we are presented with a supervisor who not only sees such behavior as optional, but challenges the professionalism of such behavior. It is unlikely that this resident would describe her tears as a supererogatory act. Most likely, she would say that she did what came naturally, sharing tears in the face of loss and tragedy. In this case, the supervisor's response is worrisome. Perhaps it speaks more of his limitations than any serious judgment about the clinical appropriateness of sharing tears with our patients.

The divider that separates obligatory advocacy for our patients from optional and ideal professional actions is broad and variable. Understanding the differences between minimum duties of our profession and patient advocacy that is beyond the call of duty are important. Compassion, along with other professional virtues, is an important element in providing good patient care, and usually guides us in defining our individual professional goals. As a teacher and psychotherapist, I have rarely seen reason to discourage other health care professionals in their cultivation of this quality. While learning to set limits on one's self and one's patients is an important component of professional development, remaining humanly connected to our patients and our work is vital. Each health care professional must find the balance between the personal and the professional, the private and the public. The fourth year medical student asks if being a doctor involves being a social worker. The answer is yes and no. Each health care professional must define the limits of his or her compassion, while applying the minimum expectations of his or her profession and of society in the caring and advocating for patients.

Note

1 Blum L. Compassion. In *Explaining Emotions*, ed. AO Rorty. University of California Press, Berkeley, 1980, pp.507–17.

COMMENTARY

Guy Micco

All the vignettes in this section question, in some fashion, the nature of the doctor–patient relationship. In the first story the question is plainly put: "Does being a doctor also involve being a social worker?" For some physicians this may rarely be a concern; for others, say those with practices in a county health clinic, it is a daily encounter. Regardless of how often it comes up in their practices, physicians all know the "revolving door" problem of patients who come into the hospital with medical and social problems, leave with the latter, and return again with both. The obvious solution to such patient "recidivism" is to help resolve *both* the medical and the social issues; thus, being a doctor requires at least a working knowledge of when and how to call for the help of a social worker (and others). Of course, resolving social issues is notoriously difficult. In Margaret Laurence's fine short story, *The Loons*, a small-town physician tries to help cure a local girl of her tuberculosis by all means available. He realizes that her social strife and deprivation is a large part of her illness and, to ameliorate this, he invites her to his family's summer vacation at the lake. But, this girl is bound to die; in the end there is nothing the good doctor can do to prevent what must be called a "social death." (1)

We cannot easily "treat" poverty, much less social isolation and loneliness. But we can understand, appreciate, acknowledge, and attempt to alleviate these conditions. *Sometimes* this means the physician – if she is able – must be a social worker or a therapist, or even a friend to her patient. When is "sometimes" necessary, when is it supererogatory, indeed, when is it inappropriate? The answer requires the best judgment and discretion of each physician, balancing how much to give his patients, his family, his community, and himself. The third year medical student who (in "I took a bus to his house on my day off") helped her "frail, elderly Chinese" patient after discharge from the hospital did the "right thing." The fact that what she did could have been done by a visiting nurse who spoke Chinese is here beside the point – the patient needed help, the student was well situated to help and did so. Bravo. A physician cannot be all to everyone – and social workers, therapists, and clergy are often, thankfully, available to help – but a physician may be "the most to as many" as she has knowledge, energy, and time to help.

My answer to the question posed in the title of this essay – "Are there limits to compassion?" – would seem to be "no," except for those limits imposed on us by time and other obligations. Yet we physicians have been brought up with the notion that too much "feeling with" our patients is dangerous – for them and for us. The crux of the argument goes like this: Physicians require equanimity (which includes, necessarily, "detachment") to be able to diagnose and treat patients optimally. Emotional attachment, thought (erroneously) to be an obligatory concomitant of compassion, can cloud the physician's judgment,

impair her hand – thus endangering the patient. As well, it may lead to a grief that will be harmful to the physician himself. Osler is credited with giving this counsel to the modern physician. In "Aequanimitas," his parting speech at the University of Pennsylvania in 1889, he says:

Imperturbability [Osler's translation of "aequanimitas"] means coolness and presence of mind under all circumstances, calmness amid storm, clearness of judgment in moments of grave peril, immobility, impassiveness, or, to use an old and expressive word, *phlegm* . . . the physician who has the misfortune to be without it, who betrays indecision and worry, and who shows that he is flustered and flurried in ordinary emergencies, loses rapidly the confidence of his patients . . . Even under the most serious circumstances, the physician or surgeon who allows "his outward action to demonstrate the native act and figure of his heart in complement extern," who shows in his face the slightest alteration, expressive of anxiety or fear, has not his medullary centres under the highest control, and is liable to disaster at any moment. (2)

Is Osler saying that the best doctors maintain their sangfroid directly in the face of a patient's suffering? I suspect so; for to be perturbed by that suffering is, perforce, to lose one's judgment. This is the basis of the supervisor's admonishing statement: "You don't help your patients by crying with them." Surely Osler would agree, for such a display would be to allow one's "outward action to demonstrate the native act and figure of ones heart in complement extern." Rachel Remen, in an essay (*Professionals Don't Cry*) in *Kitchen Table Wisdom*, recounts how she, as a pediatric intern, was admonished by her senior resident after she cried with the parents of a child killed in an automobile accident: "These people were counting on our strength . . . and [you] . . . let them down." (3) Remen stopped crying for a long time. Then she recalls, as a senior resident herself, telling a mother and father of her unsuccessful attempts to resuscitate their child. As they cried she stood "strong and silent in [her] white coat." Then the father of the child said to her:

"'I'm sorry, Doctor, I'll get ahold of myself in a

minute." Remen comments: "I remember this man, his face wet with a father's tears, and I think of his apology with shame. Convinced by then that my grief was a useless, self-indulgent waste of time, I had made myself into the sort of a person to whom one could apologize for being in pain."

Remen and others (e.g., Perri Klass in *A Not Entirely Benign Procedure* (4)) describe the pain of being forced not to cry in the presence of patients and families. I suspect this is a not-uncommon problem. In *Joshua Knew,* an emergency room physician describes her experience of having to leave the room of a child who had just died in the arms of his grief-stricken parents. Understandably, she too was grief-stricken; yet, she could not, would not, cry in front of her patient's parents: "I mumbled condolences to the parents and hurried from the room. Walking rapidly down the hall, looking neither right nor left, finally I reached the stairwell. After closing the door behind me, I sat heavily on the concrete steps. A soft wail emanated from some place deep within me. Warm tears began to flow down my cheeks as I wept quietly for Joshua." (5) Is there not something amiss when a physician must go to the stairwell to grieve?

A powerful, fictionalized version of taking compassion to the limit can be found in Susan Onthank Mates' short story *Laundry.* In it she tells the story of a pregnant 40-year-old physician and her care and caring for one particular patient, Salvadore Dantio. Mr. Dantio, Salvadore – exemplifying her not knowing how close to get to her patient, she cannot decide which to call him – is dying of cancer and wants his doctor to tell him whether to have the biopsy being recommended by the specialists. He wants to know what *she* would do. She resists, saying she is not him, and the studies show . . . "And you said please. I felt my breath clot up somewhere in my throat and I looked at your eyes your ferocious eyes and I said Mr. Dantio, Salvadore I would not do it, don't do it don't let them me do it to you no. And I couldn't stop the tears, I kissed you and waddled

out of the room and stood around the corner so your wife couldn't see me and I cried there right in the middle of the hall . . ." (6) Mates has portrayed a compassionate, emotional physician unsure of herself (in large part because of an utter lack of collegial and institutional support), yet "there" for her patient in a way we find appealing and somehow right. And this even though her judgment, as she comes to see, may have been wrong! She was being a "human being" and a physician – isn't this what we all want of our own doctor? Perhaps we would like infallibility, but given its impossibility, we'll take the compassionate doctor with all her human foibles over the Oslerian cool.

Lest I be misunderstood: I do not want to suggest that a good surgeon is one who cries into the wound of a patient whom she discovers to have metastatic cancer. Nor do I think it *always* proper to cry with one's patients. There must be some discernment in these matters within the art of the practice of medicine. In a fine essay to the point, Coulehan (borrowing from Thomas Percival's *Medical Ethics*) suggests that we strive for both compassion (tenderness) *and* calmness (steadiness). He calls for physicians to develop an "emotional resilience," not detachment, "that allows one to experience fully the emotional dynamics of patient care as an essential part of – rather than a detriment to – good medical practice." (7)

The case "How do I suffer with her?" brings up a different issue. Here, a young resident physician is referred a patient with chronic pain. The prior resident had "high praises" for him, and to prove himself "worthy," he gives his patient his beeper number saying: ". . . page me if you need me" and "We'll lick this pain." Now, two-and-a-half years later, the patient is still suffering and the resident complains: "I am at my wits' end. Sometimes I am afraid to answer her pages simply because I do not know what to tell her. Her pain has licked me . . . Her life is being ravaged by pain, and I stand helpless. How do I suffer with her?" There is not a concern here – as first it may seem – of being *too* available or *overly* compassionate. This is a problem of a young physician trying to prove himself worthy of prior praise and promising too much. The truth is – the doctor's ego notwithstanding – no one knows whether and when the source, much less the cure, of this patient's pain will be found. The physician's promise should not be "we'll lick this pain," but, rather: "I'll stick with you and try my best to help you with your pain." With that assurance, the question of how to "suffer with" the patient falls away, for compassion is not in finding the cure for a patient's illness; rather, it may be found in just what this resident is mistakenly pulling away from: empathic listening. (8) Elaine Scarry in *The Body in Pain* points out that: ". . . for the person in pain, so incontestably and unnegotiably present is it that 'having pain' may come to be thought of as the most vibrant example of what it is to 'have certainty,' while for the other person it is so elusive that 'hearing about pain' may exist as the primary model of what it is 'to have doubt.'" (9) This eloquent statement captures the problem which blocks a compassionate response to patients in chronic pain. But, the resident in this story has that problem licked – he "believe[s] that her pain is real." Compassion may then be found, paradoxically perhaps, in exactly what this resident was doing – "standing helpless" *with* the patient whose "life [was] being ravaged by pain."

Notes

1 Laurence M. *The Loons.*
2 Osler W. "Aequanimitas," in *Aequanimitas and Other Addresses*. P. Blakiston's Son & Co., Philadelphia, 1932, pp.3–11.
3 Remen RN. Professionals Don't Cry. In *Kitchen Table Wisdom: Stories That Heal*. Riverhead Books, New York, 1996, pp.51–4.
4 Klass P. Crying in the hospital. In *A Not Entirely Benign Procedure*, pp. 63–6. A Plume Book, Penguin Books, New York.
5 Clark LR. Joshua Knew. *JAMA*, 1993;270(24):2902.
6 Mates SO. Laundry. In *The Good Doctor*. University of Iowa Press, Iowa City, 1994, pp.9–14.
7 Coulehan J. Emotions in medical practice. *Lit Med* 1995;14(2):222–36.
8 Kleinman A. *The Illness Narratives: Suffering, Healing, and the Human Condition*. Basic Books, New York, 1988.
9 Scarry E. *The Body in Pain*. Oxford University Press, New York, 1985, p.4.

COMMENTARY

Mary B. Mahowald

All of these cases are about boundaries or potential boundaries between physicians in training and patients. In each situation, boundaries may be drawn by different criteria: the limitations of medical expertise, the social needs of patients, and the impact of emotion on delivery of care. As we shall see, these criteria are applicable not only to medical students and residents but also to physicians who have completed their training.

To those who view the goal of medicine as treatment of the whole person, there are no boundaries to the clinician's commitment to address all of the health needs of the patient, including those that are caused by social or personal circumstances. Nonetheless, for clinicians of any age or level of training and experience, addressing all of a patient's health needs in order to care for the whole person is not equivalent to his or her personally fulfilling all of those needs. In fact, addressing all the patient's needs demands recognition of the caregiver's own limitations, whether these be constraints of time or expertise, and willingness to refer the patient to those who have the time or expertise that can make care optimal. Doctors, for example, are not trained in social work, but they may identify circumstances in which the competence of the social worker is pivotal to amelioration of health risks and illness symptoms in people's lives. In such circumstances, the need to refer the patient to a social worker is just as great as the need to ask for a clinical consult on a specific medical problem.

Constraints on treating the whole person by addressing social health-related needs may be greater for specialists and for fully trained clinicians than for medical students because the latter usually have more time and opportunity for discussions with patients about nonmedical, health-related matters. Even then, however, it is imperative that medical students recognize the limitations of their expertise. In the first case, therefore, the answer to the question of whether physicians or physicians in training should be concerned about the separate but not medically unrelated issues of food and housing for the patient is a definite "Yes". The question of what practical interventions their concern should lead to, however, is dependent on the inevitably limited time and expertise of the particular clinician. In most cases, optimal care for these aspects of a patient's health status requires referral to those whose training has specifically prepared them for the task.

Like experts in other fields, physicians and physicians in training often have talents or skills unrelated to medicine, and occasionally these talents or skills are relevant to patient care. The medical student in the second case, for example, was fluent in Chinese and knowledgeable about Chinese culture. This enabled the student to fill an evident gap in caring for the frail, elderly Chinese man who lived alone. Other caregivers had assumed that the man understood his extensive regime of medications and would be able to take them reliably. Through familiarity with Chinese culture and greater sensitivity to the man's body language, the student knew differently. Apparently, he or she assumed correctly that this patient's care would be facilitated by more instruction from someone who understood him better than the other health care workers.

Why would the student's supervisors consider his personal concern for the patient "unwarranted and inappropriate?" Possibly they thought that the student's use of his language facility and cultural awareness was not an expression of medical expertise as such. While that is true, it does not imply that the student's use of his special skill was not, or should not be, utilized in the interest of the patient's health. Possibly the supervisors were concerned that the student's actions were based on emotional rather than professional motives. Nowadays, however, it is widely recognized that an emotional component to patient care is not only acceptable but preferable, so long as it does not impede treatment decisions or compliance.

Possibly the supervisors believed that the student should not extend care of patients beyond work hours. In general, a clinician's willingness to use time off to provide better patient care is not obligatory, but it is exemplary or supererogatory. If one of the differences between a profession and a job is that the former does not define its hours, the student showed an excellent grasp of that distinction.

The third case exemplifies not only the limits of medical expertise but also the frustrating impact those limits entail for caregivers who believe pain relief is a major goal of health practice. Although physicians often do not provide adequate pain relief, the resident in this case seems unlikely to fall within that number. He or she seems bound and determined to "fix" the pain. Given the development of a palliative care specialty within medicine, however, one would hope for consultation with a specialist on the matter. If the pain is still unrelievable, compassion is probably the best care available, and the patient should not be left bereft of it because the resident finds it so difficult to live with his or her own limitations. Acceptance of finitude befits clinicians as well as patients.

The last case is one that is unlikely to be faced by fully-trained physicians because they rarely have as much time to spend with patient's families as this medical student had. That the student had become deeply emotionally involved with the family was probably a useful learning experience for him or her. But medical students are not clinicians, and most patients and family members know that. Moreover, patients and family members often share more of what they are experiencing with nurses or medical students than they do with their physicians. This is not only because contacts with physicians are briefer and episodic, but also because patients are less likely to be intimidated by students or nurses. The student might have learned more about the impact of illness and death on patients and family members than could be learned in a residency or in subsequent practice. One hopes that that will be remembered.

Those in positions of power, whose ranks the medical student will one day join, also need to remember the constraint on patient disclosure that their positions sometimes elicit. Wise clinicians attempt to reduce this constraint by a respectful attitude towards patients and acknowledgment of their own limitations. In addition, they recognize the need to listen to patients, family members, medical students, and nurses to improve their understanding of non-medical aspects of patient care.

While it is true that clinicians do not necessarily help patients by crying with them, the student's display of feelings about the family's loss might well have been emotionally supportive to them, confirming the appropriateness of their own feelings. Such a display need not and should not interfere with judgments about care. As the medical student moves on to residency and prac-

tice, it is highly unlikely that he or she will have the opportunity to develop as close a relationship in other cases. Still, a tear in the eye and an arm around a family member who lost a loved one is not inappropriate in most cultural settings. In most cases, these expressions of feeling convey a commitment on the part of the clinician to provide not only technical care but emotional support. Caring for the whole patient requires caring by the whole clinician.

Although care *for* the whole patient may be achieved through collaborative effort by health team members, caring *by* the whole clinician demands a certain integrity, coupled with self-knowledge, on the part of the practitioner. Unfortunately, medical training tends to focus narrowly on technical expertise, neglecting the psychological development that is crucial to students becoming "whole clinicians." When psychological development is addressed in training, it is often regarded by faculty and students alike as "fluff."

Focusing on medical knowledge is necessary and useful so long as the fallacy of abstraction, i.e., interpretation of a part as whole, is avoided in practice. In other words, boundaries are not to be imposed artificially. The supposed "fluff" of nonmedical aspects of patient care and clinician conduct is not in fact separable from the experience of either party. Because of the inevitable influence of such factors on health and caregiving, they are also inseparable from effective treatment.

DISCUSSION QUESTIONS
3. Setting boundaries

1 By becoming doctors do trainees come to have different obligations? license? values? How do breaking social conventions and taboos affect a trainee's sense of self and personal identity?

2 What does establishing appropriate professional boundaries entail and do boundaries change according to the level of training?

3 Does valuing a patient's autonomy and right to self-determination require physicians to accept patient behaviors they find offensive or self-destructive?

4 Is having sex with patients ever justified? What if the person is no longer your patient? What about the argument that the patient would find it healing and rewarding?

5 How much of your personal self should you reveal to a patient?

6 How much of yourself ought you give to patients while still preserving your own health and happiness? How might the balance be achieved?

7 Should self-interest be a boundary on your altruism, or should it be the other way around?

8 In what ways can the psychological defenses that serve to protect trainees from being continually surrounded by pain and suffering not only affect their personal lives outside medicine but also affect the care of their patients?

9 When does concern for patients become over-involvement? At what point does objectivity become a kind of sterile detachment? How do you personally mediate these extremes?

On becoming a "team player"

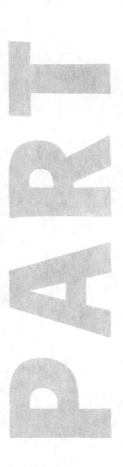

PART II

Searching for *esprit de corps* and conflicts of socialization

All relationships within a hospital are based on the authority of one person over another. When medical students first arrive on a hospital ward, they immediately find themselves enmeshed in a pre-existing, well-defined system of hierarchical work relations. Taking their place alongside (or more likely in back of) staff physicians, residents and interns, students join the medical sector of the ward community, which – apart from patients – otherwise consists almost exclusively of people whose work supports the doctors in their therapeutic activities. (1)

Part of the task for any newcomer seeking entry to an established group is to identify, and be identified with, the prevailing culture. Medical education, like other professional socialization experiences, seeks to assimilate individuals into the system by imbuing them with a sense of group solidarity, obeisance, and *esprit de corps*. The wards in which doctors in training gradually learn to be part of the medical team provide the most powerful structure for this aspect of the socialization process.

Idealistically, and perhaps naively, it is often assumed that, in addition to the acquisition of knowledge and skills, during their apprenticeship on the wards, medical trainees will be exposed to the attitudes and values of senior physicians who, through instruction and example, will nurture those attributes society expects from the medical profession, e.g., compassion, integrity, and a sense of professional ethics. Although this idealistic portrayal of life on the wards sometimes does occur, the history of the emergence of the teaching hospital attests to the hurdles to be overcome and idealism's subsequent rarity.

Paris medicine and the role of the teaching hospital

In general, leaving aside medieval hospitals which served as religious foundations dedicated to tending the poor, the aged, and the infirm, hospitals were developed as training facilities for doctors. As early as the sixteenth century, some doctors employed by Italian hospitals, such as those in Florence and Padua, were accompanied by apprentices as they went about their daily rounds, but these activities lacked systemization. The mid eighteenth century, however, saw the emergence of the idea that hospitals could become an arena for training doctors. Advanced medical students in Britain and France were brought into the hospital for training and experimenting on patients. These hospitals were explicitly not patient-centered; and academic interest began to outweigh concerns regarding the patient's more personal future. (2)

This change of priorities to pedagogy and research, came most forcefully in nineteenth century Paris where hospitals became unambiguously the center of medical school training. Hospitals turned themselves into "scientific machines" for investigating diseases and for teaching vast numbers of students. (3) Objective and analytic in spirit, hospitals became headquarters for the purpose of doing anatomical correlations and research. The specific nuances of individual patients were brushed aside. Stripping away the veneer of beneficence in "the march of knowledge," patients were largely immaterial.

This momentous change in outlook is reflected by how the sick poor in infirmaries became commodified as "clinical material." (4) Medical education everywhere followed the French initiatives and grew more systematic and scientific. (5) A fragmentation occurred that shattered interest in the body as a whole. Doctors began looking at organ systems, and this allegiance to scientific inquiry had the consequence of distancing and dehumanizing. Patients were reduced to "stomachs," "hearts," and "livers" to be studied, the legacy of which still is apparent today. Anyone who has witnessed the impersonal nature with which a patient on a gurney is wheeled into a lecture hall before a packed audience of students to serve as an illustration for a professor's description of a disease, and just as quickly wheeled out again, must face the unsettling question of the degree to which the system is still devised to produce knowledge over and above caring for patients.

The marriage of hospital and hierarchy

Along with the mantle of teaching and learning, medicine in France around the time of the Revolution took on the strict hierarchical system characteristic of academia. From the middle ages, surgeons had been arranged hierarchically according to their skills and the length of time they had practiced surgery. This system was based on the model of apprenticeships, where trainees apprenticed themselves to more experienced surgeons until, gradually, they became surgeons themselves. During the French Revolution, however, an amalgamation took place between surgeons and physicians, resulting in the same MD degree serving as certification for both areas of expertise. It was at this point, in imitation of the models of surgical hierarchies, that the whole notion of levels of stratification entered the medical picture. Additionally, the widespread affiliations between medical faculty and universities, that provided power and social position for the professors, served to support and reinforce the model of hierarchical structure in the hospital. (2)

As stratification solidified (along with the development of more precise diagnostic techniques and the movement to focus on particular anatomical parts), the patient was pushed further to the perimeter of concern. This movement accelerated in the 1850s with the development of specialty hospitals: eye hospitals, gynecological hospitals, cardiac hospitals, tuberculous hospitals, along with specialty clinics within larger hospitals, with the result that patients were seen even more as objects to be studied.

Treating patients on the periphery is a familiar theme on today's wards. A physician remembers his own internship at a prestigious Midwestern teaching hospital as ironically in contradiction to its reputation for social concerns, "What I saw made me very uncomfortable, because from the very beginning no one was paying attention to the patient. And this attitude was inculcated into our training. The primary person in the room was the physician, next in importance were other staff members, after them came the students. The patient was unmistakably last."

Power, hierarchy, and moral distress

It is this background of power emanating from the top down that frames life on the wards. Recognition of the hierarchical status of medicine – where agency for the less empowered members is frankly limited – is an ever-present reality for doctors in training.

As in any strict hierarchy, the characteristic most valued in subservient members is conformity. Deviations are not easily accommodated, and the pressures to adhere to both explicit and implicit codes of conduct can be crushing. Failure to comply can bring ridicule, alienation, shunning by group members, or even expulsion. Little wonder that the ability to "fit the mold" and "not make waves" becomes a powerful drive in the push for success as a doctor. Absorbing and exemplifying the "corporate culture" becomes equated with acceptance and team membership.

Thus, it is only to be expected that prospective trainees come to the medical situation with a built-in confusion over conflicting duties that exist between what is expected of them as individuals and what is expected of them as members who owe allegiance to a larger group. Early on, we are taught to be responsible for our own actions, that we have freedom of choice to develop individual integrity, to listen to the dictates of our own conscience, and to stand steadfast in the face of assaults to personal values. At the same time we are instructed that because "No man is an island," there is virtue in sacrificing for others, furthering the goals of the community, relating to the group's mores, and conforming to social expectations.

Weighing conflicts of conscience against power, hierarchy, and group values is an ongoing problem and is at the core of ethical decision-making for student doctors. Balancing these competing claims is made further complicated by expectations regarding the role and place of trainees in the medical hierarchy. Predictably this dichotomy of opposing claims is brought forward and becomes intensified in the medical context not only when individual integrity comes into conflict with a perceived duty to the profession, but also when dilemmas arise that trigger the less lofty and more practical concerns of self-preservation.

The ethical dilemmas of life on the wards along with the powerless position in which trainees find themselves generate what can best be described as a situation of "moral distress." (6) Moral distress differs from the task of sorting through conflicting principles to arrive at the most reasonable solution. Moral distress comes about not so much from trying to sort out what to do, but results from obstacles that stand in the way of executing what a person believes to be the right action. Thus, moral distress is the product of a two-tiered process. Initially, on one level, there is the moral problem "What should be done (or not done) in this situation?" Sometimes, after wrestling with conflicting principles, a strong sense of what is right becomes evident. At this point, however, a second, and even harder, problem emerges, "The power to decide is not in my hands, what ought I to do now?" Thus, we have a situation in which a person believes he or she knows the right thing to do but lacks the power or the authority to overcome the restraints. Nowhere is this moral distress more evident than the conflicts encountered as trainees struggle to find their place as a member of the medical team.

Team models, conceptual systems, and group identification

One of the ways people seek to become accepted and incorporated into a group is to take on as many of the trappings and behaviors of the group as possible – their language, their dress, and their mores. All of these ingredients come together on the wards as medical trainees seek to establish themselves in the hierarchy of medical teams.

The strict stratification of power and authority that governs life on the wards is understood and expressed through certain dominant cognitive models of how medical teams function. This is not surprising, since both inside and outside of medicine, there are different ways that small elite groups, needing to function together under pressure and with high stakes, can operate. Our interviews with physicians and trainees, along with the cases presented in this book, reveal three primary models of team operation: the military model (with little modification the corporation model), the sports model, and the repair model.

Systematic and consistent in what they reveal about assumptions and priorities, the influence of these models pervades the wards, not only in language but also in thought and action. By bringing this largely unconscious system to the fore, the implicit forces that drive ward relationships and decision making are made explicit for examination and evaluation in the pages that follow.

Although some of the following team models are more likely than others to fall within certain specialties, all portray the force of the conceptual systems at work in defining professional purpose and team interactions.

Military model

Although a course in military strategy is not part of the curriculum, medical trainees are constantly confronted with the nomenclature and hierarchy of a popularized military culture. In this model, doctors see themselves as heroic warriors against disease, illness, and death. Medicine is perceived as armed conflict and members of the team are part of a command unit. Under orders from their leader, they are "soldiers" "on the firing line" or "in the trenches," using their "armamentarium" to "fight the good fight." How often do you hear "No one dies on my watch?"

In order to "win the war" it is necessary to "run a tight ship" and flagging members of the team are questioned as to whether or not they are "on board." In describing the head of surgery at his institution, a physician says "He's the captain of the ship." "He does everything in the world to protect his team even when they shouldn't be protected, and he beats the hell out of them during the experience."

Like the surgeon described above, an argument is sometimes offered that surgeons are much more likely to use the military model and that, in fact, this model is appropriate because in the operating room "There needs to be a leader and there isn't time for discussion."

In contrast, others see the manifestations of military hierarchy only as a way to support the structure and maintain rigor in a disciplinary sense. In looking back on his own surgical rotation at a major American East Coast teaching hospital a physician reflects:

I question the appropriateness of the military model, even for a surgical team, especially for the junior members of the team. I think 50% of their patient-care time is not spent in the operating room. And of the time that is spent in the operating room, at least 90% is spent involved in tasks in which split-second decision-making is not relevant. In some ways I think the romanticized model of surgery as a *praxis* in which life and death always hangs by a hair only protected by the secure hand of the extremely skilled senior surgeon only serves as an excuse to reinforce this hierarchical mode.

It is certainly true that was the culture of the surgical teams of which I was a part – they were extremely hierarchical and militaristic. In fact I have a very vivid recollection of the first senior resident I worked with in surgery. He was a short, muscular man who, right from the first day, I thought of as Napoleon. He was a little balding on the top and had the Napoleonic curl on his forehead. I don't know if that impression was cultivated or not but he had a powerful persona that set the tone for the entire team. He was a commander, ready for any campaign.

The characteristics of the Napoleonic resident described above, with very little change could also be used to describe a corporate head of industry, exerting unquestioned power and authority over his subordinates. Although the values inherent in the military model (or corporation model) are pervasive throughout this book, some situations in which they are particularly apparent include cases of questioning authority regarding patient treatment, challenging a chain of command, and determining whether or not to carry out an order.

Sports model

The world of sports and the concept of the healthcare "team," with all that concept entails, exerts a powerful influence over many physicians during their training years on the wards. Whether in medicine or athletics, coveted team membership holds the promise of acceptance by an elite group, and at the same time, the peril of exclusion or marginalization if the person's performance is deemed ill-adapted by group standards. Winning or losing a place on the team hinges on such behavior as "playing by the rules," promoting "team spirit," and most of all becoming identified as a real "team player," demonstrating the ability to "move the ball forward," "stepping up to the plate," "moving it up a notch," and avoiding "whistle-blowing." A common aspiration is for the player to make a hit, hopefully a "home run" and to be avoided, at all cost, is the dreaded "strikeout." In the self-congratulatory words of one resident rating his own performance at a conference, "I knocked it out of the park."

"Rookies," be they athletes or training physicians, undergo grueling initiation rites to earn a place on the team. Hazing is an obstacle they are expected to face. Team socialization has traditionally included running the gauntlet and taking the verbal jabs and derisive remarks from superiors. As a result, medical students and interns are subordinated in ways that make them feel unworthy of being part of the team. Demonstrating team identification can also entail displacing their own feelings of inadequacy through jokes and demeaning remarks aimed at the even more vulnerable – patients. Cases such as these that exemplify inappropriate behaviors are: cases of questionable and insensitive humor, disrespectful behavior toward trainees, and the use of dehumanizing names to describe patients or their conditions.

Mechanical model

The central metaphor for other healthcare teams is the body as machine; thus, medicine is understood in terms of repairing nonfunctioning parts. Patients are seen as broken machines that need to be fixed and made "as good as new." A medical student describes how the formative early cadaver experience promotes the mechanical model of medicine:

A nonmedical student friend once asked me how I could stand to dissect a person. I responded that I felt the cadaver was not a person: "the owner just wasn't there." I went on to describe how nonetheless, I felt I knew a lot about the person just from what I knew about his body. After listening to me for a while, my friend, who had once worked as an auto mechanic, commented that it sounded much like working on someone's car. You could tell a lot about people from their car, he said; what kind of car it was, how old, how well-taken care, whether it had a stereo, how many dents it had, etc. In many ways this was an excellent comparison; it certainly sheds light on how medical students might see the body as car metaphor. In this formative first experience, our patients are absent, and we are left to deal with their damaged bodies as best we can. Small wonder we come to think of patients as broken machines, when the metaphor so aptly describes our first patient encounter. (7)

Seeing and experiencing medicine as fixing mechanical breakdowns influences how patients are treated on the wards. For example, the degree to which patients are understood as machines to be repaired permits practices that appear less than humane. Patients are awakened from sleep in the middle of the night for routine checks or record-keeping. Schedules revolve around institutional convenience rather than the patient's and family's. The patient is seen as having little to contribute to the medical encounter. The patient's perceptions are relevant, only insofar as it aids the physician, as medical mechanic and technician, to identify and fix the underlying problem.

An internist describes his experience on an obstetrics rotation in terms of the repair model, "I found the model in obstetrics like a factory assembly line, only in this case it was a dis-assembly line. We had a pregnant mother and our job as technicians was to disassemble the body as machine into two parts: the mother and the child. It was all very rote and mechanical and uninteresting, punctuated by moments of terror when you had to step in and know what to do."

Examples of cases typifying the repair model are those where procedures and educational opportunities appear to take on a life of their own, and assume a primacy beyond the patient, thus echoing the early role of the teaching hospital discussed earlier.

Inevitably, distortions created by the common conceptual metaphors described above adversely affect how members of the healthcare team view and understand their own professional roles as well as their interaction with the individual ill person. By placing a barrier, or emotional buffer, between the self and others, authentic relationships are precluded. Tying the value of physicians to being victorious combatants, or sports heroes, or even master mechanics, not only creates unrealistic standards doomed to failure, the resulting stratification of relationships dilutes the experience and expertise that could be more effectively put to the patient's benefit.

The collaborative model

The top–down pyramid models are not the only options for team organization and consequently not all ward experiences suffer from the limitations of the above described models. There is also the possibility of a collaborative model in which the appropriate metaphor is not a battlefield, corporate office, sports arena, or repair shop, but instead a wheel with spokes extending from a central hub. The team leader is basically at the center and it is understood that at the end of the spokes will be people carrying out their assigned tasks even as they "check in" with the major leadership at the center. Although hierarchy still exists, the *form* and *stylization* of the hierarchy differs, emphasizing relationship, reciprocity, and mutual sharing.

Below, a senior physician credits his own early training experience with such a model as determining not only his career direction but the way he now structures his work supervising students.

In training, I was fortunate to be introduced, almost in an accidental way, to a collaborative model on my medicine service. This chance encounter with an unfamiliar medical culture was formative for me and probably the reason I became an internist. My first rotation was with a resident newly arrived from India. He had been trained in India in the British model and although he knew everything about clinical medicine he knew nothing about the United States. He was thrilled to teach us and thrilled to have us teach him! Unlike the other teams on the ward, we became a very mutually-supportive, respectful, friendly team – a real team in the sense of collaboration. I think that team experience had more to do with his circumstances than anything else and when I am the attending physician, it is still the model to which I aspire.

In the opinion of this physician introducing a collaborative model addresses the prevailing dysfunctional models he believes are rampant in medical education:

Medical training as currently conceived is a dysfunctional model. It lacks respect for the learner and respect for the role of the poor medical student who is at the bottom of the barrel. The poor interns and residents are stuck too. I've learned as medical director of a hospice and primary care that one person cannot do everything; and for this reason, the patriarchal, hierarchical structure is just wrong. It's bad for trainees; it's bad for patients; it's bad for everyone and I refuse to do it. I like to be collaborative and create an atmosphere in which we all learn from each other. Sometimes the residents know a good bit more than I do about things; so I need to respect them and I expect them to respect me.

In describing his collaborative model he says:

The collaborative model recognizes that everyone has his or her own contribution to make. Although the responsibility for the teaching environment and the care environment is mine, everyone is involved and everyone participates. In practice on our team, I do some of the teaching, the resident does some of the teaching, and the students do some of the teaching. We are committed to listen, respect and be there, on time, for each other.

I establish some rules from the beginning as to what my goals are for our, all too brief, time together. The first thing is that we are going to provide excellent patient care. Secondly, we are going to respect each other. We are going to learn from each other. We are going to stay sane, and we are going to have a good time doing it. I make my goals explicit and then I find out what goals they have for our period of time together, what specific things they might want to accomplish. Usually they have no idea why they are there, just to get to the other side.

I try to model that in listening to cases and to what they think, then suggesting what I think and saying this is what I might have done differently. A dysfunctional model holds that there is only one way of doing things, and that's nonsense. So I never say "That's wrong," I say "Well, have you thought of this issue?" and "Here is the reason a person might choose to do it this way instead." This is the model of teaching I have in my head, even when I fall short.

However, he recognizes that the reality of what he is able to do can fall short of the ideal collaborative model, part of which involves the "patient-centered rounds":

Of course the team needs more from me than I am able to give, but that is true of my family and friends too. More and more I am trying to address this need for more of my time as a priority. Part of that time-priority is making room for more patient-centered interactions. On the wards, rather than staying in a room and talking about pathophysiology, divorced from the human being, we need to go out and spend more time talking with, and examining, patients. It's one thing to say "This is what the patient told me in the history," and "This is what the physical shows," since none of that gets challenged. But, if you actually interact with patients, then you get sometimes a completely different sense of reality – the patient's reality. So rounds have to be patient-centered.

My ideal concept of the collaborative model also involves hanging around with trainees outside of the formal time of rounds and outside of the formal things that have to be accomplished during rounds, such as hearing about the patient so that I can dictate a note to the department of medicine. Those are the realities that must be gotten through in order to get to the collaborative part of education. Sometimes I can accomplish what I want for the students, but if we get too busy I can't.

In the collaborative model, the triangular hierarchy with a broad base of underlings rising steeply to a pinnacle of power has been replaced with a circle of professionals engaged in mutual learning and teaching, benefited by the leader's guidance. Critical to the success of that enterprise is the presence of the patient's own voice as well. In such an environment would the dilemmas voiced in this book still arise? Most likely so. But an atmosphere of respect and acceptance would also be established to make bringing the problems to the team for airing and discussion a more likely occurrence.

However, as long as trainees are still taught to think of themselves as warriors, heroes, and mechanics whose primary loyalty flows up the ladder of command, any significant changes are impossible. The first step to the construction of new models of how professionals interact and think about themselves and their patients begins with a reassessment of their role expectations. Today's trainees are tomorrow's senior physicians. Changing expectations is more than an intellectual exercise, it can shape behavior and the future of medical education. Patients as well as professionals deserve no less, as the cases and discussions to follow demonstrate.

Notes

1 Shapiro M. *Getting Doctored.* New Society Publishers, Philadelphia, 1987, p.81.
2 Risse GB. *Mending Bodies, Saving Souls. A History of Hospital.* Oxford University Press, New York, 1999, Chapter 6.
3 Porter R. *The Greatest Benefit to Mankind: A Medical History of Humanity.* W.W. Norton & Company, New York, 1997, p.326.
4 Porter R. *The Greatest Benefit to Mankind: A Medical History of Humanity.* W.W. Norton & Company, New York, 1997, p.30.
5 Porter R. *The Greatest Benefit to Mankind: A Medical History of Humanity.* W.W. Norton & Company, New York, 1997, p.315.
6 Andrew Jameton, private communication, November 6, 1999.
7 Dunn E. *Winning the War, Losing the Patient: Metaphor in the Practice of Medicine,* unpublished thesis, University of California, Berkeley, 1991, p.21.

Abuse and mistreatment

A certain amount of hazing is commonly part of the treatment for newcomers joining a sports team or fraternal society. This hazing may include some form of ceremony, and sometimes these get out of hand.

In this section we examine issues of being subjected to mistreatment and abuse that can have harmful effects on multiple levels: physical health, emotional well-being, social and family life, and attitudes to becoming a physician. How much humiliation should students endure before taking their complaints to higher authorities? When does 'roughness' turn into abuse that warrants professional discipline? What constitutes sexual harrassment and what can be done about it?

12

Psychological abuse: subjected to humiliating and belittling behavior

CASE

"You idiot! What are you doing in medical school?"

Five of us were working together dissecting a cadaver in anatomy lab. It was day three of the course and there were two hours left to complete the day's assignment. The student who self-appointed herself as the group leader was assertive and eager to dissect but had botched up one dissection already, making it difficult to identify certain parts of the anatomy. Another student decided to confront her and said, "You idiot! You've completely destroyed this cadaver! What are you doing in medical school?"

I was very worried about not getting the assignments done on time and debated with myself about involving the preceptor, but I didn't know how to proceed.

CASE

"I would knock you to the floor"

I was a third year medical student on a largely surgical obstetrics and gynecology rotation. We rounded on patients at 7:00 a.m. and I was responsible for one of the four patients on the post-surgical floor. My responsibility required getting up early, checking out her vital signs, talking to her about what was going on with her, asking about any pain she might be experiencing, going over her medications and her history. I had to make sure I knew everything.

That particular morning the senior resident missed rounds and came in late just as the rounds were ending. Afterwards, I found myself in the elevator with the senior resident and one of the attendings. The senior resident asked me with regard to his own patient, "Do you remember her JP output?" – a drain to measure body fluids after surgery – I said I did not. He then asked if I remembered his patient's hemoglobin. Again, I answered "No." I had been writing notes on my own patient. At that moment the attending stepped directly in front of my face and said "If you came from my medical school I would knock you to the floor and you'd be bleeding – and I would be a hero for that." I was stunned into silence but later as I was walking down the corridor I was furious that she would suggest that I should be physically beaten. If I had made a similar suggestion about her, that would be grounds for dismissal from the clerkship. How much abuse should students be expected to take? Who, if anyone, should I have talked to about this incident?

CASE

"He treated me like a scut monkey"

I was the subintern for an ophthalmology chief resident who treated me like a "scut monkey." He expected me to do everything for him, all except examining the eyes (because he would have to do it himself anyway). He taught me nothing about ophthalmology, and I let him get away with it. The truth is that I was trying so hard to please him to get my honors. I was miserable.

It was 2 weeks before I summoned enough courage to tell him off. I threatened to take my case to the ombudsman if he did not start to teach me some ophthalmology. I had already decided at that point that I was not going into ophthalmology, and so I did not care much about his evaluation of me. But I question whether I could have done it if I had aspired all my life and worked hard to become an ophthalmologist. I would have been stuck. It would have been the dues I pay, the price of my success.

CASE

"I knew better than to spoil his fun"

The first day on my junior surgery clerkship, I witnessed the chief resident shove the intern for "walking too slow." But the intern's response was even more disturbing; he let out a wimpy, apologetic laugh and scurried along his way. The chief resident was a jerk. He was brusque with his patients and abusive to his subordinates. And he knew he could get away with it. He did. I remember one time he was making fun of a radiology file clerk, who was trying his best to retrieve a misplaced film for us. We all stood around obsequiously amused. While I resisted participation in the mockery, I knew better than to say anything to spoil his fun.

COMMENTARY

Ruth B. Purtilo

With all due respect for respect: reflections on the health care setting

How often have you heard the expression, "With all due respect . . ."? Usually the comment that follows is *disrespect* for the idea under discussion. The title of this reflection is a clue that the abuses described in the above cases require the corrective of respect in order for the professional ethic to survive and thrive.

"To respect" means to hold in high regard, with sensitivity to the well-being of the other. The Jewish philosopher Martin Buber characterized respect as the basis of the life affirming "I–thou" relationship with others (in contrast to the "I–it" encounters in which other people and objects are used for one's own ends). *Dis*respect is a theme that runs through the cases in this section. In each instance a peer or superior is breaching an appropriate regard for someone else. Sometimes the disrespect seems directed to a group of people with a hapless individual who happens to become the focus. At other times, one person is the victim. The reader does not have to read between the lines to observe the devastating effects of this indulgence of power, indifference to the feelings of another or, in some cases, imposition of outright cruelty. Anyone who has been "dissed" (as young people sometimes call it today) knows the sting of this wound.

Where do modern notions of respect arise? From a western Judeo–Christian religious point of view, respect is a compass at the center of the moral universe. It is no less than an expression of the fundamental religious *truth* that all humans are equal in the sight of God, having been made in God's image. Those who are guided by sensitive regard for other humans are believed to manifest the expressions of that truth in their everyday relationships. Historically, religious images of the physician as healer portray a person of great moral strength and self-knowledge combined with unselfish commitment to that truth.

Philosophers have most often treated the idea of respectfulness as a *virtue*. Virtue theory focuses not only on what one should do (or not do) and what kinds of good to bring about through one's action, but, more fundamentally, on what kind of character traits and attitudes a person should cultivate. In other words, respect-full is the type of person one ought to become.

Respect has become deeply incorporated into the identity of a profession as the physician's role has moved from simply healer to professional, though the religious and philosophical under-pinnings of the idea have continued to be influential too. The modern social construction of the physician *qua* professional provides him or her with a privileged role in society characterized by social esteem, self-regulation and a commitment to meet a recognized social need. The price is that the demands of the profession will take precedence over those directed to strict self-interest. To meet this high standard of social and peer expectations an appropriate moral resource is the resolve to show deep, unselfish regard for everyone with whom one interacts (i.e., show respect). Indeed the usefulness of this resource has been acknowledged at different times in society as the understanding of the health professional and patient relationship has evolved: it has been treated as a means to beneficent and kindly actions, as a bulwark against inflicting harm and, more recently, as a vehicle towards honoring patient autonomy.

From the above discussion, three governing dimensions of this notion and their moral implications can be identified.

Disrespect is intentionally harmful

Very seldom can an act be fully excused on the basis that the person was being *mis*respectful when the damaging blow was dealt. Recall that at the beginning of these reflections disrespect was characterized as indulgence, indifference, imposition of cruelty. Mistakes may occur occasionally but it is difficult to believe that the OBGYN senior resident who threatened to knock the student to the floor was miscalculating the withering effect it would have on the student. The same conclusion must be drawn of the chief resident who shoved the intern for "walking too slow." It follows that persons can and should be held accountable for the actions that fail to acknowledge others as worthy of human regard.

Because of the unevenness in power between the players in these two situations the person being treated disrespectfully is under a double jeopardy. The harm of insult is exacerbated by the

real or imagined fear that an attempt to seek comfort and justice may be punished. Being treated disrespectfully in such situations makes the already less powerful person feel more vulnerable. "I knew better than to say anything to spoil his fun. If I had worked hard to become an ophthalmologist, I would have been stuck . . ."

Disrespect undermines due care

"Due care" is the term used in medical–legal literature to describe those skills and services a patient can reasonably expect from the health professional. But a disrespectful attitude or gesture diverts attention away from the proper moral and practical goals of health care intervention that constitutes due care. An old adage says, "a hurtful word has ten times the power of the word kindly spoken." Harshness, combined with the abusers *intended* goal of demeaning or otherwise eroding self-confidence evokes a reflex response of self-protectiveness. In all the cases above the outcome is a deflection away from the patient (or the learning required to be able to care for patients) to what is happening in the disrespectful exchange. For instance, the person who was shoved for walking too slow certainly would have ceased thinking about how to approach Mrs. S's anxiety regarding her forthcoming tests or why Mr. A is on a downhill course following surgery.

Disrespect undermines team spirit

Unfortunately, disrespect spreads its ill effects beyond the victimized person. In almost all instances the cases under discussion take place in a group whose task it is to bring about a worthwhile goal that requires teamwork. The dissection "team" in the anatomy lab had to deal not only with one person's lack of skill but also with the demeaning comment, "You idiot! What are you doing in medical school?" by another student. Wherever the "blame" lay, the efficiency and effectiveness of overcoming the problem were further compromised by that disrespectful response. The story of the disrespectful physician ("team captain") who made fun of a team member with less status (the radiology file clerk) illustrates a damaging effect on *two* teams: one made up of teacher and students, the other of members of a radiology treatment team. The damage was not only to the file clerk bearing the brunt of the ridicule, it also spread to the interns who adopted a self-defensive mode of not wanting to participate, but felt afraid of the more powerful member of the team (the intern supervisor).

Disrespect destroys role modeling as a road to professionalism

The importance of role models in medical education has long been praised. From the Hippocratic oath forward, mentors have been characterized as crucial to effective learning in the exciting venture of "becoming a (good) doctor." But when role models exhibit damaging and abusive attitudes or behaviors, students have to consciously reject the model presented to them during this highly formative period, the price often being great stress and disillusionment. Their sense of betrayal all too often results in a kind of moral schizophrenia. Some students maladjust by accommodating or even adopting disrespectful attitudes and conduct themselves. In short, the disrespectful mentor becomes a negative role model with tragic consequences for the critical role that medicine plays in a community's well-being.

Concluding comment

In conclusion, respect for everyone involved in the health care environment helps nourish the appropriate moral goals of medicine. In addition to the self-discipline of individuals in the medical environment, social and organizational supports also are required. The variables for this aspect of good doctoring are set early during medical training and must be exercised and nourished throughout the physician's career. This, in turn, is everyone's task – and opportunity.

COMMENTARY

Gerrit Kimsma

Central to these cases is a tendency by students to accept abusive behavior in the context of education at medical school or the clinic. But along with this ostensible acceptance there remains an internal resistance and anger. The ethical connotations of these cases does not arise from traditional medical ethics; there is no direct patient involvement, so there is no immediate "medical ethical" dilemma. But that fact certainly does not exhaust another kind of ethical dilemma, along with its symbolism, and implications for the continued behavior of physicians within the healthcare system. On the contrary, what is at stake is the immediate message to students about the attitudes of colleagues, teachers, and preceptors.

What strong feelings and what frustration leap from these pages! Questions come up that need to be addressed in order to understand but also, and even more importantly, to prevent these recurrences. Is this tendency toward abuse part of the structure of medical training or is it incidental? Are these cases exaggerations or symptomatic examples of peer behavior one has to endure in order to pass or survive? What can we learn from it? Why is it important to pay attention to these issues? Let us try to answer these questions.

One can draw several initial observations from these cases:

1 The tendency to be abusive can be observed and experienced early in medical school and can continue throughout the course of medical training. Everyone is susceptible.
2 The relationship between teacher and student, between resident/chief of staff and intern is asymmetrical and can be described by an inequality in power.
3 These inequalities in power, when they lead to abuse, are not really confronted and thus, not countered. There is usually little or no opportunity for open discussion or for appeals to

institutional safeguards, if and when these are present.

4 Even when institutional safeguards are present, there is fear of reprisal and unjust evaluation that could affect the course of one's career path.

5 There are gender issues that sometimes emerge as well.

The case descriptions, even though some of them seem extreme, are easily recognized from the experiences of Dutch medical students. Sometimes the abuse is subtle and sometimes rude. Reflecting on their uninhibited existence offers some quite startling and inescapable presumptions. There are two presumptions that lie at the base of the problem. One is the presumption that human beings start out relatively educated and polished when they enter medical school, after their years of pubescence and before flowering into adulthood. This presumption is accompanied by a claim, some say a fact, that medical training produces, or at least does not stop producing, individuals who abuse others who depend on them.

The second presumption is that weeding out individuals with unwanted and alien behavior is impossible from the start of medical school, yet "somehow" in the course of medical training, this undesirable behavior will surface and be noticed. The individuals would then be ordered to change or be forced or advised to leave the profession.

Yet, in the end analysis neither presumption can be maintained. Understanding why some physicians behave the way they did in the case vignettes does not reflect so much on the nature of physicians and physicians-to-be as individuals. Rather it is a reflection of the nature of medical education and care in our time, though one cannot even be certain that this situation was any different or better in the past. The master was always in a power relation with the apprentice. In such an imbalanced relationship, there is always opportunity for abuse.

The exploration of poor behavior in these case descriptions invariably is curtailed by interpersonal interactions: what one person in fact did to the other and how the other person reacted, or did not react, but instead swallowed a natural response. Note that the interpersonal route is just one way of looking at it. This particular route may reflect the "color blindness" of students and interns or their "professional deformation" that has taken place even though they have participated in this game for such a short time. Thus, these cases have one trait in common: the descriptions are oblivious of the context in which they take place – the context of institutionalized medicine, where the differences between actual and professed goals of medical education and medical, institutional care are startling. Sadly, an environment is generated where "putting the patient first" invites derision because of the daily grinding mill of long hours, a million different tasks, not enough sleep, interprofessional conflicts between physicians and nursing staff, too little time for reflection, not enough time to unwind, and too little pay. If abuse in this environment is an infection, students and faculty need to be immunized. Otherwise, they will all be susceptible to these power plays.

Little wonder that coping with the strains of becoming a doctor often leads to an affliction that has been called "the toxic intern syndrome." (1) This syndrome is recognized by those physicians-to-be whose conscience has been burdened, and who want to retain some strains of self-respect, even while they recognize the almost-but-not-completely inescapable nature of the forces of medical education and medical care. "The duration, severity, and onset of the syndrome are highly variable. Some interns contract it earlier in the year, some later, and others presumably exhibit immunity. It is difficult to predict whom or when it will hit or how long it will last." "The signs and symptoms also vary: expressions of fatigue, irritability mixed with anger, recurrent irritation with support staff, residents, attending physicians, consultants, patients, and hospital systems." "The symptoms can occur in a passive-aggressive form, such as striking back at residents, nurses, and patients.''

By the next phase of the syndrome ''emphasis has shifted from helping others to conserving energy and managing time efficiently,'' leading to a cynical approach to patient management – dumping patients, too-early dismissal, and shifting patients to other institutions to avoid responsibility and complex care. The leading tenet of this behavior is not serving the interest of patients but rather to survive. Because, as one resident admitted, ''I feel abused, I am sick of answering pages, of writing endless admission notes, of feeling constantly behind, of worrying that I am missing something important, of ordering unnecessary tests for unlikely diagnoses.'' (2)

The need to survive is so well recognized that it has led to ironic and simplistic ''how to survive manuals.'' Voltaire Costeau, obviously a pseudonym – proving that the problem, although not new, is widespread – wrote a ''primer'' in 1973 on ''how to swim with sharks.'' (3) Some of his ''rules'' are quite revealing. Taken in reverse they may lead to early recognition and be part of a program of prevention of this ''toxic intern syndrome.'' Here is his list:

1 Assume unidentified fish are sharks.
2 Do not bleed.
3 Counter any aggression promptly.
4 Get out if someone is bleeding.
5 Use anticipatory retaliation.
6 Disorganize an organized attack.

If one looks at these so-called ''rules of survival'' and then reads the cases in this section again, the inherent nature of bad behavior between medical professionals becomes clear. What also becomes obvious is the opportunity to reflect upon the behavior and develop countermeasures to turn the tide and return to medicine's original goals of commitment to professionalism and patient care.

It seems undeniable that the destructive forces in institutionalized medicine and the resultant pressures put on medical and nursing staff have become stronger in recent years, especially in view of the heavy emphasis on economics in health care. Yet, in view of all these forces, there must be voices that strive to attain the values of humane care. Maybe this reflection on psychological abuse can be part of the formation of those voices.

My suggestions for intervention rest on open discussion, mutual support, and appeals mechanisms. Given the fact that anyone in medical training can succumb to belligerent behaviors, and secondly, that these behaviors if habitualized become ethically unacceptable conduct towards peers and eventually towards patients, early and prompt intervention is required by all who witness the evidence of ''living with sharks'' rules – the awareness that someone is acting out his or her frustrations. Such interventions include:

1 Immediate group response to the belligerence demonstrating ''zero tolerance'' for psychological abuse.
2 Open, nonthreatening discussions acknowledging the vulnerability and temptation of all trainees and attending physicians with regard to humiliating and belittling behavior.
3 Specifically, for medical students it should be the responsibility of the institution to have an ombudsperson available, or some other mechanism in place for eradicating instances like those presented in these cases.

Notes

1 Dyer KA. Toxic Intern Syndrome. *West J Med*, 1994;160:378–9.
2 John CC. Flogging trolls. *Ann Intern Med*, 1994;120–242.
3 Costeau V. How to swim with sharks: a primer. *Perspect Biol Med*, 1973;525–8.

13

Physical abuse: actual physical harm

CASE

"The commander"

When I was a fourth year medical student beginning a surgical rotation, I was assigned to the operating room of a chief whose reputation had earned him the name "The commander." At a certain point in the procedure, the resident was called away leaving the intern and several medical students. The surgeon singled me out and ordered me to suture the patient. I protested, explaining this was my second day and I did not feel qualified. He yelled back that "the only way to learn is to plunge in." As I hesitated he became enraged, slapped my shoulder and pushed me toward the table. I obeyed, despite serious misgivings, but when I made a minor mistake he struck my hand sharply with an instrument. For some time after I suffered with a bruised shoulder and a cut finger.

COMMENTARY

David N. Weisstub

Law schools instruct their students that any unconsented-to touching constitutes a technical battery. Any threatening gesture, even when interrupted, which was meant to produce fear in the targeted party in torts law amounts to an assault, giving rise to a potential recovery even for what is effectively an incomplete battery. These torts evolved in common law, apart from any matter deserving of criminal attention as ways of protecting dignitary interests, places where a private sphere have become the subject of dignitary violation. In such examples of torts law, no damages are required to be proven and in many instances the test can be shown to be one of a subjective nature. Therefore hypersensitivity of the wounded party is not a real defense, and potential defendants have been warned over many decades of the torts system that they must learn to live with thin-skulled individuals as they find them.

Battle sergeants and surgeons are often conflated in the public's mind as thick-skinned individuals whose attitude towards training future members of a professional cult appear to have similar aims in mind. The idea that a person must jump in, demonstrate bravery and prove that they can be adept at picking up skills rapidly with a complementary bravado produces the sort of individual, it is argued, that we can rely on to do the job. So much so that any argument about technical battery for a slap or push of a novice in the operating room might bring as much commiseration among seasoned surgeons as we might expect to find in any army barracks.

However, the commander in this example appears to have gone full steam ahead, surpassing the normal requirements and expectations of the surgery cult to have actually bruised and wounded a medical student in training. A bruised shoulder and a cut finger are beyond the rough encouragement of a professional elder who in the zealousness in taking charge might have produced a questionable push or shove.

We should accept that in professional environments, reduction of moral talk into the technical vocabulary of assault or battery language should be seen as misplaced rhetoric. There has to be some tolerance left aside for the imperfections and eccentricities of trainers. Having said this, a careful eye should be given to the presence of an evolving consensus morality about how much room to give despite the heat of the best-intentioned examples of supervision. At a certain point, roughness even in the professional context turns into abuse, which invites professional discipline if not some form of legal action. There are real moral differences that arise from surgical context. Norman Bethune running an army surgical tent in the heat of battle as a heroic figure might from a moral point of view be forgiven lapses in moral courtesy in the face of an uncooperating medical trainee. This would be so because paralysis could in that situation be interpreted as a form of moral failure where the trainer had the moral right. In such a case, the moral trainer would reserve the right to employ extraordinary means to force the assisting party back into service in the higher interest of saving lives. In so doing, the disciplined party is transformed into a moral exemplar.

The commander situation suggests a different reality. The surgeon is depicted as a self-styled macho whose need for control victimized a randomly chosen standby. Rather than choosing the person best equipped to assist the patient, the surgeon randomly chose an untrained medical student who was psychologically unprepared to do an effective medical intervention. From the medical practitioner's point of view, the defense arguably would have been made that even when called upon in unjustified or unpredictable circumstances by an authority figure, it is a value of the medical reality to respond positively and to do the job even if inadequately.

The case is interesting because even if it is true that the surgeon lost control in becoming violent and should be disciplined for such outrageous conduct, can we ever in professional environments morally defend some modest measure of physical acting-out in control situations where our aim is to socialize medical students to be on the ready in either dire or pressured circumstances? The obligation to deliver the best possible medical standard to the patient remained an issue in this example insofar as it might have been possible for the surgeon to quickly conduct an interview to find out who the best trained and best equipped psychological candidate was. However if it could be revealed that the surgeon did not have adequate time to conduct this investigation given the fact that he was in the midst of a procedure, could we morally justify what he did if he randomly chose, was verbally somewhat abusive and showed a low degree of physical aggressivity? There is decreasing tolerance for such conduct. Insofar as we can prove even in soft cases of physical abuse that we could have achieved the stated objectives bereft of such aggressivity, such behavior should never be condoned and rather should be brought under professional peer review.

Having acknowledged the necessity of peer review through an administrative procedure, it should nevertheless be stated that strong forms of legal technicalism should be circumvented. Consensual moral dialogue should be brought to bear on the episode. Since the objective would be to sensitize individuals to the harmful impact of their unwarranted aggressivity on professionals in training, persons specialized in communication and/or therapeutic exchanges should be mandatorily present. If a pattern of soft abuse after such an exchange can be shown to continue, professional discipline and penalties would be warranted. In cases where there have been bruising and cutting, a civil action for battery would be understandable, although in some circumstances regrettable if the incident can be shown to be out of character, impetuous acting-out of a medical practitioner from anxiety or extreme stress. Some form of medication, apology, exchange, special action, or accommodation should be fostered instead of adversarial proceedings. Criminal law responses should be employed only with a great caution as the stigmatization could be expected to persevere for an extended period. The commander, if there is a repeated history present in the physical abuse of residents, would be a candidate for a justified criminal law reaction. In thinking through this option, a more detailed profile of the commander and the reaction of both his peers, support staff, physicians in training, patients, and mediation observers or therapeutic practitioners should be looked at carefully before making a final determination with respect to a recommended course of action. Optimally the relevance, meaning, and effectiveness of softer measures such as dialogue, communal mediation, professional discipline, and torts remedies will have been analyzed and reflected upon before reaching the conclusion that a criminal sanction would be the most effective remedy. It should also be part of the experience and contemplation that the professional community surrounding the event should avoid stigmatizing and creating a specter of victimization of the wounded party.

Professional environments are by nature closed wherein a victim of authoritarian behavior may only be able to achieve hollow victory in the light of having made a public issue out of a private professional secret, namely a substandard pattern of professional behavior which has been subtly accommodated within the professional subculture. When this occurs, there is a double injury. Firstly, there is a double jeopardy to the wounded party, and secondly there is an accentuation of an impervious skin surrounding a professional subculture where forms of violence and abuse are tolerated because of the level of professional achievement attributed to the perpetrator. The latter lets out a signal of not only how to survive but also how to behave as a successful and revered practitioner. Creating the conditions for an open-ended and self-critical dialogue should be the first goal where morally degenerative behavior appears to be condoned or tolerated by a professional peer group. This will enhance the propensity for change and protect

and support the victim who should be reintegrated and acknowledged as a full participating member in the professional community.

COMMENTARY

Emilio Mordini

The case elucidates aspects of medical education under the heading of "symbolic training." By "symbolic training," I mean the instructions given to an apprentice regarding her profession, namely training her for her identification with her future role. I will discuss this training and show in what ways I think the "commander's" behavior was paradigmatic of a certain kind of (bad) medical education.

Symbolic training

Each profession is made up of a complex whole, a culture of knowledge and skills, many of which have symbolic meaning. They serve the purpose of pointing out how one belongs to a professional structure rather than serving the practical purposes of healing. This apparent know-how has social meaning, because it serves to identify social roles. On closer analysis it has a more individual and private meaning too, because it serves to build identities. Mainly it serves to answer the basic question: "Who am I?" which is one of the most perturbing questions human beings can pose to themselves. It certainly pertains to the struggles of medical trainees displayed throughout this book.

Symbolic training is usually characterized by three elements:

1 Most symbolic training is performed by nonverbal and suggestive communication. This step involves several elements: facial expressions, prosodic elements of speech, vocal intonation, breathing, eye contact, and gestures. These often unnoticed messages shape the

educational setting, usually below the level of conscious awareness of both the "teacher" and the "disciple."

2 Symbolic training is highly metaphorical. A metaphor is a figure of speech, which compares two things by saying that one is the other. Metaphors are currently used to describe better, with more nuance, what we mean. Each metaphor suggests a spectrum of meanings just as a note played by an instrument involves its many harmonic series. Metaphors possess a special ability to influence us and are particularly invasive psychologically. The editors detailed some of these in the introduction to this section – the military and sports models of medical teams for example.

3 As a requirement of points 1 and 2, symbolic training is largely based on interpersonal relationships. It makes use extensively of identification processes and requires highly emotional contact between the trainer and the trained.

I now can turn to medical training itself.

Physical maneuvers as a form of symbolic training

The medical profession entails the ability to perform physical procedures. Each medical student is expected to learn maneuvers that must be part of her basic professional education. These maneuvers vary from time to time, from country to country, and according to changes in the medical ethos. For instance in Italy, medical students learn how to perform a physical examination and execute some diagnostic procedures, such as measuring blood pressure, drawing blood, and doing an electrocardiogram. Medical education also includes learning some therapeutic procedures: intravenous injections, cardiac massage and resuscitation measures, emergency tracheotomy, assistance to an epileptic crisis, assistance to a normal delivery, setting of a noncomplicated fracture, executing simple surgical sutures, and the like. Yet, it is unlikely that knowledge of each of these behaviors is of any

practical utility for the majority of medical students. What is going on then? We need to go back to the origin of the medical profession to understand their symbolic meaning.

In the beginning doctors and priests were a single social figure. Hence, many gestures of "modern medicine" are likely to be the remnant expressions of this ancient conflation of roles: they are ritual gestures, symbols that affirm the individual's belonging to the "holy caste" of healers.

While technology can easily change, ways of thinking and habit are harder to replace. Technological growth in medicine has ever less to do with any change of mentalities; "modern humans" are indeed still closer to their Neolithic ancestors than one usually suspects. We are divided by no more than three or four hundred generations from them, a very short time from a biological point of view.

Physical techniques are thus charged with symbolic meaning because they are associated with the infringement of an important taboo, the interdict that concerns the body. This insight relates more directly to the case at hand.

Trespassing body boundaries

Medical students must learn how to handle bodies; no matter if they have to perform a physical examination or a surgical operation. There is a common denominator that joins all physical techniques: the infringement of body boundaries. The precondition of any learning of physical techniques is that medical students must learn to trespass boundaries between their own body and the other's body. In our culture, boundaries of body are taboo: they can be trespassed only in highly ritualized, and somehow "holy," contexts (chiefly in sex, sports, war, and medicine).

The period of medical training in which medical students are trained to perform physical behaviors is consequently one of the most stressful parts of their education, not only because of the potential for harming the patient, but also because of the inner resonances that this training can evoke in them. Students learn to perform actions that may hurt the other's body, infringe upon his or her privacy, or feelings of modesty. I think that this is the crucial moment in medical education, the moment in which the character of future doctors is formed. Young apprentices must learn how to violate a taboo regarding the body of another human being.

The ward as a metaphor of the trench

I have just pointed out the importance of metaphors in symbolic training. We are overwhelmed by films and soap operas that deal with doctors in intensive care units, or surgeons in first-aid wards and emergency rooms. Doctors seem to be replacing soldiers as heroes of popular imagination. In our society, where death is perceived more and more as an obscene event, to be hidden and denied, doctors are metaphorically compared with soldiers: they are our troops drawn up against the last enemy.

The "commander" in the case is not therefore an exception. He is the perfect instance of the metaphor I am exploring. This metaphor does not only serve to nourish popular imagery, but it has also become an important mental tool that allows doctors to survive their professional stress and, even more frequently, frustration associated with a professional life that is not at all so heroic or so gratifying. Medical students are not immune to the military metaphor and they often feel themselves to be like recruits. They employ this metaphor both to cope with their difficult hierarchic situation and to overcome their first impact with death, suffering, and illness.

As a medical intern, I spent 6 months in an intensive care unit. The common feeling was truly that of being in the trenches. Describing soldiers' conditions in a trench during World War I, the Italian poet and Nobel prize winner, Giuseppe Ungaretti, wrote: "One is like the fall/leaves on the trees." Indeed you could see a patient in the morning, speak to her, and, the day after, you could be obliged to follow her autopsy.

In this regard I still remember Agnese. Agnese was a patient suffering from a Budd–Chiani syndrome, hospitalized in our ward. She was a 19-year-old girl and she rapidly became a friend of all of us young medical students. We joked with her and she enjoyed being "our difficult case." Eventually Agnese died. On the morning after her autopsy was performed – the case was very controversial and we all participated – we all then went to the cafeteria. When I saw my colleagues and myself drinking coffee, eating sandwiches, joking, and laughing, while discussing Agnese's case, I suddenly realized what monsters we were about to become. Our internship's goal seemed at that moment to be to train us how not to perceive patients as suffering fellow beings any longer. They were just problems.

How could we, young medical students, tolerate this unbearable situation? We rapidly learned: patients became just "flesh," pure bodies, already "corpses" even before dying. That mental move allowed most of us to learn to perform intrusive and even painful maneuvers on these patients by objectifying them and their bodies.

The metaphor of the trench is actually very dangerous because it suggests the idea of two different groups of humans living in a hospital, soldiers and civilians: those who combat and those for whom one combats. In a ward, our identity – I mean the identity of doctors, nurses, and care-givers in general – is bound with our sense of who we are not: we are not patients!

Interpersonal relationships

This leads us to the last point of this short discussion: the crucial role played by interpersonal relationships in medical training. It has been said that medicine is an empirical discipline that lies between science and art, and shares some aspects of both. More correctly, we should say that medicine lies between science, art, and handicraft. Actually if medicine can be compared with art, it should be compared with the old way of making art, when artists worked in a shop, and they were both artists and artisans. The master taught the young apprentice the gestures of the art. She accompanied her disciple's hands to paint, or to carve, with the same humble, and diligent attention that a shoemaker might use to teach his apprentice how to fix a pair of shoes. Such teaching was not only technical teaching. The presence of the master was an important element of the training, because it was thanks to that presence that it was possible to transmit the capacity to feel and to understand art.

Certain knowledge must be embodied in order to be transmitted. It is a kind of knowledge based on apprehension of patterns rather than single pieces of information. The same happens when the shop boy learns an art from his master. Medicine will always require this kind of teaching. The medical teacher is always also a "master." Obviously she can be a good or a bad master, she can teach good or bad art; but she cannot pretend that her role is just to "pass on" some pieces of technical information. In any event she is forming the professional character of her apprentice.

The professional character of a doctor coincides with his ethics. Being ethical is not just a matter of following rules or laws. In the deepest and most comprehensive way, ethics is a matter of one's personal character, of what is inside a person. We can now see that the reason that the behavior of the "commander" in the case is not only an extreme example of impoliteness, but also serious misbehavior, in that his gestures were indeed teaching gestures. What did they teach?

Psychologists and psychiatrists describe a phenomenon according to which abused persons may easily become abusers in their own right. Violence and lack of respect teaches others to be violent and to be lacking in respect: that was the trenchant lesson that the "commander" taught his students.

In sum:

1 The issue at stake in the case concerns sometimes unexamined medical training and education; particularly "symbolic training" or training for a doctor's professional role.

2 An important part of the symbolic training in medicine concerns training to carry out physical behaviors.

3 These behaviors do not have great importance per se (actually most of them will not be used by future professionals) but are crucial in shaping a doctor's ethics.

4 They are important because they deal with the infringement of body boundaries.

5 This infringement implies a serious, even if often unconscious, stress.

6 The metaphor of the ward as a trench is one of the ways used to cope with this stress.

7 This metaphor, when it is used in the interpersonal relationship between medical teachers and students, has enormous potential for forming unethical habits.

14

Sexual abuse: sexist slur and sexual advances

CASE

"Homework"

A woman physician recalls, "When I was in training a urology resident said to me, "Why don't you come home with me and I'll show you how to pass a catheter." I answered that it wasn't necessary, I'd already done pediatrics."

   Was this sufficient? appropriate? Should I have reported the incident? If so, to whom?

CASE

"What do you like best?"

On one occasion, part of my training as a medical student involved observing and assisting a surgery. The surgeon in preparing the abdomen and pointing out that I was about to hold a retractor asked me pointedly, "Well, which do you like best 4″ or 6″?" Everyone around the table snickered and I was so humiliated I couldn't say a thing. What would have been the best way to handle this situation? Try to think of a witty retort? Take the surgeon to the harassment board?

CASE

"The histology lesson"

As freshmen medical students in Italy, our first lessons were about histology. The practice was for the professor to sit next to the students and explain the slides as he inserted them in the microscope. When my turn came he readied the slide and said,

"These are spermatozoa. You know how they taste, don't you?" As a young, very shy, woman from a provincial town I was stunned and humiliated. I could not raise my head to look at him or bring myself to respond.

COMMENTARY

Domeena C. Renshaw

Physician–patient sex has long been considered a felony in several U.S. states with loss of the license to practice medicine a possible outcome if a physician is charged by a patient and found guilty in a court of law. The code of medical ethics, all the way back to the ancient Hippocratic oath, pledges to protect patients from such sexual misconduct. What is confusing, complex, and less clear is the term sexual harassment. In 1991 Judge Clarence Thomas was accused by employee Anita Hill of sexual harassment. It is conduct considered illegal in the Civil Rights Act of 1964, Title VII. In 1986 the U.S. Supreme Court unanimously affirmed environmental abuse if a worker is compelled to trade sex for job survival. Also unwelcome sexual behavior (offensive flirtation, jokes in poor taste, lewd comments or innuendoes, showing sexually explicit materials) on the job with the effect that it creates an offensive or hostile work environment between someone who has power or authority over one who has less was considered improper. While men and women may interpret the term sexual harassment differently either gender may experience discomfort or humiliation from unwanted sexual comments or suggestions by one in charge. By far the majority who consider they receive sexual harassment and report it are women.

"Homework"

The urology resident was out of line and inappropriate in his response which implied a personal (home) one-to-one visit for the teaching, routinely done in the hospital setting. The line between humor and ridicule is a thin one. The woman student felt put down. She swiftly retaliated with "thanks but no thanks." The question of reporting it is complex. The urology resident may be the one who would evaluate and grade her clinical rotation. If she wished to report the incident, it should be brief, give details of date, setting, name other students present and should be handed in *after* her evaluation by the resident reached the registrar. To whom does she give her report? To the urology resident director if the program has one, or to the chairman of urology. A copy to the dean of students would perhaps be placed in her file. Could this label her a complaining feminist? That depends on the response of those in authority, and is possible.

Because the spectrum of sexual harassment is so wide, diffuse, and subjective, some have attempted to construct a hierarchy i.e.: *mild*: request for a date, whistles, staring; *moderate*: nonsexual unwanted touches, sexual remarks unrelated to work; *severe*: sex propositions related to job retention or advancement, sexual touches; repetition of the unwanted propositions, sexual threat or assault. For the first case, the context and outcome would be considered as would the abuse of power since he was senior to the student. (1)

"What do you like best?"

This is an excellent example of a "soft" sexual innuendo. Only by knowing the specific possible reference to an erection length would anyone consider this sexual. Her silence was an unintended but effective form of "extinction" or ending any sexual emphasis. Consider the six steps of the procedure of reporting this surgeon: (1) the student must write a statement with full details and sign it; (2) find the Hospital's Grievance Committee for Sexual Harassment; (3) the hospital grievance counselors will speak to the student and help her write a letter to the accused surgeon to explain why the incident was perceived as sexual harassment and request cessation and apology; (4) if it continues the student can seek an EEO (equal opportunity officer) for help; (5) if no resolution occurs she can appeal to the hospital superintendent; (6) she can litigate.

Clearly this is time-consuming and daunting to a student or average employee. Often due to lack of leadership or ineptness after a report there is so much hospital inaction that the student graduates two years later and leaves without conclusive resolution. Unfortunately the unethical harasser may continue to harass until someone litigates.

If she gave a sharp witty retort such as: "are you just a 1"? she would sink to his level of sexual innuendo, but usually she would only think of this response on the way home!

"The histology lesson"

This was blatant and cruel misuse of power in the highly unequal teacher–student public classroom setting. The perfect retort would have been, "The sperm are tasteless as is your remark. The seminal fluid is salty-sweet due to the glucose-fructose content the sperm use on their journey to find an ovum." However, the showoff unethical professor achieved his cruel humiliation goal by putting down a woman student. Italy may not yet have sexual harassment laws or grievance procedures. Bullies show up even in medical schools.

An important key element of the still vague and ill-defined issues of sexual harassment is that it makes unwanted and unwelcome remarks to its target either woman or man. They have a right to a full hearing. Making a report may be a difficult, long, and lonely journey because it is not popular to report a superior even when power has been abused. In fact the report may itself be humiliating.

None of these three cases are physician–patient sexual misconduct. They are nonetheless hurtful and memorable to the persons caught in the web of words from the mouth of a colleague who pledged "not to harm." Having a public forum for the sexual remarks that were both tasteless and inappropriate blatantly violated privacy and ethical conduct in each case.

Note

1 Council on Ethical and Judicial Affairs. Sexual misconduct in the practice of medicine. *JAMA* 1991;266:19.

COMMENTARY

Evert van Leeuwen

Ever since the days of the Hippocratic medical priesthood it has been known that the practice of medicine arouses erotic feelings on many occasions, since it involves actions which in daily life are usually related to sexual behavior. The Hippocratic oath early-on forbids physicians from engaging in intimate relationships with patients. Still many TV soaps, movies, and plays hint, speculate on, or present outright erotic feelings between physicians and patients, physicians among themselves, or physicians and other health care professionals, especially nurses. In this instance, the explicit ban is compensated for by a stimulation of fantasy and imagination. One need not be a Freudian or a Victorian to realize that these fantasies and imaginings also go through the heads of physicians and others. The

impression of the beauty of the human body, the particular dealings in the process of physical examination, as well as the reactions of shame and embarrassment, are in practice professionally dealt with usually by each physician, mostly in ways that have become routinized, demonstrating a detached professional persona that has learnt how to deal with these matters.

Besides having to learn to apply knowledge and technology, to be a physician in training means also having to develop a professional attitude. Part of that attitude has to do with any erotic feelings and the fantasies and imaginings belonging to it. To be a trainee bears some resemblance to taking part in a process that has been described as a "rite of passage." Most trainees are vulnerable with respect to their feelings and are likely to show, in spite of their student experiences, a timid and shy attitude when it comes to expressing their own attitudes and morals. The small village of the hospital is still new to them and they have to become acquainted with most of the physical particularities belonging to medical practice. They do not yet possess that detached professional skill and are not ready to employ the different escape-valves doctors use during their work.

A third aspect has to do with the "small village of the hospital," as I have called it. I believe every hospital has its own silent code of communication and action, as a matter of course. "This is how things are done in our house," or "You have to accept our established ways." In our ethics program for trainees in Amsterdam, these silent codes on wards, operating rooms, and in clinics, often form an emotional part of the discussions. "Do you have to accept everything they tell you?" "Is this normal behavior?" The last question is especially intriguing. Role-behavior requires specific attitudes and creates its own morality that can cause all manner of misunderstandings and deviant conduct. Offensive and even abusive behavior towards student doctors who do, but also do not, belong to the inner circle, belongs to the latter category. Still, without the silent code and grind, many things in a hospital would be impossible, hopelessly bureaucratic, or emotionally unbearable. Situations in which people are about to die, are severely ill, or behave awkwardly, can only be managed when the professionals can create outlets, escape valves, for the emotions and feelings which they have successfully controlled in dealing with patients.

Having made these three remarks, how shall we deal with instances of sexual insult or abuse with respect to physicians in training? First of all we have to acknowledge that even the rise of bioethics has not promoted the understanding of the moral issues at hand. The idealized ethically correct physician is not only an emotionally detached professional; she moreover has to be dominantly rational, reasonable, and efficient in ways the Prussian Kant could only dream of. This ethically correct view neglects the simple facts of communication science, in making clear that between 40 and 60% of the communication between patient and physician is not verbal, but physical, in reading attitudes, postures, and so on. (1) Moreover, many physicians never receive any training in sexology, (2) and are hardly experienced in diagnosing sexual problems with their patients, let alone insightful in seeing their own. The outlets and escape valves they create as a result of their professional career are not consciously developed, but are shaped primarily along the lines of the silent code they experienced during their own internship or residency.

The more mental and rational they have to be in their encounter with patients, the more likely they may look for an escape in meeting young, vulnerable, not-yet-colleagues, like trainees. Of course, this displacement in no way justifies offensive or abusive behavior, but it stresses that moral training of physicians should deal with persons of flesh and blood and not only with choice-oriented, politically correct, rational thinking brains. We have to analyze the hidden messages and to create a deeper understanding of the emotions involved in order to let doctors in training master their vulnerability as well as their coping behavior. Not an easy task.

On one occasion, I participated in an ethics session for interns in which there was an intelligent conversation on the balance interns have to seek between accepting and refusing different types of conduct on the part of their peers. Specific attention was paid to the fact that when your resident likes you, everything goes easier. How far should you go? One of the students kept noticeably quiet. She was paying close attention, but the discussion seemed not to involve her particular situation. In trying to facilitate her participation, I focused the issues more on how to say no. She suddenly joined in and started by saying that an attractive physical appearance can be a handicap in being accepted as a serious professional. She was hurt, not only by offensive and abusive remarks aimed at her, but also by the impression people gave that her attempts to become a good physician could not be "her real goal in life," as if she was supposed to be someone else. For her, the only solution was to be true to yourself and do not accept behavior that would make you ashamed outside the medical context.

The problem of course is that trainees do not yet have a professional self that protects them. Some clinical teachers have told me that they sometimes deliberately provoke sexual or erotic remarks. Not bothered by psychoanalytic thinking, their intention is to toughen and strengthen their students. In other words, they play with the taboo, trying to share it with their future colleagues. This approach rarely has the desired effect. Student doctors feel keenly that they must play the role of scapegoat, with all its accompanying vicarious shame. The solution is to create a level of communication at which these matters can be discussed and evaluated. Attitude, communicative behavior, and moral sense are not "natural" or a matter of course. They have to be established in practice and evaluated in practice too.

Currently in the Netherlands, the need for mutual evaluation is becoming more and more recognized in general practice, pediatrics, and internal medicine residencies. It still remains, however, only a beginning. We are only taking the first steps to create a type of medical training that takes into account the physician's behavior as a real flesh and blood person. As such, expressing feelings of hurt, disappointment, harassment, and even making witty retorts, reflect such an approach. Your peers are entitled to know your feelings and reactions, which help contribute to a mutually respectful relationship.

Notes

1 Bensing J. *Doctor–Patient Communication and the Quality of Care, An Observation Study into Affective and Instrumental Behavior in General Practice.* Netherlands Institute for Research in Medicine (NIVEL), Utrecht, 1991.
2 Slob AK, Vink CW, Moors JPC, Everaerd W. *Sexuologie voor de Arts.* Bohn Stafleu Van Loghum, Houten, 1987.

DISCUSSION QUESTIONS

Section 4. Abuse and mistreatment

1 What constitutes abuse is not always easy to define. When do "rude behavior" and "bad manners" become abuse? Where should the line be drawn?
2 Should you not accept some abuse as part of a training period, just as soldiers must accept it during boot camp?
3 When, if ever, can teacher–learner sexual behavior be justified?
4 Feeling abused or humiliated normally elicits anger, how could this be handled most appropriately? And what if the abuse continues?
5 For some people, sexual banter is offensive, while others seem to enjoy it. At what point would you say that such banter constitutes abuse?
6 If you yourself were to be accused of abuse how would you handle it?

Argot, jargon, and questionable humor: assuming the mantle at the patient's expense

In this section we explore deprecating humor. People need a release valve in highly charged emotional situations and using humor is a common way to let off steam. However, danger exists when patients are demeaned in the process. All too often, this kind of humor is used to establish distance and hierarchy as well as a way to overcome fear and anxiety. How should such depersonalizing behavior be handled?

15

Comedians: mordant humor and cynicism

CASE

"You killed one of our patients"

On my first night on call as a third year medical student on internal medicine rotation, a 52-year-old man was brought into the hospital by his son and daughter because of lumbar and bilateral hip pain so severe he could no longer get out of bed. Two months earlier he had gone to his local Emergency Department complaining of a seizure-like episode. His doctors had diagnosed lung cancer with metastasis to his brain and he had undergone surgery to remove his brain tumor.

We began to work to alleviate the pain and performed daily musculoskeletal and neurological exams. This went on for about one week; each morning arriving early to check on the vitals and physical. One morning, strangely enough, I could not locate the man's chart. When I walked into his room, he was no longer there. I was annoyed, believing that my patient had been moved to a different floor, thus wasting my preround minutes. When I approached a nurse to ask the whereabouts of my patient, I was shocked to hear that he had passed away overnight.

I felt strange. I kept thinking about my daily exams and how pointless they had been. I felt neglected; left out. Though only a student, I felt that I should have been there with the family. As I mulled over these thoughts, our team made our way to morning report. Already there, my attending came up to me with a grin on his face, and announced "You killed one of our patients." I replied with fake laughter and let the incident go.

Later that night, when driving home, I realized I

was finally alone with my thoughts. My patient had died that morning. A son and daughter had lost their father. And my attending watched over us with a wide grin on his face. I drove home, wiping away tears of grief.

What should I have done? An obvious conflict, one that all students face, is deference to senior authority. It is unwritten law that students may not talk back to attendings, question their authority or judgment. Besides, when the teacher holds the pen that writes the grade, it makes dissent much more difficult.

CASE

"Laughter and jokes at morning rounds"

In one of the Dutch hospitals where I did my surgery internship it was customary to perform laparoscopic surgeries to reduce the size of the stomach for morbidly obese patients. A patient scheduled to be operated on the next day was a 32-year-old nurse who had been dieting since childhood without success. A year and a half earlier she had given birth to a son, after which she lost a lot of weight. She underwent cosmetic surgery; but a year later she was back to her former weight.

When I presented her during morning rounds there was a lot of laughter and jokes from the residents. They doubted the effects of the upcoming operation saying, "Patients like her will gain the weight back as soon as they discover a milkshake."

Although there were legitimate questions to raise regarding the medical indication for the operation, I was shocked by the disrespect shown for this woman because of her obesity.

COMMENTARY

Barbara Supanich

Both of these cases raise very important ethical issues for the students involved in the cases, for the faculty involved in the cases and a moral challenge for the medical education system.

In the first case, "You killed one of our patients," the student is involved in the care of a man terminally ill with metastatic lung cancer. From the student's perspective, he is relegated to performing routine examinations on the patient each morning, with little sense of the overall plan of care for his patient. The student desires to be an integral part of the medical team. He has most likely participated in the admission process, wrote the order, may have spoken with family members who accompanied the patient to the hospital, and had discussions with the residents concerning the palliative management of the patient. He has invested a part of himself in the care of this patient – intellectually and emotionally. He has an expectation that the residents and the attending will continue to involve him in the care of "his" patient. He comes to work one morning and the way that he finds out about the death of his patient is that he can't find the chart! And, to add injury to insult, the attending physician makes a very pejorative comment to him – "you killed one of our patients."

In the second case, the student is presenting the case of a morbidly obese young woman. The patient has regained her former weight and will be undergoing a repeat operation for her morbid obesity. The student is shocked to hear the residents make disparaging remarks and jokes about the patient during his presentation. The student is expecting to have a professional discussion about the surgery for this patient and instead is

"barraged" by insensitive comments and jokes by the surgery residents.

Both of these cases are examples of physicians violating the ethical guidelines or principles of patient autonomy, respect for the dignity and integrity of the patient and the student, patient beneficence and well-being, and issues related to being a whistle-blower.

In the first case, the student is confronted by a system of medical education and an attending physician who is insensitive and brutalizing. From the student's perspective, he understands his obligation to his patient as providing the "best" possible care. His personal and ethical challenge is that no one on the "team" is providing any guidance to him regarding the level or type of care that this man with terminal cancer desires. Nowhere in this case presentation do we have any commentary concerning the patient's treatment choices. We do not know if the patient expressed his choices to his doctor or family members or if the team took the time to explore these issues with the man at the time of admission. And, if the man was unable to communicate with the physicians at the time of the admission, then did the doctors discuss his treatment options and ask about his preferences with his family? We do not know if he had a durable power of attorney for health care decisions or health care proxy. We do have a sense that his family was with him during this hospitalization.

My sense from reading this case experience is that neither the attending physician nor the residents on this service discussed any of these concerns. And, from the tenor of this case, this was troubling to the student. His interpretation of his experience of going through the motions of a cursory physical examination each morning as being woefully inadequate care is correct, in my opinion! Unfortunately, it is still too frequently the experience of dying patients that they are not asked about their choices for care or treatment options at the end of life and even if they are, these options are often ignored. (1) From this student's narrative, it would appear that this patient was not engaged in any conversations about his care by any of the physicians.

It is my experience that when physicians leave the rounding and examinations of patients with terminal illnesses to the students or residents, it is because the attending physician is very uncomfortable with issues related to death and dying. They have made up their mind that "there is nothing more that they can do," and so in a very real sense, they abandon their patient. Beneficence is a moral obligation that we have to our patients to promote their best interests. This means that we have a duty to understand the patient's values and choices regarding treatment options or approaches. We, as medical educators, also have an obligation to model this type of behavior with our medical students and residents. The physicians in this case did not fulfill this obligation to this patient or the student.

One of the common defense mechanisms that physicians use when they find themselves in very stressful or uncomfortable situations, is "black humor." Black humor is most commonly utilized by residents and attending physicians when they are uncomfortable with certain issues like death, or have strong biases against certain types of people, such as certain racial groups, religions, women, poor people, or morbidly obese individuals. The humor always dehumanizes the groups or person, and tries to take the pressure off of the doctor to confront the issues raised by the situation by scapegoating the patient. This is what happened in the second case – the residents found it easier to be irreverent and disrespectful of the female patient with morbid obesity than to directly discuss the concerns raised by the student regarding a second surgery or the concerns of the patient. I think that cultivating an awareness and deepening the sensitivity of medical students and physicians to the implications of our own prejudices and social biases is crucial to the moral and professional development of the medical profession. (2)

In the first case, the critical moral challenges for the student, I think, are to come to a better understanding of what beneficence means for this patient and for himself, to recapture his sense of self-respect and to demythologize in a safe environment the myth that the attending is "always right." What does beneficence mean for this patient? We really don't know from this scenario. But, I think most human persons, when they are experiencing a critical illness or are near death, want an opportunity to discuss with family and/or their physician their crucial or defining values, concerns, and personal treatment decisions. We need to create environments for our patients and students that will invite and support such conversations.

This student also needs to be treated with respect by his teaching attending and residents. Psychological mistreatment of medical students is unfortunately an all too common experience of students in the U.S. and throughout the world. One study showed that up to 75% of medical students experienced some type of slur by faculty, other clinicians, nurses, or other medical students or residents at least once during their four years of medical education. (3) The challenge of this case is clear – all of us need to create environments in our teaching settings which allow students to feel comfortable sharing their observations and concerns regarding patient care and treatment issues.

In the first case, we also need to demythologize the myth surrounding the medical culture that maintains that the attending physician is "always" right. It is a wiser and more realistic culture, which maintains a *learning* environment for all of us – attendings, professors, students, residents, and patients! Since this is the ideal and certainly not the case for this student, what are his realistic options? I would offer the following strategies. First of all, he needs to identify a safe environment for himself that will afford him an opportunity to openly discuss these ethical issues. This could be with peers, a trusted faculty member, or an outside confidant. Secondly, he needs to identify a trusted senior physician with whom they can discuss such troubling cases and concerns. This can be helpful to them in several ways – they can have their feelings validated, they can verify the ethical issues of the case with a "neutral" third party, and they can obtain clinical and ethical wisdom from a more senior clinician or ethicist. Third, he can explore with the trusted senior faculty member appropriate future strategies for dealing with this particular attending. The faculty member may be very helpful in sorting out personality conflicts from a clear breach of ethics or student abuse.

In the second case, the primary ethical issues for the student are the lack of respect for the patient and blatant stereotyping of this patient; the neglect of the residents to address the risks and benefits of the surgery or other treatment options for this patient; and the issue of how this student can effectively counter such disrespectful comments by more senior clinicians.

Stereotyping of patients and other forms of prejudicial or biased comments are all too common in the morning report room. Terms such as "gomers," "scumbags," and "losers" are all too frequently used by residents and attendings who excuse the behavior due to heavy workloads or minimal sleep or scapegoat the patient. All of us bring who we are into medical school and into the practice of medicine. It is not sufficient to state that your behavior and comments can be explained by the remark: "this is who I am, accept it." We do need to understand each others' background and beliefs, but I would submit that our moral development is as much a part of our continuing medical education as CME topics in cardiology or more effective patient education methods. A physician has an obligation to assure that the best interest of their patient is honored. This cannot be accomplished if the physician holds a very negative viewpoint or bias concerning certain characteristics of patients. Too often the bias can evolve into a moral judgment such as – *all obese patients* are lazy or have no self-control or self-respect. I think that it is a critically important aspect of medical education to assist medical students and residents in under-

standing that their unconscious biases can and do affect their interactions with patients. (2) The medical student is relatively powerless to influence the residency curriculum at this stage of his career. However, he may have influence through curriculum evaluation forms to anonymously make suggestions about this aspect of medical education.

An additional slant to this case is that this is a female patient with morbid obesity. There is literature to support that male physicians are much less tolerant of female patients with a variety of lifestyle issues than men with the same issues. (2) These prejudicial and sexist attitudes need to be consistently addressed in medical school curricula at both the preclinical level and in clerkships. I think that it is less likely that such comments would have been made if the patient were male rather than female.

This student also has the option of choosing to confide in a trusted senior faculty member, in order to discuss his concerns and frustrations and to discuss strategies for coping with attitudes that are personally unacceptable to him. A key part of maturing as a person and as a professional is knowing how to interact with individuals who have values or attitudes that are very different from your own and when and where to challenge them. Students need to have a setting in which they can make such choices and choose which strategy will be of greatest benefit to the patient and themselves. An immediate strategy that the student could use in this case is to not laugh at any of the biased jokes or comments, and redirect the discussion to issues like – what are the proper indications for this surgery; does this patient meet those criteria; what are the risks and benefits for her; does anybody know what her goals are for having the surgery again?

Respect for the patient and her treatment goals are critical to providing her good medical/surgical care. It is our obligation as medical educators to assure that our training programs have zero tolerance for sexist, racist, or any other forms of offensive behavior towards patients or peers.

Notes

1 Solomon MZ, O'Donnell LO, Jennings B, et al. Decisions near the end of life: professional views on life-sustaining treatments. *Am J Public Health* 1993;83:14–23.
2 Kurtz ME, Johnson SM, Tomlinson T, et al. Teaching medical students the effects of values and stereotyping on the doctor/patient relationship. *Social Sci Med* 1985;21(9):1043–7.
3 Uhari M, Kokkonen J, Nuutinen M, et al. Medical student abuse: an international phenomenon. *JAMA* 1994;271(13):1049–51.

COMMENTARY

David N. Weisstub

Some forms of humor are not funny. To sensitive persons, humor at the expense of others should not be encouraged. In child rearing, there are many moments when parents and teachers have to draw the line between the sort of humor where persons share in a perception or find through an experience that the collective reaction is simply to roar in good fun. What is problematic about humor is where to draw the line between sharing and victimizing, between seeing some things as amusing because the object or the brunt of our fun is to turn a person into the other, thereby objectifying, minimizing, and degrading. Oftentimes a member of our community or indeed another community who looks different is simply regarded as marginal because of the current fashion, or bonding which has occurred.

Any well-integrated society must, by the very nature of being a community (Gemeinschaft) develop a humor of its own where persons who are socially adjusted learn the cues of the humor games that are played. So much so that humor often leads to rituals. There is no greater pleasure among the middle-aged or the elderly than to recall with deep nostalgia and gladness those life incidents which are part of collective humorous memory. Having acknowledged this, it is equally important to pay attention to what should be termed the "dark side of humor," and to understand that groups of communities often take the turn in social encounters and historical events where humor becomes black, deviant, and/or punitive.

Socialization within professional education is particularly fascinating with its attendant rituals in respective humor because many of the authority structures, at least in Western society, associated with professionalized humor play a significant role in the creation of what could be termed a professional "skin." Part of profession building in the established professions of law and medicine is to train students, both in forms of distancing and in how to network, interact, and react in achieving a professional persona. Even in the more accommodating and professional institutionalized environments produced by liberal movements in the twentieth century, deep structural forms of paternalism and elitism still persist and are endemic to our very strongly cultural notions of professionalism. Part of becoming a professional is to be able to hear the unspeakable, for example, to be told "you killed one of our patients" and be able to resist such a verbal-emotional attack and bounce back through a form of professional coping mechanism in order to go on performing professional tasks. This is akin to becoming a soldier, to leave the ranks of ordinary citizens, thereby becoming part of a fraternity of hard-nosed survivors, a group known for its capacity to push on in the face of adversity, insults, attacks on ego, even incursions into what are perceived to be the private spheres of emotional or moral life, encompassing race, gender, and ethnicism.

What typifies end-of-century thinking is that our cultural threshold for tolerating attacks on, and even participating in the humor about minorities, oddities, or defects has profoundly diminished. This is sometimes referred to as the culture of political correctness. We currently have a long list of no-nos which arguably have been or should be incorporated even into the corridors of engineering faculties and hospital wards. Put simply, demeaning behavior by professionals towards their clients, particularly when it includes members of a vulnerable population is now perceived as unacceptable, and deserving of admonition, and even social 'ostracization' and penalty or professional discipline.

In the past few decades, there has been heightened awareness, in our post-Holocaust and post-Freudian universe, that Millgram-type experiments tell an important story about how the dark side of humor becomes amalgamated with hierarchical structures to produce beastly or deadly outcomes. In softer forms, black professional humor is often connected to a line of authority where the weaker or dependent members of the social ladder learn the appropriate cues on how to prove that they have stood the test and have, in fact, become one of the boys. This reality can conjure up a feminist debate stating that traditional or establishment male behavior has a tougher or more demeaning manner than any equivalent manifestations in bonding examples of female humor. Equally, charges are made that "majorities" are often smug in their joke-telling and humorous descriptions of the behavior, appearances, or customs of "minorities." In a similar vein, social critics have made the point that frequently it is an earmark or attribute of minority communities that they develop a ghetto mentality which is a euphemism for specializing in inside jokes which target the threatening, often perceived as aggressive, majority group. If these patterns are real, then humor is intrinsic to the fluid functioning of all groups, big or small, male or female, and even if the variances can sometimes depict certain recurrent mores, gender-based attitudes, or profound intergenerational outlooks (mother's milk) there is still the basic, moral question in every case of where lie the moral limits of humor.

Certain negative experiences, that is, desensitizing aspects of professional socialization, seem to have been part of all professions or elites. The relevant question is, whether it is either timely from the point of view of changing social attitudes and/or shared notions of how to educate ourselves, families, and students in the moral life, to put an end to any form of humor that unnecessarily defers to authority and/or builds solidarity on the backs of vulnerable persons. On the one hand, there is the lure to toughen-up young professionals, even if it may lead to some moral infractions. Because it is hoped that the net gain will be to encourage strength and tenacity over fragility and hypersensitivity. The calculation is made that moral adjustments can be made later. The wager is that decent folk will return to their moral upbringing and respected virtues of the moral life appreciated in the culture at large to temper elitism with humility and paternalism with caring. Unfortunately, there is limited evidence, if any, to suggest that with years of socialization, professionals that have been trained in mordant humor subdue cynicism with mercy. Rather, the evidence is more universally present that professionals, like most well-situated citizens, find it difficult to identify with their imperfect clients and/or victims-at-large and more easily accommodate to comfortable associations, either in imagination or the real world, with members of their own social class or inner circle. This raises the point about whether our held beliefs are in fact misguided about how to produce real soldiers, capable doctors, and effective lawyers.

Is it a sign of social weakness and social deterioration for us to outlaw or socially combat strong examples of ethnic jokes, racial slurs, etc.? Positioning ourselves in a world of such questions is part of a larger framework of inquiry, which touches professional socialization. Should we confront medical education in the universe of ward ethics; that is, shocks delivered by authority figures to dependent persons in training about matters of life and death, love, compassion, and integrity? Indeed by training or asking the trainers to become the subject of scrutiny with regard to humor, are we on the right path, or do we rather intrude into the protective sphere of a skewed but justifiable professional morality which builds and rebuilds on its own, reproducing moral narrative? The answer to this question should be the subject of a serious ongoing debate in setting limits for humor-rituals in professional settings.

What we find in the hospital example before us is a situation where resistance against the unwarranted humor of an authority figure may not only lead to a loss of status or professional retaliation, but as well to the rejection of one's peers. They might view "moral seriousness" as a signification of weakness: professionals generally object to any strong form of moral Puritanism. Professionalism brings with it a certain rhythm of daily life such that those who step out of tune are quickly regarded as maladjusted or unsuited to the pressures and strains of professional battle. If this description is correct, then any effective moral solution should lie in a top-down scrutiny of how to improve conditions for a nonthreatening dialogue where standards of respect can be elevated and rewarded in the hierarchy. Until now, the idea that a wide-reaching moral maximization or humanism is the gold standard for professional socialization is naive at best. It therefore is a real challenge for medical educators to try to find the ways in which to improve professional moral standards alongside technological advancement. If anything, the dissociation of doctors from patients, elite professionals from novices has been exacerbated by the propensity of the machine to become the reference point for what matters, works, and attracts approbation. Regrouping the forces of a caring morality in the face of widespread medical technocracy appears like a weak foot in the view of many acclaimed professionals.

Is the case of "you killed one of our patients" a clear example of crossing the line? What if it could be shown that an accompanying reality to the psychopathic grinning of the attending physician in our example was that he had an extraordinary history of a high standard of medical practice over a period of 25 years? Would such

evidence require of us that we should temper our criticisms directly or indirectly, the desire for an actualizing of complaints and even possible organization of collective reprisal?

Sometimes offensive and insensitive conduct in professional training reside in the very same person who is held out by the institutional environment as a celebrated teacher or even a closet grandfather type or humanist. We have all had the experience of a frightening ogre to freshmen being redefined by more senior students as more bark than bite or theater rather than reality. How should we as students, colleagues, or supervisors apply the test of the limits of moral tolerance where there are mitigating or redeeming features? Surely we cannot set the limit to include perversion. The image presented in this case is of a professional who appears to be fearlessly testing and mocking the sensitivity of physicians in training. Short of overwhelming data to support the notion that there is a double or conflicting story being told, resistance against such behavior should be supported, enhanced, and collectively shared. Nevertheless, we must bear in mind there are constructive ways of re-educating authoritarian professionals who have repeatedly tested the limits of black humor, victored there and who have followed the dark corridors where tragedy is treated with mob applause and gaiety. When professional environments begin to show such signs of moral acceptability, there should not be time set aside to reflect on the appropriateness of resistance. In such instances, the reactions should be immediate and swift.

Laughter and jokes at morning rounds

Wellness and health is a state which professional healers see as the object of their interventions. For a long period education has been directed to the end result of applying a technique based upon a ground of knowledge that can defeat what is perceived as a counterforce, illness, a defective appearance, or indeed a genetic handicap. Persons who cannot respond beneficially are quickly regarded as losers in the system, poor invest-ments, or even worse, underline the fact that science and related professionalism are proven inadequate to restructure or realign the course of nature which has been revealed in some inad-equate form. The challenge is so great to match capacity with outcome that poor candidates for healing are sometimes turned into objects of disdain. They are, so to speak, not even worthy of taking risks or making investments because ap-pearance or health-wise they have been shown to be failures in the making, not unlike the presenta-tion of a criminal recidivist before a panel of even would-be penal reformers. Health failures seen in this way are walking embarrassments to health professionals.

It is axiomatic that professionals in training quickly pick up on what is worthy of so-called professional investment. Patients who thwart the system by their inability or incapacitation with respect to benefiting or maximizing their service provisions of any given health system are either avoided or shunted away. The most extreme examples are to be found in terminal chronic wards or in places where social embarrassment has become the effective measuring stick of where medical overseers have been given the right of sustained guardianship. Nursing homes of poor quality and the asylums of yesteryears are notable references. Such sad images are further emotionally stressed when we add to them statis-tical facts that certain populations are dispropor-tionately represented in closed institutions and within the profiles of specific diseases.

Given the fiscal restraints that are currently being experienced in Western industrial states, we have become very reactive to how to prioritize our medical and surgical interventions. This is also true in contexts where the issue is the avail-ability of social or supportive services to medi-cally needy populations. Sadly, in the course of training students or colleagues on how to make difficult choices in health delivery systems, the point is made in the spirit of black humor. In getting persons to distance from the "defective

object," one of the techniques utilized is to bring laughter to the situation where the dismissal of the abandoned person is part of the humorous idea that the chronic, defective, or terminal indi-vidual is actually an enemy of the good practice of medicine or responsible government. That is, the patient is redefined in images captured which lures us to see the person as playing with the system, exploiting resources to the point where we as professionals would be foolish to indulge such behavior. Our tendency towards charity is trumped by the cold water pragmatism, which informs us that the medical user is in fact an abuser.

Examples of cosmetic surgery are telling be-cause here we have a blatant exchange of images between a client and professional. In cases of extreme obesity, the professional is still likely to be left with the reality that the patient will always look like an aesthetic-medical failure. Why treat freaks if real ordinary citizens can be restored to what is perceived from a professional point of view to be a standard of acceptable health? Cases of obesity can also bring highly derisive reactions because one might term these as falling into a mid-level category where laughter still for profes-sionals may appear safe, albeit mean-spirited. Such cases differ from examples where people are born with extreme genetic deformities, are con-fined to wheelchairs, or are in states of depend-ency with an appeal being made on the part of society to administer care to all and any beings born of human parents. Even though persons committed to theological belief systems may find themselves failing morally in participating in laughter about fatness because there is somehow the belief that this condition is brought on by ingratitude with regard to potential health and is self-induced. So viewed obesity is looked upon as a state distinguishable from cases of true depend-ency and/or misery. In this way, fat persons even when unjustified are often condemned for their state of ugliness or weakness. This has certainly not been helped by our body-building cultures which have accentuated the beauty of leanness in this century, nor by the advertising images portrayed by the divergent cultures which have trained populations to eye beauty within highly defined parameters. Medical professionals who are part of a larger culture will inevitably reflect the values, images, and attitudes of prevailing mind-sets. Although an uphill battle, medical educators must take it upon themselves with the assistance of persons who specialize in image-making to re-educate how we approach symbols of medical failure or ugliness and the way in which we respond to these images in medical decision making in diversified contexts and environments. Laughing about obesity is part of a larger trajectory that stretches to include how we look upon elderly persons who have begun to regress into infantile patterns of behavior. Our social intolerance for situations which "do not look good" and where we think even with a great deal of investment there is little prospect for improvement are just those arenas where the level of civility of a society is tested. Every effort should be made in professional settings to control and to lead to the conditions of social judgment, appropriate dialogue, and even confrontation when members of such professional communities from students to respected elders participate in mockery and mirth in the face of ugliness and despondency.

16

What's in a name? Derogatory references

CASE

"Goombah"

As a medical student on the wards one of the things that startled me quite a bit was the amount of questionable humor that surrounds interactions between physicians. I admit that I also find the use of certain "nonclinical" terms funny; although sometimes I wonder if I would laugh as hard under different circumstances. For instance, referring to a mass on an X-ray or a growth subcutaneously as a "goombah" occurs fairly frequently. When describing a case to the floor consultant I have heard phrases, and repeated them myself, such as "This is a 34-year-old white male with a big ol'goombah on the left side of his neck." I then proceed to describe the mass and the location in more detail. It sets the tone of the interaction as one of both interesting pathophysiology and some degree of lightheartedness. Would the patient take offense at my description? Would he care? What if he were an inpatient and we were standing outside his room and he could overhear us discussing his case?

I am reminded of the time an 83-year-old woman was admitted with a basal cell cancer that had eroded through her nose. It was such a sight that many physicians on the floor (on other inpatient teams and from other consult services) were alerted to the severity of her mass and the rarity of the physical diagnosis opportunity. When we were rounding in the morning outside her door our leader said with the appropriate hand gesture to the face, "And what's up with our little old lady with the thing on her nose?" When I asked why we couldn't move a few doors down to discuss her he

said, "It's not as if she doesn't know why she's here." Does the fact that it was sort of funny and we, as a team, snickered a little, mean I am truly a horrible person for finding humor in the way a patient is presented?

CASE

"Shooter with a fever"

As a medical student on the wards I found that describing an intravenous drug addict with a high temperature as "shooter with a fever" failed to draw pangs of astonishment because the categorization was used by *everyone* there. "Shooter with a fever" brings to mind a specific course of treatment, specific antibiotics used, and a range of microbes to worry about. Does using that description lessen the patient's status any more than "IV drug user with a fever?"

CASE

"The 'gorked gomer'"

It was 3:00 a.m. and an elderly homeless person had just been admitted to the emergency room. At the bedside I started to wash up with the residents. One resident seemed tired and angry and said, "I can't believe we got beeped out of bed for this gomer." The other resident nodded in agreement and said, "Hopefully this won't take too long. The patient is gorked-out already."

Knowing that "gomer" stands for "get out of my

emergency room," and refers to patients who require a huge amount of care that is thought not worth the effort, and "gork" means "God only knows," describing patients who are unresponsive and out of it, what should I have done? What might I have said?

CASE

"FOB"

During rounds one morning a patient who was brought in the night before was described as "FOB." I was a medical student and unfamiliar with the term. When I asked what "FOB" meant there was a lot of laughing as the resident said, "fresh off the boat." I was so stricken I said nothing. Later, I wondered what they would have said if I had told them my parents escaped to this country on a boat.

COMMENTARY

Jacquelyn Slomka

Goombahs and gomers: the ethics of biomedical slang

Most third year medical students enter the clinical world armed with scientific knowledge and idealism. They soon discover that clinical education is not simply an application of scientific principles to the correct medical situations, nor is clinical practice always the compassionate endeavor they might have expected. Clinical training involves a socialization into the work group of the medical team, which has its own norms and standards. Clinical training also involves socialization into the "subculture" of medicine, which has a particular language and set of values. Like the foreign language student who, upon arriving overseas, is dismayed to discover that the natives do not speak the language according to the textbook, so too the medical student, upon beginning

his or her clinical rotations, may be surprised to find that his or her professional colleagues fail to speak perfect scientific "medicalese." The student instead discovers that the language of the hospital is full of slang expressions and new idioms that he or she must learn in order to function and survive. Unexpectedly, medical slang often reflects negative values derived from the realities of the hospital setting. To those uninitiated into the clinical world, these values challenge their idealism.

These four cases contain examples of what linguistic anthropologists and folklorists refer to as "speech play," a playful, often humorous, and consciously artful manipulation of language. (1) These cases evoke an uneasiness for the students on several levels. The students have endured two years of intense study of scientific terms and concepts, yet in the language of the clinical setting, certain scientific terms are seemingly devalued. In fact, using the nonscientific term paradoxically demonstrates the clinical experience of the speaker – the slang term is used not because the speaker lacks knowledge, but precisely because he/she is very knowledgeable, to the point that he or she can "play" with the medical language. At the same time some of the nonscientific terms sound mildly flippant or disrespectful, while others are frankly insulting or offensive. The student may experience conflict in admiring the speech play because it connotes clinical expertise of the speaker, yet condemning it for its aura of disrespect to the patient.

Occasionally, terms that may have originated as speech play are used in an angry or abusive manner and neophyte students receive another blow to their idealism: physicians can become angry at patients. Not only do they become angry, but the power differential within the physician–patient relationship and medicine's assumed aura of beneficence enable physicians to act out their anger within a socially accepted context. "The dammed little brat must be protected against her own idiocy . . ." says William Carlos Williams in "The Use of Force," as he forcibly tries to pry open a child's mouth to examine her throat. (2) In a setting where the lines between "doing good" and "doing harm" are often blurred, the student may learn that the only difference between necessary harm and patient abuse lies in his or her own internal sense of professionalism.

In the first case, the term "goombah" is used in contrast to the medical–scientific description of the patient's neck mass. The term is one that an adult might use with a child, just as parents might describe urination to a toddler as "going wee-wee." But the patient is not a child and herein lies the uneasiness of the student. While physicians are often admonished for using technical language in speaking with patients, the term "goombah" seems to go to the other extreme and infantilizes the patient. Would the patient take offense at the term? It would depend perhaps on how well the physician knows the patient and on how the physician presented it. Words may have powerful meanings. The term "tumor" or "mass" could invoke fears of cancer and death for some patients. In such a fearful patient, if the mass is benign, the use of the playful term could convey to the patient the nonserious nature of the mass. On the other hand, if a malignancy were suspected, the use of the term might convey a falsely benign impression to the patient. If clinicians are unsure about whether a patient would find a phrase or word play humorous, the safest course may be to err on the side of formality and avoid the slang expression.

The description of the woman with the cancer eroding through her nose could be viewed as "gallows humor." Noses can be funny – recall Samantha the Witch making magic by wriggling her nose, or Jimmy Durante's "schnoz." Contrast the horror of this woman's disfiguring cancer. Humor is often used in clinical settings to cope with the helplessness, anger, fear and other strong emotions that disease, death and uncertainty evoke. (3) Gallows humor can be forgiven. But gallows humor and the comment, "It's not as if she doesn't know . . ." within earshot of the patient, suggests an insensitivity to the patient's

plight that is less easy to forgive. Is the indifference displayed by the team leader a result of the proverbial harshness of medical training that robs future physicians of the capacity for empathy? Or do the leader's comments reflect a general lack of respect for elderly persons, a seemingly common phenomenon in today's society? The use of the term "little old lady" (sometime abbreviated as "LOL") has moved from speech play to political incorrectness in its image of both age and gender bias. (Furthermore, the closer this writer gets to becoming a "little old lady," the more offensive she finds this term!)

"Shooter," on the other hand, is an adoption of street language for the medical description of "IV drug user," and to some extent this term has entered our popular culture through television and film. The fact that "everyone" was using the term may simply suggest a knowledge and adoption of the latest slang expressions. An aspect of speech play is evident here as both "shooter" and "fever" are two-syllable words and both end in "-er." Short-hand expressions are useful in case presentations, and objectification of the patient ("IV drug user"; "shooter") occurs in the course of case reporting. However, the danger lies in extending this objectification to the interpersonal aspects of the therapeutic relationship. Henry notes that what makes individuals "persons" is that they are connected to the social system by symbolic attachments. (4) A name is such a symbolic attachment. When Mr. Smith or Ms. Jones becomes "the IV drug user" or "the shooter," or when Ms. Brown becomes the "little old lady with the thing on her nose," they are depersonalized, treated as less than persons, because they are not accorded the symbols of attachment that keep all of us connected to our social system. It is often argued that objectification and emotional distance are necessary for the good mental health of clinicians. The challenge for professionals is finding the appropriate balance between a self-protective psychological distance and an emotional closeness that permits a therapeutic empathy with the patient.

Physicians in other countries probably use speech play, but the extent to which it occurs in other medical systems is not known. One example, however, comes from the Moroccan health care system. In Morocco, biomedical physicians are trained in the French system, and biomedicine coexists with a traditional medical system. The scientific medical language of the physician is French, while the language of the average lay person is Arabic. As in the American system, Moroccan biomedicine deals with organic disease as separate from the psychological and emotional aspects of illness. Moroccan biomedical physicians frequently encounter patients who complain that "everything hurts." Because no disease concept ideally fits this phenomenon, biomedicine assigns a psychological label – usually a form of depression. When a patient enters the clinic complaining that "everything hurts," physicians facetiously refer to the patient's illness as "la kollshite." This term is a combining of the Arabic word for "everything" ("koll shi") with the French suffix "-ite," which designates a word as an illness. (In English, the "-ite" suffix corresponds to "-itis." For example, "bronchitis" and "laryngitis" become "la bronchite" and "la laryngite" in French.) The word is politically loaded in that it represents the power of biomedicine to define what is and what is not an illness. The patient knows he or she is "sick all over," but no syndrome exists in biomedicine for a totality of symptoms. The term "la kollshite" is intentionally facetious and reflects the physician's frustration and inability to deal with the patient's symptoms. But speech play also can work to underscore the social, political, and cultural dimensions of illness. The French/Arabic linguistic dichotomy of "la kollshite" parallels the cultural and social dichotomies of Moroccan society – modern/traditional, educated/illiterate, rich/poor, urban/rural – between the physician and patient, between traditional medicine and biomedicine, and between urban and rural segments of Moroccan society.

The speech play of American biomedicine likewise may emphasize political, social, and cultural differences between professionals and their patients. In the fourth case, the acronym FOB rhymes with the common acronym used for shortness of breath (SOB), and could therefore be considered to be speech play. The fact that the term was viewed negatively by this student, implies that the patient described as FOB either was an immigrant or a foreigner. Without more contextual information, the use of this term is difficult to assess. However, the scenario suggests the term was used to underscore the patient's differentness in a negative, possibly derogatory way.

The insidious notion that some patients are more deserving of medical care than others appears to be fairly prevalent among some clinicians, but perhaps should not be unexpected given the profit-oriented nature of health care today. In the case of the "gorked gomer," it is not simply fatigue that drives the residents' behavior; they are also judging the "social worth" of this elderly, homeless patient. Would they react the same way to the elderly parent of one of their friends or a retired medical school faculty member? Does their hasty judgment of the patient as "gorked out" suggest the patient will not get an adequate work-up of a mental status change or other problems for which he was admitted? In Samuel Shem's novel, *The House of God*, the term "gomer" was used in frustration by the residents, but still had the character of speech play, as in their construction of the feminine form, "gomere." (5) Certainly residents who are sleep-deprived and overworked are going to be less able to cope with complicated medical situations and may be less able to be empathetic with patients. But in the above scenario, the terms are not used as speech play, but as verbal abuse. The import of the residents' statements is that the patient is not worthy of their time and lost sleep, nor of the knowledge and skills over which they are supposed to act as society's stewards.

What can the student do? Because the residents are in a supervisory role, it would be difficult for the student to challenge their behavior. Perhaps one solution is for the student simply to recognize the behavior for what it is and to resolve not to emulate it. But the student should also recognize the wider implications of verbal abuse and inappropriate use of medical slang – that they are symptomatic of a less caring health care system in a less caring society.

Clinicians will continue to use medical slang. As a general rule, speech play should remain "backstage," out of hearing of patients. Speech play is inappropriate when it becomes verbally abusive, or when it is used maliciously to denigrate the social worth of a person or class of persons.

Students can use informal meetings, ethics case discussions, or medical student meetings as arenas for talking about the uses and abuses of medical slang. As a group, students could address the issue of patient abuse with program directors, or with individual mentors as a means of changing behaviors. Ultimately, change at a higher level of the organization may be necessary as verbal abuse will continue to exist in a system that tolerates it. The idealism that students bring to the clinical setting is a foundation for their future professionalism. Words and meanings can shape the way this sense of professionalism develops. Students and other clinicians should choose their words carefully.

Notes

1 Burson-Tolpin A. Fracturing the language of bio-medicine: The speech play of U.S. physicians. *Med Anthropol Q* 1989;3(3):283–93.

2 Williams WC. The use of force. In *One Doctoring: Stories, Poems, Essays*, ed. R. Reynolds & J. Stone. Simon and Schuster, New York, 1991, pp.92–5.

3 Bosk CL. Occupational rituals in patient management. *N Engl J Med* 1980;303(2):71–6.

4 Henry J. *On Sham, Vulnerability and Other Forms of Self-Destruction*. Vintage Books, New York, 1973.

5 Shem S. *The House of God*. Dell Publishing Co., New York, 1978.

COMMENTARY

Harvey M. Weinstein

What's in a name? Derogatory references

The first article of the 1948 Universal Declaration of Human Rights states that "All human beings are born free and equal in dignity and rights." The concept of dignity underlies human rights thinking and law as it has evolved in the last 50 years. For me, it is useful to think about my role as a physician in terms of how I respect the dignity of my patients, the dignity of my profession, and my own dignity as a human being. Dignity is a complex concept – it involves a recognition that another person has worth; that compassion for others honors them because they are alive and because whatever their life circumstances, they are entitled to the same rights, privileges, and respect as everyone else. Underlying this basic concept of human rights is the acceptance of difference, whether it is racial or ethnic, gender or age, able or disabled, familiar or foreign. If we take seriously the physician's adage to "do no harm," then openness to difference and acceptance of basic human dignity will require that we treat equally all who come under our care.

Humor is a critical aspect of healing. It is also a significant coping mechanism when we are faced with stress, pain, and fear. Humor ought to be part of every physician's lexicon, of the repertoire used to deal with death, decay, and even depravity. Humor can help our patients face the future; it can help us face the death of a child or the frustrations of being unable to ameliorate suffering. Humor can also distance us from those who seek our skills, guidance, and knowledge. It may, however, become a suit of armor – protecting us and ensuring that we do not feel compassion; it allows us to so dehumanize those in need that they become organs or lumps and bumps, less than human but safe to treat as long as the interaction is constrained and emotions controlled.

I have long wondered about the distance we are

taught to maintain. I remember being told in medical school, "Don't get overinvolved." But what does that mean? How can I not be involved with the young woman who is paralyzed following an automobile accident? How can I not be involved with the teenager who has just overdosed on drugs? How can I not feel for the alcoholic man who has lost everything and now sits in the emergency room with no one to care for him? I have also wondered about the awesome power that physicians are granted by society. To be dying, to be in pain, to face loss – these are the times of greatest vulnerability. And it is the physician who is there, counseling about treatment options, advising about life styles, keeping people out of the country, allowing others to enter. Without the acknowledgement of human dignity, then we become mere technicians, processors of life and death. We abuse our power and we are the poorer for that.

In recent years, I have been working in Bosnia. I have also worked with refugees in America. I have heard about ethnic cleansing; I have listened to stories of torture and genocide. I have heard of doctors who travel the world providing humanitarian aid to those in greatest need. However, I have also heard about physicians who participate in torture, who advise the torturers or falsify death certificates. There are physicians who cut off hands and carry out the state's will. Under the guise of patriotism, physicians heal the state and sacrifice the individual. Under the guise of science, physicians participate in unethical human experimentation. In Bosnia, physicians made choices about who to treat based on ethnic difference. When people become dehumanized and those in power support their humiliation, the line between distancing and active destruction becomes blurred.

What does this have to do with medicine in the United States or other Western countries? Although not as blatant, we do provide discriminatory care. We only need ask who has access to coronary artery bypass surgery, renal transplants, or hip surgery? When we label someone as a "gomer" or "FOB," are we not placing them in a category of the unwanted? By ignoring the whole person, the powerful self-fulfilling prophecy ensures that they will live up to our diminished expectations. If they become "the other," are we fulfilling our trust or are we contributing to the dehumanization of those who seek assistance and betraying our ideals? Distancing is a slippery slope for those on whom society confers such power.

The vignettes suggest that the "humorous" language of medicine forces medical students and house officers to examine its effect on their peers, themselves, and most importantly, their patients. Do patients resent being labeled as someone with a "thing" or a "goombah?" Most likely, they will say nothing. When someone is vulnerable and depending on the other for care, the power imbalance is so profound that questioning the authority becomes too frightening. And yet, powerless and afraid, the patient's sense of being human is further eroded by such flippant allusions. So too, we question ourselves when we use these words, "Am I truly a horrible person?" No. We act to protect ourselves and to fit in with our peers. The challenge is to discover how to use humor to benefit both patients and ourselves while maintaining the dignity that all are entitled to. I would also say that a "shooter with a fever" and "an IV drug user with a fever" both dehumanize. The patient is more than a drug user. He is a man, perhaps a father or husband, a son, an engineer, a lover, and a friend. Labels narrow the focus and lose the humanity. Finally, the peer pressure to use these words is great. For students to stand up to house staff or attendings is difficult. But these are "teachable moments" – opportunities to support our profession by restoring to it the compassion and respect for basic dignity that earned it society's trust.

DISCUSSION QUESTIONS

Section 5. Argot, jargon, and questionable humor: assuming the mantle at the patient's expense

1 How do the slang and jargon that permeate professional conversations on the wards provide insights to the speaker's values as well as his or her fear, anger, and frustration?
2 What clues about these fears and anger have you picked up in your training?
3 What have you done with those clues, if anything?
4 What are appropriate responses to slang and jargon used by your peers? By your superiors? By those who evaluate you?
5 Is remaining silent when others refer to patients in disparaging or derogatory ways complying with that behavior? What type of response is called for?
6 Would it make a difference, and if so how, if an offending remark regarding a patient is made by: a fellow medical student? an intern? chief resident? attending? chief of service?
7 What words about patients offend you the most? Why?
8 Have you ever caught yourself using jargon or slang about patients' suffering? How did you feel about it afterwards – like "an insider," "one of the in-group," or did you feel badly that you succumbed to the temptation?

Making waves: questioning authority and the status quo

Perhaps the most looming obstacle for trainees trying to act morally is the perception of medical hierarchy and struggling to find their place in that hierarchy. Challenging the decisions and actions of someone higher in authority can be the most threatening and unsettling of dilemmas. Inevitably moments arise when trainees question the decisions of their superiors. This raises tremendous conflicts. Should they press to question authority, or stifle their objections in respectful silence? To what extent should they perhaps put their career in jeopardy by challenging the system? What should the response be, for example, if the student is asked to do a procedure a superior does not want to do, on for example an AIDS patient? At the same time, positioning oneself for a more favorable place in the hierarchy, even to the detriment of peers, becomes difficult to resist. This problem of accepting the status quo is amplified when influence is peddled by drug companies and other outside forces.

17

Personal identity

CASE

"Who am I"

As medical students we were not discouraged from introducing ourselves by saying "Hello, I'm Dr. So and so," as opposed to identifying ourselves as students. If we happened to be doing rounds with an intern or resident, the physician would introduce himself or herself as "Dr. X and over here is Dr. Y" – indicating a student. When I introduced myself as a medical student, I got the feeling people thought it was silly or unnecessary.

CASE

"Don't tell her you are a medical student"

As a medical student I overheard an intern tell a fellow third year student to get a history from a patient, "But, don't tell her you are a medical student because she won't talk to you."

CASE

"Premature description"

As medical students we were given no instructions as to the proper way to identify ourselves to patients. I saw classmates introducing themselves as "Dr." and one student even secured a credit card with "MD" after his name. I was uneasy about this less than honest self-description, but the practice was common and the perpetrators were never corrected by faculty.

CASE

"The anonymous greeter"

The first morning of my internship in ophthalmology I arrived at the Amsterdam office of the specialist to whom I was assigned. He was a gruff, authoritarian man, and I was a bit afraid. I introduced myself and repeated what I understood to be my function. I would meet the patients and escort them to his office where I would observe the consultation.

After I shook hands and introduced myself to the first patient, the doctor called me aside and told me I was supposed to greet his patients anonymously and without hand shaking. His reason was that interactions wasted time and spread bacteria. I was aghast. I thought his instructions were impolite and undignified and would leave patients wondering what I was doing there.

Up until that time in my training I had acquired a certain understanding of how patients should be treated which included an introduction and some description of the role of their health care personnel. Was I wrong?

CASE

"Without portfolio"

At the end of my second year as a medical student, I received an externship at a hospital and was looking forward to an important learning experience before I started my clinical rotations. When I arrived, I was shocked to find myself responsible for a ward of 30 patients. Theoretically, there was supposed to be attending supervision; but in reality there was none. There was no one to rely on and I had no clinical experience. I carry many awful memories of that time, but the worst was when one of the patients had a cardiac arrest. With only another medical student (also without clinical experience), and myself to attend to him, he died.

COMMENTARY

Griffin Trotter

"Who am I?" Our question from the first case would fit rather comfortably in a primer for adolescents. We might also expect to hear it issuing from the bluish lips of an inebriated, chain-smoking existentialist. But the question in question seems a little oblique to practical medical ethics. Shouldn't we stick to the basics and concentrate on articulating medical values that enjoy consensus support?

I believe, to the contrary, that questions of personal identity constitute a central moral problem for students of medicine. Training to be a doctor is a process of self-transformation where success is measured largely by the ability to reengineer one's personhood in a manner that integrates values and norms of a new, physician identity. By invoking the concept of an identity crisis, and exploring its moral and psychological dimensions, we can shed light on a number of ethical dilemmas that confront medical students. From the standpoint of descriptive ethics, the identity crisis may be an appropriate model for understanding the genesis of these dilemmas. From the normative standpoint, insights about the resolution of identity crises (coupled with the assumption that a functional, integrated sense of personal identity is morally desirable) can provide guidance for the cultivation of clinical virtues and for critical appraisal of the moral tradition in medicine.

The identity crisis, often misunderstood as

solely a problem of adolescence or middle age, is a ubiquitous aspect of human experience, occurring at any age. Roy Baumeister and his associates have distinguished two varieties of such crises. (1) The first – identity deficit crisis – occurs when personal identity is not sufficiently developed to meet current demands. Identity conflict crisis, the second form, occurs when various components of personal identity generate conflicting demands.

The circumstances of medical training provide a perfect medium for identity deficit crisis. In the effort to become doctors, medical students strive to establish a radically new and thoroughgoing component of personal identity. In early clinical years, they are often asked and expected to do the things that doctors do, as if they were, in fact, already doctors. They approach patients in white coats, asking serious questions and examining exposed flesh. They are frequently expected – by patients, nurses, fellow students, and attending physicians alike – to generate sophisticated diagnoses and treatment plans, and to impart medical wisdom seamlessly to patients. Of course, if they were up to these tasks, there would be no need for medical training. Hence, there is fertile ground for an identity deficit crisis. Medical students never know enough, never exhibit enough skill, and never harbor enough experience in the ways of clinical medicine to meet the demands of full service doctoring. This failure to measure up is acutely painful and, at times, debilitating. However, it is also a stimulus to moral and personal growth.

Several maladaptive ways of coping with identity deficit are illustrated in our cases. It may be reassuring or even exhilarating for medical students to introduce themselves as "Doctor." Getting a credit card with "MD" on it could have a similar effect. However, these practices strongly countervail one of medicine's core values – honesty. As such, they fail not merely because they are objectionable, but also because they do not succeed in ameliorating the identity crisis. Calling oneself "Doctor" isn't a very effective way of alleviating anxiety about insufficient knowledge or skill. A more likely result is a magnification of feelings of inadequacy and guilt. Not only is the student who calls herself "Doctor" not a real doctor, but now she is also a liar. Trust is the cornerstone of patient–physician relationships and honesty is the medium of trust. Any attempt to establish one's professional identity by sacrificing these values will be counterproductive – heaping an identity conflict on the already inevitable identity deficit.

Faculty members and residents may be culpable for creating ethical dilemmas of this nature. In our first case ("Who am I?"), faculty members apparently engage in a habit of introducing students as doctors. If students later explain to patients that they are actually students, then the faculty members' deceptions are exposed and confidence undermined. Students may also be vulnerable to the wrath of attending physicians. On the other hand, if students acquiesce to the charade, they are cooperating with dishonesty and undermining one of medicine's pivotal values. In the second case ("Don't tell her you are a medical student"), a resident advises a student to deceive the patient. Here the student will also be vulnerable to recriminations if he or she insists on being fully honest to the patient.

Regrettably, the practice of introducing medical students as doctors or pretending that they are doctors is common. This practice is based ostensibly on concern for the well-being and comfort of patients. The reasoning seems to be that if patients believe real doctors rather than students are attending them, they will remain sanguine. The patient, thus deceived, will be more likely to trust the student and will not suffer uncomfortable doubts about the quality of medical care. Hence, the strategy is based on the paradoxical notion that we should cultivate trust through deception. As such, it is a classic instance of beneficence twisted into paternalism.

The assumption that patients will be unable to handle the generally benign presence of medical students is ungrounded. Certainly some patients will have misgivings about students in certain situations. Often, these misgivings can be corrected with frank discussion. I frequently tell patients that having a medical student involved in their care is a distinct advantage. Since the case load for medical students is much smaller than for residents and attending physicians, the patient gets more attention from the student than would normally be available from attending physicians. Often a diligent student will uncover crucial historical information or pursue fruitful lines of inquiry just because he or she has the additional time that is required for these efforts. Meanwhile, double doses of attention are garnered from the attending, who must assess the patient herself while also addressing the medical student's assessment. The vast majority of patients will acknowledge this benefit.

And what if patients staunchly refuse to be examined by students? No doubt, this situation will arise. But it is uncommon. After explaining possible disadvantages that patients will suffer under such an arrangement, it is probably best in these cases to excuse the medical students. Of course, there is an ethical issue about whether patients have a right to expect competent medical care when they will not cooperate in establishing the necessary conditions for such a right (namely, the education of physicians). However, this issue is not a central concern, since most patients are very willing to be seen by medical students.

Perhaps the practice of deceiving patients about the status of medical students is ultimately motivated more by a desire to avoid discomfort to physicians and students than it is for the benefit of patients. If so, the practice is clearly unjustified. As the testimony of medical students in our cases illustrates, this deception is (and should be) a source of moral anxiety for students. Further, even if students and faculty feel better in the long run when they execute such deceptions, the moral imperative in medicine is primarily to benefit patients. The duty of beneficence, in turn, requires honesty and the cultivation of trust. If a certain amount of embarrassment or other personal discomfort is required in order to preserve integrity, then so be it.

"The anonymous greeter" and "Without portfolio" are also examples of how insecurity about one's clinical identity can be exacerbated by irresponsible medical educators. In the latter case, absent medical supervision is particularly grievous because of the endangerment to patients. How students should respond when thrust into such unfair situations is a difficult issue. It would be simple in theory to endorse a zero tolerance policy, advising students to revolt at every unjustified deception and every instance of unethical behavior on the part of attending physicians or residents. However, the policy of prudently choosing one's battles is a more defensible strategy. For instance, the intern in the ophthalmology clinic would be justified in acquiescing to the "anonymous greeter" protocol if he or she judged that there was little hope of making headway by discussing it with the attending physician. The student in the unsupervised ward would have a greater responsibility for opposing the status quo, since it poses a serious and direct threat to patient welfare. Even here, however, there are several factors that would lessen the obligation to confront the problem directly. There could be limitations in medical resources that make such lapses temporarily inevitable; or an authoritarian power structure might make it patently impossible and inherently self-destructive for students to attempt to initiate meaningful reform.

Cases where students are asked to misrepresent themselves as physicians may be more straightforward. Lying and dishonesty are rarely if ever justified. Not only do such practices undermine legitimate trust, but they are considered by some moral philosophers to be inherently immoral even apart from the bad consequences. They fall awry of moral standards by failing to respect the dignity of patients as relatively autonomous moral agents who deserve and need to know the truth about their medical care. Students should refrain from calling themselves "doctor" and they should refuse to participate in such deceptions. If a student is introduced as "Dr. Y," he should generally respond at the earliest practical moment with something like, "actually, I am a medical student here at Hometown University."

Once again, however, there is an element of moral nuance. It is possible in unusual circumstances that a student would produce severely negative repercussions for herself or for the care of her patient by exposing such a deception. More often, however, acquiescence betrays lack of courage or resolve. No doubt, medical educators and supervisors are more culpable for such evils than medical students, but students also bear responsibility when they cooperate. One of the oldest and most important moral insights is the notion that every decision, no matter how small, is an act of self-construction. If we repeatedly cooperate with seemingly trivial deceptions, we eventually become habituated to deception. We become dishonest people and, in this case, untrustworthy physicians.

Medical students are faced with the daunting task of establishing a strong sense of personal identity and professional integrity in an environment that challenges them from every angle. This challenge may become almost unbearable when role models upon whom students depend ask them to participate in practices that undermine core professional values. In the long run, students will be able to overcome such obstacles only if they develop a vivid image of the ideal physician they hope to become. Three strategies may help: (i) Establish one or more attending physicians as special mentors or exemplars of professional virtue. When other supervisors exhibit morally culpable behavior, these bad examples can be countered with mental images of how the chosen mentor would behave differently under similar circumstances. Students may then attempt to be true to this higher standard. (ii) Identify medicine's core values – the values that every great physician supports. Think seriously about these values and periodically reflect on how they are (or aren't) manifested in clinical practices. Interestingly, even medical rebels like Hawkeye Pierce (from the film MASH) and George Clooney's character in "ER" exhibit fidelity to core values, such as compassion and honesty, and they are honored just insofar as they are loyal to these values. (iii) Create a personal strategy for cultivating core values. Each medical student should be honest about his or her strengths and weaknesses. The chosen specialty should be a means of accentuating strengths and of developing a personally inspired and unique way of serving. But there should also be an effort to target important personal weaknesses for improvement. For instance, students who lack empathy should go to special lengths in order to cultivate this capacity, attempting to be even more empathetic than ordinary virtue would require.

Note

1 Baumeister RF, Shapiro JP, Tice DM. Two kinds of identity crisis. *Pers* 1985; 53:407–24.

COMMENTARY

Kate Christensen

What do we call ourselves, when we are not yet doctors but are caring for patients? Will patients think less of us if we introduce ourselves as students or residents; will they feel less confident in our care and less likely to follow our recommendations? Every medical student and resident faces this issue at some point in their training. I faced it in my first month as a medical student. One of my fellow students passed out his new business cards, which said "Doctor John __" and urged us to call each other doctor, for practice. This bit of deception, even if it was only self-deception, disturbed many of us, and we persuaded him to stop.

The temptation to deceive arose again when we started our hospital duties with patients in our third year of medical school. We were still students, with no MD after our names, but the real physicians supervising us introduced us to patients as "doctors." Were we to object to this, risking embarrassment for our attending phys-

icians and possible reprimand for ourselves? And anyway, after so many years of thankless toil to get where we were, wasn't it about time we were given a little respect, even if it was a bit premature? The truth was, most of us secretly liked it. It gave us a taste of the respect and power we knew would soon be rightfully ours.

Are there any legitimate reasons for this deception? Most patients do feel more comfortable and comforted in the hands of a doctor than those of a student, and might be more apt to comply with the treatment plan. A more compelling argument is efficiency; when introducing a team of students, residents and attendings on hospital rounds it becomes quite cumbersome to describe the training status of each. Doing so can also be bewildering for the patients. And in the broader scheme of things, patients are contributing (although often unknowingly) to the greater good by serving as teaching material for future doctors.

There may be another reason for calling students "doctor" in public hospitals, where most of the patient care is provided by physicians in training. I trained as a medical student in a county hospital and at a Veteran's Administration hospital. The unspoken concern was that if a patient was told their "doctor" wasn't a doctor, they might demand to be cared for by a real doctor, and the system was not set up to provide this. Furthermore, I doubt that most patients realized that 90 per cent of their care was provided by trainees and that at night, there was no board-certified doctor in the hospital at all.

What was wrong with this? From our perspective, very little, aside from some qualms about the slight dishonesty involved. The problem becomes obvious when we change places with the patient – now how does this slight dishonesty look? I am being introduced to the physician who has my health in her hands, and am informed that she is "Doctor Jones." I have no reason to think she is not. I have every reason to think she has some experience with my illness, with the medications she is prescribing, with the tests she is ordering. If and when I find out that she is still two years away from even having a license to practice medicine, that she has in fact never treated my illness before, I am apt to feel angry, afraid, and betrayed. I have been deceived, and not for my own benefit but for the ego of the "doctor" or for the financial benefit of the hospital.

When looked at from the patient's perspective, we can see that the right to know the training status of those providing our care is part and parcel of the informed consent process. Informed consent is not just a form to be signed. It is the process of giving patients all of the information relevant to their care, all the information they need to say yes or no to a given course of therapy. If a patient is being cared for in a teaching setting by physicians in training, the identities and roles of the members of the care team can be very relevant. Patients should have a right to say no to this arrangement, as well as a right to agree to it.

Is there any benefit to the trainees in divulging to patients their true status as students or physicians in training? When faced with questions about whether or not to be honest with a patient about anything related to their care, I first assume that they will find out somehow. So then the question becomes: what will be the consequences when the patient finds out the truth, and do the benefits of the deception outweigh those consequences? I believe the negative effects, the sense of betrayal and distrust, that occur when a patient finds out that she has been deceived far outweigh any perceived benefits of the deception. On the other hand, disclosing one's training status up front can have some positive effects. Most patients appreciate the respect shown by an honest explanation of who is who on the care team. Some are too ill to care, and want to believe that everyone in a white coat has expertise to bear on their illness. But I believe most do not want to be treated in a patronizing manner, and would like to know the qualifications of those caring for them.

Divulging one's training status can have a di-

rect beneficial effect for the student or resident as well. It can be very uncomfortable pretending to be something one is not. Once the patient knows what our training status is, their expectations are likely to be more in line with what we are in fact able to do. We will then be more comfortable admitting when we do not know the answer or cannot perform a procedure and need to ask for help.

In the United States the organization that accredits hospitals has now mandated honesty. The Joint Commission for the Accreditation of Healthcare Organizations (JCAHO) 1998 standard for informed consent contains the following:

In addition to an explanation to the patient of potential drawbacks, problems, and likelihood of success, possible results of non-treatment and any significant alternatives, staff members also inform the patient of the name of the physician or other practitioner who has primary responsibility for authorizing & performing procedures or treatments; any professional relationship to another health care provider or institution that might suggest a conflict of interest; their relationship to educational institutions involved in the patient's care; any business relationships between individuals treating the patient, or between the organization & any other health care, service, or educational institutions involved in the patient's care. This information should either be documented in the progress notes or as on a consent form. (Standard RI. 1.2.1)

Although some may find this mandate intrusive, I think it helps to overcome the resistance to change established by many decades of tradition. It will force us to be honest, and to learn how to deal with any negative consequences that arise out of that honesty. An honest introduction of care providers will eventually become a seamless part of the informed consent process, as it should be.

18

Duties to treat?

CASE

"Unnecessary personal risk"

I was a medical student when I observed the following case scenario. A 38-year-old woman came into the Emergency Department complaining of a "terrible headache." She had not been feeling well the previous week and admitted to having a cough, fever, chills, and occasional bouts of nausea and vomiting. She was accompanied by her boyfriend who said she had been "acting funny" in the days prior to admission. The patient was a regular heroin and cocaine user and had been using the drugs over the past few days.

Lab tests revealed that the patient was HIV positive. Her prognosis was grim, the attending speculated she would only live another 6 to 12 months.

The patient was admitted to the General Medicine Service. Over the next few days the patient underwent extensive testing to determine if she had any other diseases likely to affect an immunocompromised patient. She was treated with a variety of IV medications. During the course of her stay, she began to complain of shortness of breath. After examining the patient, the medical resident asked the medical student to draw an arterial blood gas (ABG) from the patient.

The medical student had not been following this patient, and though he had successfully performed previous ABGs in the past, he asked to be allowed to abstain from drawing blood from this patient who was known to have AIDS. He said he was uncomfortable at being put in a situation that he felt put him at unnecessary personal risk. Seemingly surprised by the medical student's response, the resident said nothing and proceeded to perform the ABG himself without mishap.

For me, this case raises a number of questions: Do medical students have an obligation to treat persons with AIDS? When do students assume professional duties? Should the resident have insisted that the student perform the procedure?

CASE

"He was telling me to take a risk he wasn't willing to take"

When I was a third year medical student, treatment for AIDS was just beginning and no one knew how the disease was transmitted. During my medical clerkship we had a patient with AIDS. He was kept in isolation and whenever we went in to see him everyone wore gloves, masks, and gowns. During the rounds, I noticed that the intern remained in the doorway and never entered the room.

During the patient's hospitalization, he developed a fever and needed blood cultures drawn. The intern told me to draw them. I had never done blood cultures. In addition to my own insecurities about doing the procedure, ensuring a good evaluation, and being seen as a team player, there was an additional pressure. I felt I was witnessing someone else's unethical behavior. He was telling me to take a risk he wasn't willing to take himself. I didn't know what to do.

CASE

"I said I might be pregnant"

One morning before rounds, during my internship in cardiology in a Dutch hospital, I was called before the department secretary and told to go to the CT scan room. I was informed I was needed to hold the hand of a very agitated patient to help calm her so the test could proceed. Almost immediately after entering the CT room I realized what was happening and that, in my view, I was being used improperly. I found myself wearing a lead apron and standing next to the patient while the four senior members of the department were sitting in a room next door. The plan was for me to hold the patient's hand throughout the entire CT exam. Both our hands would be exposed for a test that could last half an hour.

Just before the exam started, I heard someone ask if I were pregnant. At first I said "No" but a second later I changed my mind. Knowing the situation was not right, and to be able to leave, I said that I might be pregnant after all. That answer provoked a considerable consternation and a stern inquiry, "How can that be? Are you pregnant or not?" My possible pregnancy was receiving more attention than the poor patient who was lying on the table throughout all this commotion. The response made it easier for me to decide to get out of there. To my astonishment the patient was sent back to the ward with the excuse that the exam could not proceed because of her agitation.

I believed the situation to be unjustifiably dangerous for me. Was there a better way for me to handle it?

COMMENTARY

Gerrit Kimsma

These three cases have a common denominator: a risk of abuse. The root of this risk is located in the relationship of teachers and medical students. This relationship is by definition one of inequality – inequality in status, in knowledge, and in experience. The intention of medical training is to reduce these inequalities. For this reduction to succeed, students need their peers. This need means a dependency between teaching doctors and students. This dependency can provide an open door to abuse. This risk of abuse is heightened by the old-fashioned aspect of the teaching relationship (usually without a clear job description) with rights and duties but without clear guidelines to recognize the student's development from relative inexperience towards growing sophistication. This risk is also present because students are dependent on the evaluation of their immediate peers, usually the residents who they have to work with in close collaboration. In addition, given the fact that students are at the lowest level of responsibility, it is often not clear who their immediate peers are and to whom they are responsible: the interns, the residents, or the chiefs of staff.

In order to receive a good evaluation students tend to go out of their way to please residents and others who are involved in their assessment. Students also tend to underestimate their lack of experience. They show inclinations to perform medical duties without adequate guidance in order to become sophisticated as soon as possible to reduce the inequalities and become recognized as an equal. This mix of sometimes misguided aspirations and ambitions make students especially vulnerable targets for the type of abuse that the above cases describe.

Each case highlights one particular aspect of abuse in the theater of teaching.

The first case describes a refusal of a medical student to perform an ABG. The resident subsequently proceeded to perform this intervention himself. This case does not contain a description of the story afterwards. What the case description does contain is the formulation of an event, a difference of opinion between student and teacher, and the question whether medical students have an obligation to treat persons with AIDS.

This final question comes too fast for comfort. What should have been asked is: are there rules and regulations about students performing blood drawing procedures in situations of potential risk? And the second question is: if students are required to perform these interventions, what is the level of experience they must possess? How are these interventions being guided by their peers in order to prevent unwanted risk?

The silent response by the intern suggests that there are no rules and regulations. Taking over of the intervention without further discussion means that a chance to clarify the reason for the refusal (lack of experience in this particular situation of risk, emotions of anxiety) and the opportunity to teach a procedure in a situation of some risk, has not been used. In short, the teacher has not taught and the student has not learned. In general the answer to the question: "does a student have an obligation to treat persons with AIDS?" thus depends on the level of experience, especially in situations of risk, and the adequacy of supervision on the part of the teacher in guiding the student to perform the intervention well.

If it becomes clear through observation that a student may have enough relevant experience, then a student cannot refuse an intervention that is part of normal medical procedures, as should be stipulated in any "rules and regulations" developed about patient care.

The bad attitude of the intern in the second case becomes clear when we have the above "frame of reference" in mind. Here the student did not have experience at all in drawing blood for cultures. This inexperience makes the intern's attitude inexcusable. It demonstrates an attitude of cowardice. The emotional dependence of the student on the intern means that the student is manipulated into performing an intervention without the necessary experience, and does not even feel free to object or to discuss the unethical behavior of the teacher.

The third case highlights the aspect of abuse in an extreme form. Here the student is asked to take risks that no staff member apparently is willing to take, while the procedure is even canceled when the student discovers a lie that allows her to ungracefully withdraw. Here the absence of a fair job description is the cause of a demand to participate in an intervention: the student does not know whether this is normal procedure or not. She discovers the unusual nature of the request only after she realizes what is being asked of her and the risks she has to take, and observes her lack of protection when staff retreat to a different room. This case also highlights a lack of procedures for reporting these events. This procedure should teach everyone who is involved in education of students that abuse should not go unchecked, or certainly without consequences.

COMMENTARY

Neal Cohen

Every physician is expected to treat every patient who seeks his or her help, addressing all clinical problems thoroughly and effectively. In doing so, most physicians acknowledge the personal sacrifice which accompanies the responsibility incumbent upon them. At the same time, each physician is an individual and has personal rights and responsibilities that should not be ignored. The three cases included in this chapter identify some of the challenges associated with balancing patient and personal needs and risks. When caring for a patient, a physician assumes responsibilities to thoroughly assess the clinical problems and treat them. In essence the physician has established a contract with the patient to do whatever is necessary to address their clinical problems and concerns. At the same time, the physician is not obligated to do things that would harm the patient, nor put himself or herself at undue risk. The question for each physician then is to assess the degree of personal risk and define ways to minimize it.

The cases included in this chapter identify some of the problems associated with evaluating personal risk, minimizing it, and at the same time providing appropriate patient care. The two cases that describe the challenges associated with caring for an AIDS patient emphasize some important lessons for residents, students, and any other health care provider. First, each physician should understand the potential personal risks associated with caring for a patient and ways in which to minimize the risk. When caring for AIDS patients, for example, the risk of contracting the disease, while small, is real. The same thing can be said for risks associated with caring for patients with hepatitis, probably the two most commonly acquired infectious diseases. As we have gained a better understanding of the epidemiology of AIDS and hepatitis, we are aware of routes of transmission and the impact of personal protection on patient care.

For the medical student or resident, education is the key to appropriate patient care and personal protection. The student, unlike the attending physician, does not have the same level of responsibility, nor obligation to treat a patient. The student and resident must fulfill the responsibilities within the educational program. Their responsibilities do include direct patient care, but under supervision. The student should expect to be trained in methods for performing procedures as well as ways to reduce risks associated with each intervention. In the case of "unnecessary personal risks" the student can expect to learn to perform an arterial puncture, but only after appropriate training. The training should include methods to perform the procedure, appropriate equipment and its use, and techniques to provide personal protection. If a student has not had experience with an arterial puncture, he or she should not be asked to perform the procedure in a patient with an infectious disease that could be transmitted to the student. The student should first be trained to perform the procedure using a

manikin or other simulated method. After successfully completing the simulation, the student should be expected to perform the procedure *under direct supervision* on a patient who does not have a disease process that could be transmitted to the student.

Although the expectations of the student are clear, fulfilling the requirement of appropriate training can be challenging and put the student in a difficult position. In a busy, stressful clinical environment, the student may be encouraged to assist in the management of patients in order to ensure that care is provided in a timely manner. Even under these circumstances, the student should be expected to ask for assistance in completing procedures for which he or she is not familiar and to obtain appropriate guidance and supervision. While the student may be reluctant to ask for assistance, he or she should be willing to do so, to ensure that the patient's management is appropriate and that both the patients and the student's risks are minimized.

The third case in this chapter raises some additional issues related to personal risk. The risks associated with radiological procedures, such as CT scans are more difficult to define than those associated with transmission of HIV from patient to provider. In evaluating the personal risk associated with any procedure, the student should first try to define the magnitude of risk and the timing of which it might be manifest. In the case of an infectious disease, for example, the infection may occur quickly. The manifestations of the infection, however, may be delayed. Infection with hepatitis C virus can occur after needlestick or contaminated transfusion. The liver failure associated with hepatitis C virus, however, may not occur for years and the clinical presentation be indolent. The same can be said for radiation exposure. The risk the student is being subjected to may have been small, but the student was not appropriately educated about the risks, nor provided with adequate protection. Once the risk is known, the student should be given information about how to minimize the risk or protect against it. In the case of radiation exposure, a lead apron may help protect the torso, but would be of no benefit to hand exposure. While a lead mitten may have provided adequate protection, alternative methods may have been more appropriate to keep the patient comfortable during the procedure and allow its completion without putting any provider at risk. In some cases, continuous sedation or general anesthesia may be required to safely complete a diagnostic procedure in an otherwise agitated patient.

Finally, this case raises an additional concern. In response to a potential risk, no practitioner should lie to get out of a situation in which they feel uncomfortable. The medical student should expect that the risk will be defined and that appropriate protective methods offered. If they are not, the student should decline participation and, if necessary, discuss the concerns raised by the case with a supervisor. The student should be willing to describe their discomfort and discuss ways in which to ensure that the patient's care is optimized, while their own personal risk is minimized.

While it is important to recognize that the physician has a responsibility to treat a patient who presents himself, the physician is not obligated to provide care that is of no benefit or inappropriate. In some cases, the physician will recommend treatment that may turn out to be more harmful than beneficial. When doing so, the physician and patient should have a discussion about the potential risks and benefits and the patient given sufficient information to make an informed decision. In those situations in which a patient requests care that is inappropriate, the physician is not required to provide it. In an emergency situation, the physician cannot abandon the patient, but must use his or her judgment to provide the care that is clinically indicated. In an elective situation, however, the physician can deny care to a patient if he or she thinks it is not clinically indicated. When such a disagreement occurs between the patient and provider, the physician should try to identify an alternative provider who can assume responsibility for the patient's care. The patient cannot be abandoned, but the physician cannot be required to provide care that is not indicated and can decline participation in care if he or she thinks it is not medically appropriate. When balancing patients' needs and personal risk, the physician has to make the same risk–benefit analysis that is required in any clinical situation. When the personal risks seem to outweigh the patient benefit, the provider should explain the reason for withholding the intervention and the diagnostic or therapeutic alternatives. If the patient disagrees with the physician's assessment, he or she is then free to request referral to an alternative provider.

19

Hierarchy and the dynamics of rank

Questioning authority

CASE

"Just a consult"

The other day I saw a patient being treated for hyponatremia with salt tablets. Between the morning and afternoon rounds, he went from being arousable to barely responsive to pain. I talked to my attending about my observations but he was uninterested since, as he indicated, we were not the medicine team, but just a consult. We did not notify any of the doctors about the patient's decreased level of consciousness. The next day he was in the ICU on a ventilator.

CASE

"Don't mess with the chain of command"

During rounds with the chief resident and the attending, the attending laid out a course of treatment for the patient. Rather than question the attending's judgment, out of her earshot the chief resident said "No one does it that way, but we're just going to let this go and it's going to bite her in the ass." There seemed to be no concern for the impact on the patient, and I asked, "Can't we talk to another attending?" The chief resident responded with an emphatic, "No way! There is a strict hierarchy here. You only go through your attending and if you mess with that chain of command by

going around her, you'll get it!" I was left with the question, "Where does the patient figure in this chain of command?"

CASE

"Why use that medication?"

As an intern, while making rounds on the cardiac unit, we were presented with a patient who had been admitted for an inoperable descending aortic aneurysm. He had a history of hypertension, coronary heart disease, and arrhythmia. The attending, who had a reputation for being "hands off" and typically less involved with house staff and patients, was using a newer beta blocker which carried with it a risk of arrhythmia. I, along with other interns, questioned the choice since there were other effective medications in controlling blood pressure, without that risk. In response to our question, "Why use that medication?" the attending responded vaguely, "Let's go with it." Our teaching cardiologist and cardiology fellow also said the medication didn't sound like the best choice. Although we continued to feel uneasy, we kept our concern to ourselves and the attending's decision was not seriously challenged.

I checked the patient at 11:00 p.m., after he had been receiving the medication for 36 hours. His blood pressure was low, but not alarmingly so. Thirty minutes later he experienced arrhythmia and died.

As an individual I know I can refuse to carry out an order that I believe to be a mistake, and thus protect myself. However, the more important question is how to protect the patient?

CASE

"Level with me"

As an intern at a large teaching hospital, I established what I perceived to be a trusting relationship with an elderly man who had no family. He confided in me that he feared he had cancer, mistrusted doctors to tell him the truth, and asked me to "level with him" whatever the results might be from the tests he was undergoing. The lab tests confirmed that his illness was indeed terminal and that he probably had a limited time to live. I wanted to go to the patient directly and tell him what he was facing, but the chief resident said that to do so would cause undue harm. He said such a delicate situation required a more experienced approach and he would be responsible for informing the patient. The resident's explanation was so jargon-filled and obtuse that I was sure the patient did not get the full picture. I wanted to discuss his situation with him more openly but at the same time I didn't want to go behind the resident's back or undermine his position.

CASE

"Why couldn't the patient be premedicated?"

We were nearing the end of rounds about 6:30 in the morning when the surgery team stopped at the door of a patient who had been admitted the night before. Before entering, the patient was introduced to us as "An addict with a huge abscess over left thigh that was drained last night. A dressing change now and two later by the nurses and we should have him out of here by tonight." When we walked into the room the patient was sleeping. We said "Good morning, we have to look at your wound and change the dressing." The patient was suddenly surrounded by seven people with a very bright light shining on his body. We all reached for different equipment, rolled gauze, sterile water, etc. He seemed startled as two sets of hands busily unwrapped his leg. Soon his skin was exposed showing a longitudinal incision about 7 inches long in the middle of his thigh bursting with gauze padding. As the team started to take the gauze out the patient began to scream. Not a regular scream but a bone chilling "I am in as much agony as I can possibly imagine" scream. Those of us who were students looked at each other bewildered, could they be doing this wrong? The third year resident continued undaunted with a terse comment for the patient, "We are almost done." The patient was writhing in pain and reached for the resident's arms pleading "Please stop, don't do any more." The resident answered, "Mr. Jones just one more piece, we have to do this to help it heal." With one final pull, the resident removed the last gauze, the one stuck to the most amount of bare muscle, and the patient let out a final ear piercing scream and dissolved into tears because he could do nothing to stop the pain.

On the way to the cafeteria I asked why they couldn't call ahead and premedicate so the patient would feel less pain as the gauze was taken out. The residents snickered a little and said, "Not enough time, we move too fast."

I wondered if this patient's status as a "shooter with an abscess" influenced the treatment he received. Also, I believed that as a medical student any challenge to how things were done would not only have been disregarded, but would have been seen as being a poor team player or "weak" medical student, a term that precludes the possibility of receiving "honors."

CASE

"I followed orders even though I thought they were wrong"

As interns in France we are very close to our patients, almost as close as the nurses. In a sense, we almost live our patients' pain. In one instance, the patient was a man in terrible pain with metastatic bone cancer. A decision needed to be made regarding increasing the patient's dose of major drugs for better pain control; and a consult was called with the attending. The meeting took place, not on the ward but in the attending's office as he sat behind his desk. The attending, who saw the patient only infrequently, saw no compelling reason to increase the dose. He said, "We can live with pain, let's wait a few hours." Distance from a patient makes people think differently than if they were close to the person. I had to go back and deal with a patient for whom I had enormous empathy and I could do nothing to alleviate his pain without directly disobeying my attending. I followed orders even though I thought the orders were wrong.

CASE

"Help! My senior registrar has gone fishing"

In Denmark you have to do 6 months of surgery, 6 months of internal medicine and 6 months of general practice immediately after graduation in order to get your license to practice independently as a doctor. The available places in this compulsory rotation are distributed by a lottery, and because I had drawn a fairly bad number in the lottery I ended up in one of the provincial hospitals, about as far away from my home town of Copenhagen as it is possible to get in Denmark.

My first 6 months were to be spent in the Department of Orthopedic Surgery, which was also responsible for the Accident and Emergency Department. The town was a coastal town, with a large fishing fleet and a very active nightlife, and because there was only one hospital in the town, the A & E Department was usually very busy (actually the third busiest in Denmark in number of patients).

Now during the weekends the total medical staff of the Department of Orthopedic Surgery consisted of a senior registrar with specialist qualifications in orthopedic surgery and a house officer. The senior

registrar did the ward rounds and the emergency operations, whereas the house officer managed the A & E Department and minor things on the wards. The senior registrar was supposed to be in the hospital from 9:00 a.m.–3:00 p.m. and be on call from home the rest of the weekend.

Towards the end of my second month in the department, I had my first Saturday as house officer in charge of the A & E Department. I had, of course, been doing A & E work on weekdays, but this was the first time when I was supposed to "go it alone" without anybody senior in the hospital, but as the consultant in charge of the department had told me: "Don't worry. If you have even the slightest doubt, or if there is something you don't know how to do, then call the senior registrar, and he will come in to help you out."

Well, everything went smoothly in the morning and early afternoon. There were the usual lacerations, distortions, broken fingers and toes and other minor things, but nothing that I couldn't handle. But around 4:30 in the afternoon this suddenly changed. The injury wasn't very complicated, just a dislocated right thumb, and even though I had never treated such an injury before, the treatment method was well described in the departmental instruction book and in the major Danish textbook on orthopedic surgery. So, I administered the local anesthetic and when it worked, I performed the reposition without problems, but the thumb wouldn't stay repositioned. The books had no solution for this problem, so I decided to call the senior registrar and ask him to come in and help. His home phone had an answering machine on which redirected me to his mobile phone. I called the mobile, and got him on the phone immediately. He was not very pleased. As he explained to me this was one of the best angling days of the year. The weather was perfect, and the sea-trout had just started their spring run for their spawning places. He was standing with his waders on in the best trout and salmon river in Denmark, and he wasn't very keen on doing the 20 mile drive back to the hospital and spoil his angling. He then proceeded to tell me what to do, and

I tried to impress on him, that what he had just told me to do, was what I already had been doing, and that this didn't work. I was however ordered to try again and duly did so, with no better result than before. I called him again, but he said that the patient could wait until Sunday morning, when he himself would see to this simple matter. I argued that this was unacceptable. He couldn't really mean that a patient should wait for 12 hours, just because of his fishing. At this point he made it very clear that he was a senior registrar, and I was just a house officer, and that he wasn't coming in.

COMMENTARY

Søren Holm

For all seven cases in this chapter there are two easy solutions that immediately spring to mind:
1 The insensible and unethical superior should mend his or her ways.
2 The junior doctor should be courageous and do what is right,whatever the personal consequences.

Both these solutions are obvious and attractive from the point of view of ethical theory, but at the same time problematic as practical solutions to the problems. I therefore want to use this commentary to try to analyze in more detail why this (apparent) conflict between the ethical and the pragmatic occurs.

In all seven cases we have a conflict between the orders or actions of a superior in the medical hierarchy and the line of action which the junior doctor in the case believes to be best for the patient, and also the morally right thing to do. It seems obvious that the only right action to take is to overrule the order of the superior either directly and openly, or in some hidden, not so easily detectable way. This seems to follow on a consequentialist analysis of the cases, focusing on the possible consequences of the actions, on a deontological analysis focusing on rights and duties, and on an analysis focusing on the meaning of the doctor–patient relationship. There may be reasons to suspect that the obvious answer does not tell the whole story. One of the things the simplistic analysis above leaves out, is that all these cases occur in a very complex social setting, i.e., the modern hospital.

In the stories we only hear of a few persons, but in reality there are of course also nurses, nurses aids, relatives, and a number of representatives of other groups of people involved in these cases. The story format also disguises that for many of the actors this is neither the first nor the last time they will meet each other. It may well be the case that they will continue to meet many times a day for years to come.

The stories do not hide that there are power relationships, but they do not tell us enough of the context to enable us to decide whether these power relationships are legitimate or illegitimate. That some persons have power over other persons, and that they use this power in certain circumstances, is not in itself illegitimate. Power is a necessary part of human organizations. So we have to distinguish three kinds of situation: (1) the power relationship is illegitimate, (2) the power relationship is legitimate but the use of power in this specific case is illegitimate, and (3) both the power relationship and the specific use of power is legitimate. Although both situation one and two involve illegitimate use of power, they do so in very different ways.

To bring out these features we have to look at the seven cases within the richer context of the hospital organization. In the basic theory of organizations it is commonplace that all organizations can be characterized by three interacting factors that influence decisions and decision making:
Structure
Process
Culture

If we look at these one at a time, we will find that consideration of each factor illuminates certain ethically relevant aspects of the cases.

"Don't mess with the chain of command" – the importance of structure

There are many ways in which one could structure medical work in hospitals, but the traditional structure is a strict hierarchical structure with an attending (consultant) at the top of the pyramid and several levels below with a gradually decreasing level of expertise and decision-making power. In some kinds of hospital organization these different structural pyramids are fairly clearly separated, so that every patient, and every junior doctor "belongs" to a specific attending, whereas in other systems each department has a layer of attendings who are jointly responsible for the patients in the department, and for the several layers of junior doctors.

Seen from an organizational point of view this structure is thus a close approximation to the ideal bureaucratic structure described by the German sociologist Max Weber. The reasons for choosing this structure are clear, at least at the idealized theoretical level. This structure creates a clear designation of responsibility. Everybody knows his or her place in the organization, knows which cases (in this context, patients) belong within his or her responsibility, and knows which superior to refer to in cases which exceed the predetermined level of decision-making capacity assigned to each level of the organization. What the seven cases so clearly demonstrate is, however, that the ideal bureaucratic structure can also create problems, if it is populated by nonideal decision makers (and this will almost always be the case).

It is, however, also important to realize that the hierarchical medical structure outlined here also differs from the ideal bureaucratic system in several respects. First there are many more totally separate "pyramids" in a hospital than in most other organizations, and there are within each "pyramid" far fewer formalized decision-making procedures than in most other organizations. If we talk about "chains of command" in medicine – which is an interesting military metaphor in its own right redolent with connotations of the "fight against disease" – it is fairly obvious that these are much more localized and parochial than in most other organizations. In the military even the "biggest" attending would be no more than a captain or a major and would have many controlling levels of command above him or her, deciding on policy and procedures. In medicine such an attending is the supreme commander, only controlled by forces outside of the hierarchical structure. The medical hierarchy, and its "chain of command," is thus much more vulnerable to aberrant or idiosyncratic commanders than most other organizations (a theme which is illustrated in a number of the cases).

One specific problem which recurs in all seven cases is, that because there is a linear chain of command (i.e., a junior doctor only refers to one senior doctor with regard to a specific patient), there is no legitimate way to bring in a "second opinion" in cases of disagreement. The usual justification for maintaining such a linear chain of command is that (i) it is the most efficient structure, (ii) it promotes increased responsibility by making responsibility clear and minimizing the risk of dangerous diffusion of responsibility and concomitant lack of decision making, and (iii) it enables fast decision making in acute situations. All three characteristics are undoubtedly true, but it is important to note that the same goals can be reached within organizational structures that are more open to exploring disagreement and uncertainty.

In a structure where patients, for instance, belong to a department, and not to an individual attending, it is possible for junior doctors (and to some degree for patients) to "exploit" different points of view among attendings, by ensuring that a given decision is discussed in a forum where no attending has absolute decision-making power. This may lead to a small loss of efficiency, but it does not necessarily lead to a dangerous diffusion of responsibility, or to a loss of quick decision-making capacity. In the acute context the structure simply reverts to a linear structure.

A number of the cases in this chapter could potentially have been resolved in a more satisfactory manner if the chain of command had not been strictly linear. It has been shown that in medical structures with greater possibility for the open discussion of decisions made by superiors, junior doctors assess their influence on ethically important decisions as larger than their influence on purely technical decisions. It has also been shown that junior doctors do actually utilize mechanisms for the discussion of decisions if such mechanisms are available.

Seen from the patient's point of view there is, however, one significant drawback in a system with a nonlinear chain of command. In the linear system you know the person who is your attending, and in the majority of cases where this relationship works out all right this may be of great benefit to you.

The linear system is also the only system where there is an obvious way to remunerate attendings on a fee-for-patient or fee-for-service scale, and this probably adds to its popularity in countries without well-developed public health care systems, although it is not limited to such countries.

The importance of process

The second important factor in understanding decision making in organizations is process. How are decisions supposed to be made, and how are they actually made within the organization?

Within health care the official view is usually that there are clear guidelines for which types of decisions can be made at which level in the hierarchy, and clear guidelines to ensure that decisions made at higher levels are also implemented at lower levels. This naive view is, however, easily dispelled by just brief exposure to actual health care organizations. Decisions are often made at the "wrong level" or they are not made at all. Those decisions that are made are often not communicated effectively, and decisions made at higher levels may be effectively blocked or circumvented at lower levels. It is also important to

remember that the medical hierarchy is not the only game in town, and if one of the other powerful hierarchies in the hospital organization (e.g., in some countries the nursing hierarchy) does not agree with a certain decision it may also be blocked or circumvented. In many countries it will, for instance, be impossible to keep a patient in ignorance about his or her prognosis, if there is not a prior agreement between all groups that this is the right course of action. There are simply too many ways in which a, deniable, slip of the tongue may be used to give the patient correct information.

In some of the cases in this chapter we see basic flaws in process that could easily be rectified. In "Just a consult" the consult process, or the attending's understanding of this process, is obviously defective because it effectively precludes the passing on of important information. In "Why couldn't the patient be premedicated?" it is also obvious that there is a basic procedural error. The unacceptable scenario which is described is one which is likely to occur repeatedly, if premedication is never used in similar cases. What is needed in such cases is not deep ethical reflection, but simply some fairly simple changes in procedure.

In other cases the problems in the process are more difficult to spot, and perhaps also more difficult to do something about.

One of the reasons that attendings are given the final say in decision making about patients is that they are believed to be the persons who are best qualified and most competent to make these decisions. They do not just lead by right or by force, but they lead because they are best suited to lead. In the real world this presumption of qualification and competence may, however, not hold up to scrutiny in specific instances. There may be a lack of professional knowledge; there may be idiosyncratic views; or there may be various forms of personal incompetence which indicate that this is a case where this specific attending is not best placed to make a decision. Several of the cases illustrate this problem, and they also illustrate that it is a problem that the hospital organization is ill-suited to deal with. There are very few ways in which the decision-making process allows for subordinates to express their belief that a superior may not have absolutely up-to-date medical knowledge or may use slightly idiosyncratic techniques. This is partly so because this is most often seen not as an objective comment, but as an attempt to impugn the personality of the superior. Attendings often seem to believe that they have risen to their present elevated position purely on the grounds of their personal merits, and this leads to a state of mind where any criticism is interpreted as personal.

Cases like "Why use that medication?" or "Don't mess with the chain of command" perfectly illustrate how problematic decisions are made because the attending (presumably) has less than perfect medical knowledge in a specific field. Similarly, a case like "I followed orders even though I thought the orders were wrong" illustrates what may happen when the attending does not have the necessary personal knowledge about the patient.

The possibility that such cases can be resolved with a more appropriate outcome can be improved by looking at the decision-making processes and changing them in ways that minimize the risk of blocks in the information flow, and maximize the opportunity for all voices to be heard and taken into consideration.

The importance of culture

Even in perfect organizations with perfect structure and perfect process things do not always work as they should. By contrast, in many imperfect organizations things work much better than should be expected. This has led organizational researchers to look at the importance of organizational culture. All organizations have an organizational culture, even those where nothing has been done to foster such a culture. The culture is important in many ways, and two of its functions

are especially important in the present context: (i) the culture supplies (at least some) of the values that are fed into the decision-making algorithm, and (ii) the culture fills in the "holes" in decision-making processes by specifying who can make decisions and on what basis of knowledge, in those cases where the formal procedures do not provide the necessary specification.

Most of the cases in this chapter exemplify the same very serious problem in organizational culture. Namely, it is obvious that they could not have taken place in a culture that did not allow a certain level of callous behavior towards patients, and a certain amount of abuse of power towards junior doctors. A culture which allows attendings to make binding decisions about patients without seeing the patient, which allows senior registrars to put angling before patients, or which allows doctors to change dressings on patients in the most painful way imaginable, is very simply a deficient culture. It is also a culture that is totally unsuitable for the education of future health care professionals because of its disregard for important human and professional values.

Now, organizational cultures can be changed, but such a change requires a diagnosis of the problems and a leadership that is willing to put effort into the process of change. Change in a culture does not happen just by itself (except in the very long run), and it is very difficult to bring about if the persons in positions of power do not support such change. What would be necessary in many of the cases in this chapter is thus a sustained effort aimed at making it clear to everybody in the organization that certain kinds of behavior will not be tolerated in the future.

Exit, voice and loyalty

I have discussed some organizational changes which can help to prevent the occurrence of situations like those described in the cases in this chapter. But what should a junior doctor do, if he or she is in an organization where no such changes seem to be forthcoming?

In his seminal book *Exit, Voice and Loyalty* Hirschman discusses the options open to those within an organization who are dissatisfied with some aspect of the function of the organization. (1) He shows that the three main options are loyalty (i.e., stay within the organization and suppress your dissatisfaction), voice (i.e., voice your dissatisfaction internally, or in some cases externally), and exit (i.e., leave the organization). In the previous sections of this commentary we have already looked at some of the problems caused by the option of voice for junior doctors within the medical hierarchy, and here I just want to add a few comments on the option of exit.

There may be cases when a junior doctor is working in an environment where the interests of patients are repeatedly and/or systematically neglected, and where all attempts at having this state of affairs discussed have been unsuccessful. In such situations there are only two options left for a person who wants to maintain his or her integrity as a moral person: (i) complain to an external authority (external voice), or (ii) exit from the organization. Both options are likely to be extremely costly at the personal level. The position of junior doctors is complicated by the fact that most of them are in training. They need their jobs, not only as a way to make money, but also as a necessary step on the way to becoming fully fledged specialists. Doing anything that can jeopardize the place in a training scheme is thus much more costly in the long run than is immediately apparent to most outside observers. This is one of the factors that give senior medical doctors much more power over their subordinates than superiors in many other hierarchies.

One solution to the problem of the cost of exit could be to establish confidential complaint mechanisms where junior doctors could voice their concerns about the actions of attendings, and expect that something would be done. Such a system would, however, require a radical overhaul of our present ideas about the status of attendings within medical care and postgraduate medical education.

Note

1 Hirschman AO. *Exit, Voice and Loyalty: Responses to Decline in Firms, Organizations and States.* Harvard University Press, Cambridge, MA, 1970.

COMMENTARY

Griffin Trotter

The cases in this chapter bring to mind the 1992 Columbia Pictures film, *A Few Good Men*, where two soldiers are tried for murder. The defendants in this movie had been ordered by their lieutenant to "haze" a weak and inept fellow soldier. During the hazing, the other soldier coughs up blood. Though the tormentors desist at this point and call an ambulance, the victim dies in the hospital. These facts eventually come out in the courtroom. It also becomes evident that hazing, though illegal, is frequently practiced at the soldiers' station. On this basis, the soldiers are acquitted of murder. However, they are dishonorably discharged for "conduct unbecoming a Marine." Near the conclusion of the movie, one of the befuddled soldiers asks the other why they have been convicted of "conduct unbecoming" when they were merely following orders. The wiser soldier replies that the Marine Corps have an ideal that trumps obedience to orders: Marines are supposed to protect the weak. (1)

Medical students and physicians also have an ideal that supersedes the chain of command. They are supposed to act in the best interests of patients. True loyalty – i.e., the form of loyalty that is morally required for medical professionals – consists of willing, practical, and thoroughgoing dedication to this ideal. Loyalty (as here defined) should not be confused with obedience because (as per the Marines in *A Few Good Men*) it may require disobedience. When there is serious concern that carrying out orders will significantly compromise patient care, medical students have a moral responsibility to question those orders. Attending physicians and residents, by virtue of their role as educators, should be ready and willing to address such questions.

On the other hand, the chain of command in medicine is not an arbitrary restraint. It exists for a purpose, and should not be violated cavalierly. There are a variety of ways to adequately deal with most clinical problems. Often conflicts about competing clinical strategies amount to little more than disagreements about which of several adequate approaches is best. In such circumstances, it is reasonable that the person with the most training, the most experience, and the most legal and moral responsibility be the one who has the final say. Hence, attending physicians generally have more decision-making authority than residents do, and residents have more than students do. Allowing students to disobey instructions whenever they feel they have a better idea would endanger patients. Further, there are situations in which the necessity for rapid intervention will preclude extensive discussion about the wisdom of a supervising doctor's orders.

Two pressing issues emerge for medical students: (1) When should students question the orders of a clinical supervisor? (2) When should students violate the chain of command? The first issue is easiest. Medical education and patient care are both enhanced when students ask questions. Hence, students should ordinarily feel free to question mentors. Further, students are obligated to ask questions when they have good reason to believe that adequate patient care hangs in the balance.

Questions should be timed appropriately. For instance, students should avoid challenging a supervising physician at the bedside if it will come across as a threat to the supervisor's authority. Also, there are occasionally circumstances where questions can distract a physician from adequately performing a demanding or delicate procedure. If possible, such questions should be deferred. These exceptional circumstances notwithstanding, any attending physician or resident who routinely punishes or humiliates students for asking questions has no business working in a teaching hospital.

In "Don't mess with the chain of command," the primary issue isn't about the chain of command. It is about asking questions. For some reason, the resident physician in this case is reluctant to discuss treatment options with the attending physician. Instead, the resident expresses glee over prospects that the attending physician's bad decision is "going to bite her in the ass." If (contrary to the situation portrayed in our brief narrative) the resident was unreasonably brushed off by the attending physician, then suggestions about consulting another attending physician might be appropriate. In any case, the medical student ends with precisely the right question: "Where does the patient figure in this chain of command?"

"Just a consult" involves an interesting variation on the reluctance to ask questions. Here, an attending physician fails to question another attending physician after the student observes that a patient is receiving substandard therapy for hyponatremia. Patient care and medical education are both compromised because of this failure to communicate. Apparently, the consulting physician in this case honored misguided notions of good manners and/or a rigid division of clinical responsibility over the ideal of helping patients.

Unfortunately, the moral tradition in medicine is stained by a long heritage of such preoccupation with internal harmony over serving patients. For instance, when it first appeared, physicians reviled the clinico-pathological conference because they were more concerned with upholding a strong public image than with becoming better doctors by learning from their mistakes. Thomas Percival's early treatise on medical ethics reflects a similar mentality. (2) It comes across more as advice about good manners than as an analysis of moral responsibility. The attending physician in "Just a consult" represents this "Miss Manners" strand of professional morality.

The second issue – When should students violate the chain of command? – is difficult. Violations of the chain of command can endanger patients, they can seriously undermine relationships with supervisors, they can expose students to severe disciplinary action, and they have a potentially negative effect on the cohesive function of the medical team. In order to address this issue, we need to flesh out the concept of clinical loyalty a little further.

Two distinctions will help. The first is a distinction between the task and the goal of medicine. Medicine's task is the role it fills for society. It is what makes medicine a beneficial and important service to the larger community. Medicine's goal, on the other hand, is what medical professionals are aiming at.

Note that the task of medicine is defined from the standpoint of society at large. Anyone with a stake in good health care has a degree of authority in determining it. The goal of medicine, on the other hand, is largely a function of physicians. It is the professional objective that for them holds primary importance.

Roughly speaking, there is agreement that the task of medicine is to promote human flourishing by addressing human disease, disability, and human suffering with the tools of medical knowledge and medical technology. (3) This amounts to serving the best interests of patients. When physicians are motivated primarily by the objective of achieving this task, then the task and the goal of medicine are in harmony. When physicians afford a higher priority to their own reputations, or to profitability, or to the maintenance of professional decorum than to the accomplishment of medicine's task, then the goal and task of medicine are out of harmony.

The morally obligatory form of loyalty consists of a commitment to aligning medicine's goal with medicine's task. When loyalties are directed elsewhere, they are moral liabilities rather than virtues. Of course, this is not to say that earning a living, supporting a family and getting along with colleagues is not important. Each physician is a person with a multitude of loyalties. But our actions as physicians should reflect primary concern for our task as physicians. When we don our white coats, we should aim, above all else, to serve our patients.

For some readers, the term "loyalty" may imply single-minded devotion to particular individuals or groups at the expense of more universal moral considerations or competing moral claims. This is a very serious and important objection that must be worked out in the lives of every physician. We must take care that our commitment to patient care does not blind us to the reality and importance of potentially competing values such as responsible stewardship of health care resources and maintenance of social order. It is helpful in this regard to remember that our clinical responsibility extends to all patients, actual and potential, who depend on our services. Our task is not exhausted by care rendered to the patient sitting on our exam table. We are also beholden to the people in the waiting room, and to everyone who trusted in our expertise, availability, and cooperation when they arranged health care provisions for themselves, their families, and the community. Thus, when we treat a gunshot wound, we are morally and legally obliged to notify police – regardless of whether our GSW patient perceives this act to be in his best interests. Likewise, we have an obligation to withhold certain broad-spectrum antibiotics from all but the sickest patients.

A second useful distinction is between authority and power. Power is an ability to affect worldly affairs. Medical knowledge constitutes a kind of power, since it helps us optimize certain health-related outcomes. Attending physicians are powerful individuals, not merely by virtue of their clinical knowledge, but also because they have considerable ability to influence the decisions and circumstances of other persons. They can make life very good or very difficult for medical students. Attending physicians control most aspects of medical training and they profoundly influence medical students' future prospects through evaluations of their performance.

Authority is the ability to wield power legitimately. The key to understanding this concept resides in the notion of legitimacy. When Orion (my 12-year-old son) uses threats of physical pain to force his younger brother to accept responsibility for the dead fish in the dirty clothes hamper, he is wielding power but not authority. On the other hand, when I threaten Orion with the loss of TV rights if he fails to tell the truth, then I exhibit power *and* authority.

When attending physicians and residents use their powers to accomplish the task of medicine, they exhibit authority. The medical chain of command is structured, or should be structured, to enhance this form of authority. When clinicians intentionally (or occasionally unintentionally) use the chain of command to thwart the task of medicine, they lack authority. In these instances medical students and others should consider violating the chain of command.

Not all abuses of power warrant breaches of the chain of command. Sometimes the abuse will be minor and the repercussions of rebellion severe. For instance, no student should be expected to jeopardize her career by defying a powerful attending physician who insists on using suboptimal analgesia for a preoperative patient. In such a situation it would be reasonable to study and report on the latest data about pain relief for preoperative patients. But to directly disobey orders by administering unauthorized narcotic analgesics would undermine legal and clinical structures that function, in the long run, to protect patients. Such an act would also prevent the student from helping future patients, as disciplinary measures would probably involve a permanent loss of clinical authority for the student. Prudence, that most fundamental yet elusive of moral virtues, demands that medical students weigh risks, benefits, and burdens of any possible decision to violate orders from a supervisor. Will the patient really benefit? Will clinical care for this patient or other patients be enhanced in the long run? Will I jeopardize my career in order to provide a relatively trivial service?

The importance of orderly and responsible decision making demands that the chain of command be violated only in the most extreme cases and only when other avenues have been exhausted. In "Why use that medication?" the interns should have protested more vehemently about the use of the new beta blocker. If such protests failed, they would be warranted in discussing the matter with another attending physician. However, the scenario, as presented, does not suggest a need for directly violating the chain of command.

In "Level with me," the resident fails to inform the patient adequately about clinical findings because the truth is obscured in jargon. This approach is especially inappropriate due to the fact that the patient has clearly expressed a desire to be informed fully about his diagnosis. The resident exhibits gross incompetence, and the results of his blunder are potentially devastating for the patient. The intern should take necessary steps to ensure that the patient gets the full story. This might be accomplished by explaining the technical jargon used by the resident. It is not likely that an intern would be criticized or punished merely for explaining the meaning of medical terms.

"Why couldn't the patient be premedicated?" is a very disturbing case. Here the problem appears to be system-wide. Several residents snicker at the suggestion that a patient be premedicated before a painful procedure. They justify their lousy patient care with the paltry observation that "we move too fast." A resident or medical student forced to work on such a team faces a huge obstacle. Though every reasonable effort should be made in such circumstances to provide conscientious patient care, it is unrealistic to expect a medical student or intern to transform such a seriously flawed medical culture. Perhaps the best advice in such cases is to nurture a strong sense of medicine's legitimate goals, and to refuse to be taken in by the cynicism and selfishness that seem to have infused the given clinical service.

Finally, in "Help! My senior registrar has gone fishing" there is dereliction of duty by the senior registrar. In such instances, the only alternatives are to try to find another physician who is willing and able to help the patient or to proceed as well as possible with the given resources.

Notes

1 I discuss this example and its ramifications for the understanding of loyalty at greater length in *The Loyal Physician*. Vanderbilt University Press, Nashville, 1997, pp.78–81.
2 Percival T. *Medical Ethics*. Classics of Medicine Library, Birmingham, Alabama, 1985. [Percival's book appeared in 1803.]
3 Jonsen AR, Siegler M, Winslade WJ. *Clinical Ethics*, 4th edn. McGraw-Hill, New York, 1998, pp.15–22.

Acting against authority

CASE

"When I speak you must follow"

We were very busy in the ICU one morning when I was an intern in Paris. There were many problems and only a few doctors and we had to triage patients. I was faced with two situations. One patient was a young man in respiratory distress for whom the probability of successful treatment was very high. The other patient was an elderly man in a coma, a cancer patient in acute renal failure. The determination had just been made that the man had suffered a severe cerebral hemorrhage and indications were that nothing further could be done for him. For me the choice was clear, all attention should be turned to saving the young salvageable patient.

At noon the director of the unit arrived – a man with a reputation as a very difficult personality. He decided to focus on the elderly patient who was almost dead. The director wanted to use the occasion for a teaching experience and began to explain all the aspects of the patient's condition. I said, "Never mind why this man is going to die, give me help in saving the other patient." He took great offense and shouted, "Go into my office, we have to talk." I took care of the young patient and then I went to his office. He was furious that I had challenged him in front of the nurses and demanded, "When I speak you must follow."

The coma patient died two hours later.

From my perspective, we were in a situation where we had to establish priority. It was an act of conscience for me to not take any time away from a patient we could save in order to discuss the medical details of a patient we most certainly could not save. I do not know how I could have handled the situation better – how to pay proper obeisance to my superior and at the same time care for my patient.

CASE

"The patient is dead, leave him dead"

I was just finishing a residency when an 18-year-old stabbing victim was brought to the Emergency Department with blunt force trauma to his chest. When I saw the patient, he had no vital signs, although one of the medics said he lost vital signs just before he came through the Emergency Department doors. I was faced with the question whether or not to do a thoracotomy. Established protocol dictates that thoracotomies are not performed on patients who present with no vital signs and injuries of this kind. Everyone in the Emergency Department agreed, "The patient is dead, leave him dead." Over the strong advice of my colleagues, I chose not to listen. If he had lost vital signs just moments before, that was good enough for me. When his chest was open we found that he had a pulmonary laceration, his heart was intact. We were able to cross clamp the laceration and the patient was taken to the operating room. I heard later that he survived and lived to walk out of the hospital neurologically intact.

Although I gambled and won, when the case was presented in grand rounds at the morning report, there was much heated discussion. I was admonished and told that in the future I should adhere to accepted practice. I was reminded of the huge outlay of monetary and human resources in every thoracotomy, including respiratory, X-ray, and nursing personnel, as well as the 15 or so members of the trauma team who are immediately activated. Keeping in mind that 99 percent of thoracotomy patients do not survive, and of those who do many are not neurologically intact, it is understandable why my decision was viewed as perhaps cavalier. However, I was operating under the principle of doing what I thought was in the best interest of the patient. I deviated from a protocol and had to endure professional reprimand. What should guide me in the future?

COMMENTARY

John Harris

The two cases entitled "When I speak you must follow" and "The patient is dead, leave him dead" raise interesting issues although they are not, I believe, in themselves very complex and I doubt that there will be many who are in doubt as to what the right thing to do was in each case. Indeed, one might think it a sad commentary on the medical profession that although in each case the principal doctor concerned did what was clearly the right thing, he or she appears to have been censured by medical colleagues for so doing. We will look at the cases separately.

"When I speak you must follow"

This case superficially presents the form of a particular dilemma; namely whether younger or older patients or patients with greater or lesser life expectancy are entitled to priority in virtue of either their better prognosis or the possibly longer life expectancy awaiting them after successful treatment. This dilemma is a real one and while many think that priority should be give to those either with better prognosis or with longer life expectancy or indeed, with better quality of life to be gained from treatment, I do not in fact think that that is the right solution. I have argued strongly over the years that neither their prognosis nor life expectancy nor quality of life should give one person advantage over another when, by hypothesis, each is entitled to *the same concerned respect* as any other person and therefore each is entitled to the same chance or opportunity of what life expectancy remains to them. (1–4) Thus, had the director of the unit been exemplifying this magisterial impartiality, when he decided to focus on the elderly patient, I would have supported his decision at least if it had been the result of a fair unbiased decision procedure establishing which of the two patients should be treated first. One such procedure might simply have been to toss a coin thus giving each the same chance of the treatment that might benefit them (albeit to a different degree). The justification for such impartiality would be that on the assumption that each had something worthwhile to gain from treatment and each would likely die without treatment, the moral reasons for saving each were equal since each stood to lose and gain the same thing at least on one conception of sameness. Each stood to lose his life; each stood to gain the chance to live the rest of their life. The fact that the quantum and the quality of rest of life to be gained was different in each case is of course necessarily true of all patients since in most cases no two lives are of exactly the same duration and of exactly the same quality. The incommensurability of the values involved can be illustrated by the following case. If a millionaire and a pauper both lose everything they have, on one measure each has lost a vastly different amount, the millionaire has lost millions, the pauper has lost a very small amount of money. But on another method of measurement each has lost everything, therefore each has lost the same.

These measures of what has been lost are incommensurable and there is no way of showing that one measure of loss is superior to the other. This being the case it can never be obviously right to have a rule of rescue, which demands that the person with the best prognosis or the longest life expectancy or the better quality of life should automatically have preference. All of that said, none of those interesting issues arise in this case. We are told, and we must accept, that literally "nothing further could be done" for the older patient and therefore there was absolutely no reason to prefer that patient. We must conclude that the doctor in this case acted rightly in challenging his superior.

The only remaining issue is whether medical hierarchies in which "obeisance" must be shown to superiors serves a useful function in medicine and whether in cases like this it should be maintained even if at some risk to patients. It seems doubtful that it serves any useful purpose and equally doubtful that it should be maintained at the cost of the rights and interests of patients. This is not to say that senior doctors should not have authority over junior doctors, simply that their position of authority does not have to be maintained by elaborate rituals of respect and politeness. Senior doctors should certainly be challenged and ultimately each doctor must answer first to his conscience and only second to his medical superiors, for if he or she does wrong and as a result a patient dies, the junior will also be responsible.

"The patient is dead, leave him dead"

Here the doctor had moral luck on her side. She made a choice that turned out to be the best. There seem to be two principal issues here. Should there be protocols designed principally to save resources and should these protocols be followed even when there is a chance of saving a worthwhile life? The protocol that seems to have been in force in this hospital would, I think, be regarded as eccentric. We are here in a case suitable for the rule of rescue. This is not simply a decision about how to allocate scarce resources but a decision about whether rescues, even expensive ones, should be attempted in emergency situations. Most protocols would take the view that it is worth attempting a rescue if there is a chance of success. For example, nobody says that cardiopulmonary resuscitation should not be attempted at the curb side following an accident even though the chances of success are poor. It is true that such a rescue is economical of resources immediately deployed (although of course a successful resuscitation will commit subsequent resources) but at least this shows that the chances of success are not the relevant consideration. The next question to address is whether the costs of the attempt are relevant. They would be in circumstances where the deployment of those resources for this patient means that other equally or more deserving patients will not be treated. This does not seem to have been the risk here since it is not stated that the 15 or so members of the trauma team were urgently required elsewhere. If they were, then a triage type decision would have to be taken and as I indicated in discussion of the case above the basis of any triage rule should be carefully considered.

In the present case then the doctor acted rightly and fortune blessed her. Fortune also blessed her patient. The only remaining issue is as to whether the rightness of her action and its fortunate outcome justify her contravening accepted practice. We know that accepted practice changes and hopefully changes for the better. It is therefore always in principle possible that accepted practice may be wrong and that the proposed breach of it constitutes a change for the better. This may not be known in advance and so no general principles can be produced as to whether contravening accepted practice is right or not in particular cases. All that can be said is that it is not clearly always wrong to go against accepted practice. The question should always be not "What is accepted practice?" but "What should be accepted as good practice?"

The principle appealed to by the doctor, in this case "doing what I thought was in the best interests of the patient," is also not always the best principle to follow. What is in the best interests of the patient in front of you may not be in the best interests of one or more other patients not in front of you. For example, where the patients are in competition for the scarce resources to be deployed, appeal to that principle is unreliable. However, in the absence of any respectable evidence that other patients, by hypothesis equally or more deserving, are in real and present danger, if the patient before you is in danger, you have good reasons to treat that patient. I conclude that in this case also the doctor did the right thing although not for the reasons that she gives.

Notes

1 Unprincipled QALYs. *J Med Ethics* 1991;17(4):185–8.
2 QALYfying The Value of Life. *J Med Ethics* 1987; September: 117–23. [Reprinted in *Medical Ethics*, ed. RS Downie. Aldershot, Dartmouth, 1996.]
3 What is the good of health care? *Bioethics* 1996;10(4):269–92.
4 Harris J. What the principal objective of the NHS should *really* be. *BMJ* 1997;314:669–72. [Reprinted in *Rationing: Talk and Action in Health Care*, ed. B. New. BMJ Publishing Group, London, 1997, pp.100–6.]

COMMENTARY

Alan Steinbach

Once upon a time, you were all there was in the world. Then maybe you recognized your mother, then dad, then others. Once upon a time, there was no authority, just your own actions. Then mom made rules. At first the rules are simple; don't bite the nipple. Then more complex. They tell us there are rules. They know the rules, often they make the rules; they are authority.

Once upon a time, not so long ago, you learned about authority beyond your parents. Now you know lots and lots of rules. Some rules involve a degree of paradox. Rules protect us from violence; there are violent punishments for breaking rules. We learn respect of the authority that enforces the rules. We learn about governors and presidents, about coaches and captains, about sergeants and generals. We learn that good students obey the rules, and to become a medical student, you must have been particularly good. So, you know a lot about rules and authority, and must have demonstrated your respect for authority on many many occasions.

And yet our folk stories are full of revolution and defiance of authority, or perhaps answering to a higher authority. The brave student who espoused the patient's cause and defied the blood-sucking administrator is a St Elsewhere legend. Doctors who defend patients' rights are respected, if not universally trusted by other doctors. Authority, we are told, must be challenged if it is found to be in error. How do we know when it is time to challenge? The purpose of this section is to explore acting against authority.

The two examples given should be considered against the magnificent expanse of the glory of modern medicine. We know so much! In school, college, university, and graduate medical education we learn chapters, books, and huge piles of information. In clinical settings we then learn ways to use this information to diagnose and treat medical problems. We learn that medical authority is properly based on information, not just on faith or belief. We swear oaths to do no harm, to save life, and also, to care for our fellow physicians. Although we generally respect authority, we hope that authority has all the information well in hand.

What happens when authority is wrong? What is wrong-ness, anyway? When the entire movie leads up to the moment of moral decision, and the trumpets blare, it is easy to second-guess the hero. But in our personal movies, with events unfolding at 3 in the morning and no sound track except vomiting; when the resident is asleep, it's hard to tell that a moment of decision has arrived. Is what you were just told to do really as wrong as it feels, or are you just too tired to know? When no one else at morning rounds seems to notice, what should you think? What should you do?

There can be conflicts of authority; of course, authority doesn't like to admit that happens, so the problem is often identifying the conflict in an ostensibly routine "this is a minor problem" situation. There are limits to authority, and authority doesn't like that much, either, so it is sometimes hard to realize that something happening is way out of the area of the authority claiming to be involved. And there are levels of authority, which authority doesn't like to be reminded of. Sometimes if you take the time to think things through, getting the right level is the most critical step to resolving an authority problem.

This underscores the need to be as sure as possible of the situation. This is why ethics committees spend so much time on hearing various opinions about the "facts" of a case. Although as individuals with a job to do, we may not be able to devote this much time to each case, we can try to pursue a decision-making tree that parallels the decision-making process of the ethics committee. First, what is authority? Second, what are the facts of the case?

We recognize many different levels of authority in our lives as human beings. Usually, the list comes down to this:

Me (or my patient) first, then
My kin (or my patient's family), then,
My friends (and colleagues), then
My society (or nation), then
Humankind

Some people feel there is a divine or natural law that somehow emanates from a higher authority. They might add, "then God," or "then the planet."

Business, professional, and institutional authority want each of us to recognize its regency, usually somewhere between friends and society. So, putting that in, the whole "ruler" of authority levels might look like this:

Me/My Patient   Family   Professional   Institutional Business   Society   Humankind

In any situation of real-life complexity, there may be many apparent conflicts with authority. A version of the ruler illustrated above might come in handy at those 3:00 a.m. Code E events that this book is intended to be helpful in.

In "When I speak you must follow," the director of the unit decided to refocus the team's time on a moribund patient with academically interesting findings. The intern takes direct exception to this, apparently in a very confrontative way. Whose issues are involved? Let's do it by the levels:

Me/my patient . . . the intern wants to care for the more deserving respiratory case. We don't know if the patient(s) have opinions; at least one is comatose.

Family . . . we don't know what the family of the patient wanted . . . a commonly missing piece of information.

Professional . . . the director wants to focus on the moribund patient who apparently is "interesting" for teaching.

Institutional . . . the director is de facto representative, but it isn't clear that the institutional views are in evidence yet.

Business . . . not raised as a consideration here. Probably wants to minimize expenses, and should be explicitly considered to avoid implicit influences.

Society . . . Some societies have very specific laws or customs regarding futility that may be helpful here. There is a general priority to save productive lives.

Humankind . . . the 10 commandments, or 10 precepts, or whatever forms you prefer them generally state humanity's higher goals. If you find yourself doing something that violates one of these, think again.

Using the authority level ruler, some things are clear. If there are families their opinions should be sought.

Also, the institution is probably on record as

valuing patient care and saving life over teaching opportunity, something that any team member can present to the group. In this case, on the information presented, it seems clear that if a triage must be done, the man in a coma (M. Moribunde) must be triaged, and attention turned to the more viable respiratory failure (M. LeRespiratoir). The families may both be the house officer's allies; the one urging comfort care only, the other wishing for maximal attention.

Thus, if the intern wanted to best serve his patients, his agenda should be to clearly and yet politely remind the director of his responsibilities to both patients, both families, and, in the choice he must make, to the institution. If this information is before the director and he persists in directing care to M. Moribunde, the intern might draw on societal authority ("why not let M. Moribunde die in peace; we can save M. Respiratoir for years of service to society if we act now . . .").

In the example, the intern describes actions that did not best serve his patients. It seems that he precipitated a Code E situation by a confrontational statement when he realized that the Director intended to focus on M. Moribunde. It seems to me that an equally impassioned but more politically astute intervention would have produced a less traumatic result.

In the second case presented, the situation develops in an instant with the arrival of a patient who is dead (no vital signs, trauma victim). The rules (institutional level authority) say nothing should be done. The senior resident (personal level authority) second guesses the rules by deciding that a *recent* loss of vital signs is different than *no* vital signs, intervenes, and restores life, at the usual enormous cost in institutional/societal resources. Although he had the personal status to do what he wanted to do, he is held accountable to the rules. In thinking about this case, it may be critical to understand the apparent facts, which depend on an understanding of what being dead is. In most apparently absolute situations, there are actually gradations of status. For example, with death, you might create a ruler like this:

Decaying Long dead Just dead Might be dead
Dying Unstable Living

Using this "ruler," it can be seen that the patient in the example was reclassified by the resident as a Might be dead or Just dead. Does he have the authority to do this? Yes, as long as he can point a straight path to the general principle of "Everyone deserves resuscitation." A Decaying or Long dead person clearly is an exception, but Just dead is the borderline unless specific experience has proven the borderline is elsewhere. Societal and institutional authorities generally agree that borderline cases should be treated at the level above. According to that, the resident was right to resuscitate.

However, suppose what the resident has chosen not to tell us is that a study had already shown that "Just dead" is really the same as "Long dead," for trauma cases, and that all house officers including himself were fully oriented to this study, and agreed, as a group, not to make "Just dead" into "Might be dead," but rather into "Long dead." In that case, the resident has no right to commit institutional resources to resuscitation, because a policy is already in place, and as a team member, the resident has made an error based on the facts (not knowing the apparently Just dead patient is Long dead for purposes of resuscitation).

In other words, in this case whose authority to follow depends critically on what are accepted as facts. If there is a question, go to the "best for the individual" criteria. In this case, the resident is right. If not, follow the rules. In this case, the resident is wrong.

Sometimes evidence-based medicine runs counter to individual intuition or societal hopes. For example, current outcome studies suggest that although the use of high dose adrenaline in advanced cardiac life support (ACLS) or in CPR can get a "live" patient out of the ER, most people resuscitated this way are severely brain damaged or die. An institution could not adopt a policy that said don't resuscitate *any* ACLS patients arriving from the field with no vital signs, because it has been shown that *some* (not many) of such patients will survive to a meaningful life. But it *could* adopt a rule against the use of resuscitation in the "Just dead" and residents working in that institution would then be expected to follow the rule. An institution cannot adopt a procedural rule that is significantly at odds with a general societal principle. But if there is accepted evidence available, and the profession or institution has taken note of it, each individual is responsible for upholding the course of action dictated by the evidence.

Does that mean that a doctor must resuscitate *all* patients arriving with vital signs from a traumatic accident? Yes. Certainly the patient's membership in a gang, skin color, age, and attitude are not relevant. It may be a major effort of will to set aside personal biases, but you must do it quickly and completely. Possibly concurrent major disease is a mitigating factor, but trauma treatment needs very simple rules, because it evolves so rapidly. That's why the Pre-Hospital Do Not Resuscitate (DNR) form is very short. As a member of an emergency team, it's your responsibility to know about the existence of authority such as the DNR, and defend that authority in all cases. Knowing the rules is important, just like your mom told you.

Sometimes in thinking about a specific case, the wrong level of authority may seem to be involved. For example, from the financial (business and society) point of view, the cost of the resuscitation is very high. The societal value of the specific individual may appear to be low (55-year-old male with adult onset diabetes mellitus and a below knee amputation from county jail). Perhaps the individual (e.g., living will, DNR order) has already given you a rule to follow, if you know to look for it. Perhaps someday, society will decide that 58-year-old white males with vasectomies making under $150,000 should not be resuscitated, and make a rule to that effect. In the absence of such authority, the P test is useful. ("If Mr. Nifeangun was the president/your parent,

what would you do?") Triage the individual to the best case scenario you can; in this case, imagining him to be your parent, to avoid making a decision based on incorrect authority.

Authority is easier to act against when you happen to represent the authority, as the senior resident did in "The patient is dead, leave him dead." But you cannot act this way without expecting repercussions, particularly if it becomes clear that your own considerations are at odds with the institution's. Unless there was at least an ambiguity in the rule of nonresuscitation, the resident acted incorrectly. For example, the house officer who has strong views against abortion must not endanger a patient's life when an abortion would save her. One who believes in the power of prayer must not delay protocol intervention to pray with the patient. Just because you feel a 75-year-old with cancer has no real life does not entitle you to enter them as No Code without their explicit acceptance.

One of the most important parts in the successful management of a Code Blue situation is remembering to call the Code. Similarly, Code E situations are easier to manage if you at least recognize that a situation exists. Learn to rely on your instincts, and then follow a simple plan.

Code Blue
Patient unresponsive
Check airway
Check breathing
Check circulation
Call code Blue and begin CPR

Code E
Feel uncomfortable with what happened
    Excuse me, what just happened?
Conflict with what I know is right?
    Explanatory information
Conflict of authority?
    Explain authorities and rank order
Continued wrong action?
    Escalate verbal intervention
Call Code E
The intervention in Code E situations is primar-

ily verbal. There are some basic dialogue pathways that I have overheard and adopted, or tested myself and found helpful. Here are some examples, in order of how deep the doodoo is getting.

> "Sir, perhaps I didn't hear right. What have you decided to do?"
>
> "Doctor, could I briefly review the clinical situation(s) involved here?"
>
> "M. le Directeur, perhaps the lecture could wait until the (other) patient is treated?"
>
> "If I understand what you are saying, I am not sure that I agree with your plan. Could I say why?"
>
> "I don't agree. Could we take a moment as a team to discuss the plan?"
>
> "If you insist, I must say clearly that I will have to file an incident report. I really disagree with your plan, and don't feel comfortable participating or even just standing by."
>
> "No. I won't do that."

In the example "The patient is dead," there is no time for much dialogue, but a fellow team member might have said, "remember we all read the study about Just dead patients and agreed to treat them as Long dead." Thus reminded, the senior resident might have realized that his efforts were out of line with rules, and paused to check with other team members. He might then have been more able to modulate his own desire to save life with the evidence, and the abilities of the team.

When such rapidly evolving situations are likely, some institutions conduct scenario drills to help avoid conflict and ethical dilemmas. During World War 2, truck drivers read cartoon books showing them how to run down a child in the road to avoid swerving over a cliff and endangering their load of soldiers. ACLS protocols indicate that resuscitation efforts should be terminated after a certain point in the algorithm. This kind of practice, or for that matter, institutional rules of any kind don't eliminate dilemmas. For example, a family may not recognize brain death as the criteria for Dead. But at least members of a team can practice working in evolving situations, and try to reach agreement on basic principles before the situation is in their faces.

Does it matter that the patient in the example "The patient is dead, leave him dead" survived the resuscitation and surgery? Of course, it matters to the patient. And it should matter to the institution. Perhaps the rule is wrong, and some trauma victims without vital signs *should* be resuscitated. Yet the senior resident's actions must be judged by the circumstances at the time, not those proven by later study. When he asks what should guide him in the future, the answer is the same that should have guided him at the time; a clear understanding of authority concerned with the case, and an ability to communicate effectively, plus knowledge of all the relevant information possible.

From what level does authority draw its validation? For example, in "When I speak you must follow," the Parisian intern presumes that the director is drawing on the needs of the educational institution, and perhaps his own interest in stroke, in choosing to spend time with the moribund patient. Similarly, the intern believes he is drawing on the immediate needs of both patients in deciding to attend to the patient in respiratory distress. First there is the need of an elderly man in a coma resulting from renal failure related to cancer. Medical treatment other than comfort care would seem to be futile. In the U.S., a durable power document might exist instructing practitioners to provide no further treatment. In contrast, the young patient with respiratory failure presented to the intern an obvious need for triage to immediate intensive care. If this patient also had a terminal diagnosis (advanced AIDS, hepatitis C, cancer, etc.) then from the original meaning of the term "triage," he as well as the patient in a coma might be assigned a category of *futile/will die despite treatment*. Then there is the need of a younger presumably healthy individual with a treatable emergent problem. The intern clearly believes this patient must be triaged to top priority.

In this case, the ethical dilemma becomes simply a problem of communication (between a brash intern and a stuffy director). A politically astute intern might have been able to resolve the issue by reminding the director that a duty to save the patient's life no longer existed, and that the requirement of the practitioner was thus congruent with institutional needs (don't waste resources) and professional codes (provide comfort and relief of pain).

The intern has to know that the authority he wants to challenge does not have better clinical judgment. Perhaps the director knows something the intern does not. If the situation degenerates into anger, critical information may be lost. In other words, the contrast between the two patients must be real, and the best possible information must be clearly considered in deciding which of the patients is the most deserving. Anything less will give a bad outcome.

Let's assume instead that no durable power exists for either patient, or even that a family is at the bedside of the comatose man demanding medical attention. They want "everything" done. Would this change the situation? It would certainly emphasize the need for good information about the patients' condition, but society defends the right of medical personnel to triage patients when necessary. I believe that M. LeRespiratoir should be treated, and M. Moribunde triaged to comfort care.

Most landscapes make more sense when you are walking slowly through them. Rapidly evolving situations create more chaotic images, and are thus harder to cope with. In such situations, authority is most valuable and most vulnerable. Valuable because something must be done quickly, and if several opinions exist, some process must take place rapidly to decide on actions. It is the responsibility of the authority to create such process. But authority is vulnerable, because the pressure to act creates a higher potential for error.

When the process is mysterious, when no explanation is offered, and no chance to discuss decisions is provided, authority is most vulnerable. But this is also true for a challenge to authority. In the case "When I speak you must follow" the director is presented with a confrontational intern, perhaps before the director realized there were other patients who needed care, or that the duty roster was thin. Perhaps understandably, the situation immediately becomes a struggle for control, apparently without an exchange of information. Perhaps the director is not really aware of the shortage of doctors, and thus the need for triage. Perhaps the intern is not aware of circumstances that make treatment of the respiratory failure patient more difficult, perhaps even futile, and the coma patient more reasonable. Without a chance to exchange views, the challenge to authority may actually result in harm to *both* patients, since the angry exchange obviously takes time from medical treatment.

It seems a general principle that many ethical dilemmas arise primarily because of failures to communicate. Optimally, when such a difference emerged, a process would ensue that resulted in the best decision possible. Instead, the intern challenges authority by throwing back on the director the intern's opinion that the director has misused his authority, when in fact he may just not have all the facts.

Ultimately, real differences of opinion may coexist. In this case, if the director is impelled by a desire to teach, and the intern by a desire to save lives, there is no ethical dilemma. The director is wrong, the intern is right. No ethics committee would have to convene to consider the case once this situation was clear, although members of the committee might want to spend time counseling the parties. Saving the patient's life clearly outweighs any curricular (institutional) needs. The efforts of the house officer should be directed at moving any apparent disagreement to a level of testable reality (teaching vs. saving lives).

Suppose the director "doesn't get it," and despite the most astute political intervention, flatly says that teaching takes priority over saving life.

This clearly represents a situation when one may literally stand in the door.

One of my fellow medical students was assigned to help prep for surgery a 16-year-old patient with developmental delay due to prenatal rubella scheduled for a TAH-BSO (hysterectomy and oophorectomy). As she reviewed the chart, the student understood that the operation was being performed because the patient's mother worried about her affectionate nature, and didn't want her to become pregnant. It seemed clear to the student that informed consent regarding alternatives had not really been obtained, and that the 16-year-old did not know what was happening. After briefly presenting the situation to her intern and resident, and getting shrugs, the student recruited me to join her in physically blocking the door to prevent the patient from being wheeled to surgery, having sent a third student to the dean. Eventually someone from the dean's office arrived, there were whispered consultations, and the surgery was postponed, and later cancelled.

A simple checklist, comparable to that read before operating an aircraft, might be helpful in rapidly evolving situations. The outlined Code E procedure presented earlier might be a starting point for such a checklist. Additionally, consider the following:

Are the facts in evidence and agreed upon?
(Try to describe/jot down the facts and see if you can make them make sense.)
Is there a reasonable doubt as to the best decision?
(That is, reasonable scientific doubt, or no real science/outcome experience.)
Which authority is involved?

Me/My patient Family Professional Institutional
Business Society Humankind

Have I got the situation right?

Decaying Long dead Just dead Might be dead
Dying Unstable Stable

Striving to stay on top: competing with peers

CASE

"He would always arrange to have the easiest cases for himself"

A fellow intern treated the rest of us in a particularly unfair manner. He was willing and eager to advance himself at our expense. When he was on call, instead of waiting for the "hit list" of patient assignments, he would go to the Emergency Department and always arrange to have the easiest cases for himself. The more complicated cases were then given out to the rest of us. I hated him for it. If I complained, I was afraid I would be seen as weak or a "wimp."

CASE

"Just another cut-throat medical student"

On the first day of gross anatomy, I was assigned to a team of four medical students. The cadavers were submerged in vats and it was a tense time for all of us as the bodies were hoisted up to table level and we began dissection on the back. As we worked, trying to follow the text instructions, myself and two other members of our team noticed a low persistent murmuring nearby. Our fourth team member was standing by the cadaver's side, holding his hand and rocking back and forth as she whispered, "It will be OK, this won't hurt, you'll be all right." Her seemingly bizarre behavior continued throughout the following weeks as subsequently she insisted that the cadaver's toes be covered with a cloth to prevent chill as he was lowered into the preservation vat at the end of each class. I had serious concerns regarding my classmate's emotional stability, but did not know if it were my place to take my concerns to a faculty member. Should I leave it to chance that her behavior would be noticed by someone in authority? Did I have a responsibility to the medical profession and/or her future patients? Our class was scheduled to begin clinical assignments later in the semester and she would soon be in contact with live patients. I was also worried that if I did alert others, I might be viewed as just another cut-throat medical student trying to eliminate the competition.

CASE

"The new arrival was the ideal 'victim'"

I was a resident in one of the best ICUs in Paris. In the midst of always being very busy caring for patients, the atmosphere in the unit was heavy with conflicts between the heads and the residents.

A doctor arrived from a distant provincial town. He was understandably anxious about coming to our highly regarded unit, and he arrived with great misgivings. What happened after he joined the unit reminded me of ancient Greece where in times of conflict an ugly man living in the suburbs was chosen as a victim and conflicts were displaced onto him.

Every problem in the ICU became the fault of this new addition. The other residents criticized his treatment of patients and his explanations. Actually, he was a very good doctor, but because he was less sophisticated, he became the object of everyone's derision.

I, like others in the unit, benefited from his status as scapegoat since the focus on him took the pressure off of us. I was aware that I was "safe" because he got the admonishment. I felt guilty and even though the treatment he received was unfair, I did nothing to stop it. I benefited from his misfortune and I took refuge in that fact. I am not sure what I could have done, but I still feel ambivalent about the situation, I never came to his defense.

COMMENTARY

David N. Weisstub

In all hierarchies in workplaces, there is a division of labor, but unlike what is found in nature, or in the kibbutz, questions of fairness according to theories of wants and needs persist. Humans seem to specialize in examples of the bad apple, where greed and exploitation are attributes that alas can lead to success in political and corporate life. So much so that soft or weak forms of psychology are often congratulated and rewarded, even when advancement and success are at the expense of peers. The philosophy of getting ahead at any price, although officially decried in public morality, seems to still find a home in the most competitive worlds and especially in our libertarian economies. One could argue that this phenomenon is most pronounced in elite institutions, including medical schools. Where an individual truly stands out as an exploiter and is uniformly admonished by his or her peer group, the matter is less subtle and simply deserving of group intervention based on an equitable demand. There are notable examples where the cleverest of a bunch find the vehicles to avoid dog work and locate the most efficacious route for career upgrading and the accumulation of prestige. Excessive examples of such exploitation lead to failure as we well know from our routine observations in films and novels where the real manipulator loses in the end. The problem however rests with the successful manipulator, the one who is not cast aside because he is reduced to the definition of a con-man, bringing on the revolt of peers. Rather we should place our attention on the well-honed socially smooth individual who has enough going for him or herself that they are able to escape social reprimand, in the course of seeking out mobility within a professional hierarchy. Are we to discourage morally sound individuals who come forward to complain against social systems which indulge opportunism? How are we to cope with instances where the wimp attribute is pinned on the worker bees who are caught by their own morality of purpose? If the immorality of indulging mobility tactics is found to be endemic, then there remains a serious moral job of reflection to be conducted in professional environments.

The process of distancing from morally unacceptable or deviant behavior within a peer group is complex. There is the moral obligation to evolve communally in accumulation of professional experience. Flowing from this, it is a self-evident objective that there is an optimization of the best level of group achievement. It is understood that turning against a peer in such a situation should only be based on the gravest of information where bringing a third party is connected to a higher duty to forewarn that one's peer is a potential risk to the safety of those placed under professional care. A blurring of reality, an aura of mental disturbance, deeply ingrained prejudices, or desire for vengeance are examples where a duty to warn and protect can justifiably be set off within a peer group.

One of the sensitivities surrounding medical students is that there is a built-in pressure within the survival game to allow defectives to be crushed under the weight of the bell curve. After having struggled so valiantly to enter what is perceived by many to be a pressure cooker, morally aware individuals are hesitant to be reduced to the role of tattler. Paradoxically, those individuals who share an intense moral sensibility towards the protection of patients should be the strongest candidates for policing the training environment. Bad examples of such interventions however, are do-gooders who have such an impulse towards self-righteousness and a presumptive arrogance about knowing what the correct standards are for behavior, that they are given to premature judgment short of the aforementioned extreme examples which should give rise to dutiful recognition and reporting of unwarranted risks to potential subjects. Early warning signals of such behavior are not only morally justifiable,

but should be part of the responsibility of institutional morality at the highest level. It is not possible to balance the benefits to clinical subjects in a favorable light when bizarreness is part of the moral equation. When samaritanship is an excuse for currying favor with superiors, it should not be condoned, but when it is part of a well-thought-through professional duty, even among novices to protect the values of the professional environment, it should be accepted and dealt with in a discreet and responsible fashion by the authorities. A proper moral response should also include a tolerant handling of the perceived disorder such that there should be institutional support for therapeutic review of a situation where every attempt is made to make it possible for the trainee to return to the function of professional services.

Short of real mental disorders, there are a wide range of conditions where groups initiate a convenient displacement vehicle for releasing tensions or enhancing an elite style with which it is particularly comfortable. In large urban centers, where teaching hospitals are usually located, the concept of a country bumpkin is a familiar point of reference, especially in places where there is a strong sense of cultural centralization. In certain countries, coming from the provinces is a burden which can follow even the most talented professional throughout a long career cycle. This often translates as the inability of social hierarchies to separate style from substance.

The unfairness of such attitudes is very apparent when the skill set is technical rather than discretionary or judgmental. Since much of instruction and leadership is part and parcel of what we see as attractive professional style, there is inevitable blurring throughout the range of activities found in training centers of our inability to dissect reality from fiction, unwarranted praise from unjustified criticism. Often it is only with the benefit of hindsight that a vast life experience recasts the victims of early education or indeed professional training as unsung heroes lost on a specific time and place where the events occurred. Without expecting to perfect these built-in inadequacies in every social hierarchy, it is still a moral necessity that we fight against a natural instinct to sing the songs of the winners and to gain acceptance through participating in the silence that turns the underdog into a nonbeing.

We are all familiar with the popular fiction that has depicted the grammar school boy who was tormented by being outclassed in an Oxbridge common room or where the farmer's son or daughter found their way by trial and humiliation to the upper echelon institutions in the time of Franz Josef. These nineteenth-century images bring both tears and laughter in our viewing of a Chekhov play, so much so that we often fail to realize that there are persistent forms of social institutional hierarchy that make it possible for every generation to redefine its underdogs. Even in politically correct environments if we look carefully there are even ways of being accepted as a member of a minority or as a person raised below the poverty line. There are cues for knowing the rights and wrongs within any acquired professional-style rhetoric. Persons who carry with them socially unacceptable styles in any given environment are ripe for being pushed aside. Even within minority populations, there are persons whose social skill set can be found annoying or threatening to the socially advancing group. Within educational institutions, there are recognizable subcultures, and even when we regard ourselves as cosmopolitan or liberal, such official statements of self-recognition or definition can be elusive or misleading. In so doing, we fail to admit that there are boundaries and styles of behavior which are correct and other forms which are unacceptable to the group at large or to subcultures within it. Sometimes it can be within a minority population that there is a deep infliction of being cast as an outsider. Excessive intensity about political ideals, sensitivity with regard to racial slurs, heroizing an unpopular symbol, a commitment to a religious set of beliefs, a provocative manner of dress, obesity, sexual prefer-

ences, having a particular handicap or disease, a perceived poor manner of accent or speech may all give rise to conditions for precipitating social denigration. The internal conflict and hurt created by further diminution within the minority group with which one is identified may be the most violative encounter to be experienced. Therefore, all groups existing in institutions, both majority and minority, should be familiarized in the initiation phase of higher learning with the needs for mutual support.

COMMENTARY

Jean-Christophe Mino

All three of the cases presented here illustrate the difficult psychological context in medical training that engenders competition. The tension and anxiety to distinguish oneself and perform well can have the positive effect of stimulating personal growth and self-improvement. But, this is not the whole picture. It is the darker, or more perverse, side of competition that concerns us here.

Competition is not special to the world of medicine; competition is a general fact of social organization. However, there is a notable difference between competition in medicine and other settings, such as business. Competition among medical professionals may carry with it deleterious consequences for patients. If medical personnel are unduly concerned with their status within the organization and how they rank with their supervisors (who they believe have the power to control their destiny), then it seems inevitable that there will be a conflict between what is in their own best interest and the best interest of the patient.

I believe the roots of competition can be found in a system of medical training that fosters both individualism and isolation. Typically, students spend much of their time studying alone; and little, or no, encouragement is given to group efforts. The fact that individual performance is so highly valued, exaggerates the competitive aspects of the process. This pattern which promotes individualism is an integral part of the structure and organization of medical education.

In France, for example, medical training involves three levels of stiff competition where trainees are pitted against their peers. Initially, after the first year of study there is an exam which is only passed by approximately 10 percent of students (the 90 percent who fail are given one additional opportunity to succeed). There is a second culling, approximately five years later, for those who wish to go on for specialist training. Only about one-third of those taking the exam are accepted to continue. Finally, after specialization and residency, there is another competition for the prestigious few "chef de clinique" positions – a necessity for those wanting to work in academic hospitals.

It is not surprising after years of fierce competition during training years, that physicians have difficulty working cooperatively as members of a team. Yet team membership is exactly what modern medicine requires. A hundred years ago one doctor took care of one patient, but today's rapid escalation of information necessitates a wider approach. Unless the direction of medical education changes to allow a comfortable participation in the group-oriented procedures required by modern medicine, there will continue to be an ongoing conflict in the student's functioning, with the possibility of detriment to the patient.

When I was a new resident and on call for the first time, I felt very much alone. Technically,

there was a "chef de clinique" whom I could call; but I was keenly aware that she would not be pleased to hear from me. On the ward was a foreign physician functioning as a nurse until he could gain French certification. He was a pulmonologist and one of my patients had pneumonia. I asked his opinion as to treatments and we discussed the case. The next morning when I recounted the incident to the chief of the department I was severely rebuked: "It does not matter what he thinks. Your patient is your responsibility *alone.*"

Although I was criticized for my early efforts at collaboration, I was reminded of an important reality – even when seeking counsel (as more and more we are required to do in medicine), you still must make your own decisions. In the end, you alone are responsible for your patient and you rely on yourself.

In Paris during my residency, I had an opportunity to participate in a demonstration project which consisted of a group of approximately a half dozen medical students who met monthly with a resident for several years to discuss issues that were meaningful to them, both of a personal and professional nature. This was a marked deviation from the usual solitary and conventional activities characteristic of medical training. These sessions allowed the participants to receive support, and to identify with a close group who all had some emotional investment in each other.

The question to be addressed is: Must competition in the pursuit of professional goals always involve the stress of loneliness and isolation, or can medical education incorporate structural means to allow students to grow and develop in a more congenial atmosphere?

20

Conflicts of interest

CASE

"Should I accept drug company goodies?"

It is no secret that throughout all the years of training, and beyond, drug companies court doctors. Also obvious is the fact that the companies lavish more attention on us as residents than when we were medical students; but in my experience, from the very beginning the lure of drug company offerings has been an ever-present enticement. There are all those free pens, writing pads and, more temptingly, weekly lunches in the conference room cosponsored by a department and a drug company. Knowing there is no such thing as a truly "free lunch," and these perks are being offered for a purpose, should I accept drug company goodies? I do not feel that I am selling my soul by accepting hospitality and marketing gifts, but at the same time I do not feel entirely comfortable. Is my integrity necessarily compromised by enjoying such benefits? Would it be morally permissible to accept some perks but not others?

COMMENTARY

James Weber

Gifts from industry

The universal practice of pharmaceutical companies bestowing gifts on physicians is well documented. (1–6) However, this practice is controversial because gifts cost money, and the cost is ultimately passed on to their patients without their explicit knowledge. (7) Approximately 25 percent of the dollars patients spend on prescription drugs are devoted to pharmaceutical marketing, with part of this budget returned to physicians in the form of gifts, food, hospitality, and promotional campaigns. (8) In the United States, drug companies spend over $10 billion per year on promotional gifts ranging from tickets to sporting events and 5-star meals to weekend golf and ski vacations. (9) Despite serious abuses regarding gift giving, the pharmaceutical industry has made outstanding contributions to the advancement of modern scientific medicine. (7) However, some gifts that reflect customary industry practices are inconsistent with the basic principles of medical ethics. Furthermore, an obvious conflict of interest occurs when physicians accept personal gifts that have no benefit to their patients.

The acceptance of gifts assumes that a relationship between industry representative and physician has taken place, accompanied by an inherent sense of obligation. Despite the contention that acceptable pharmaceutical gifts do not adversely impact prescribing practices and the promotional materials provided have educational merit, physicians are now armed with compelling data that suggests otherwise. McKinney recently surveyed physicians from seven hospitals affiliated with three academic training programs and found that 67 percent of faculty members indicated that their objectivity could be compromised by accepting industry-sponsored gifts. (10) More recently, Chren determined that physicians

Table 20.1. *Gifts from industry*

Acceptable	Not acceptable
Medical textbooks	Cash
Modest meals (educationally related)	Direct subsidies for time, lodging, and personal expenses
Gifts related to clinical practice	Personal or family use of drug samples
Underwriting CME costs	Obligatory strings attached
Medical student, resident, and fellow scholarships	

Modified from: Gifts to physicians from industry, *JAMA* 1991;265(4):501.

who had interacted with, or accepted money from pharmaceutical representatives were almost five times more likely to request the company's product as a hospital formulary addition than those who did not. (7) Many physicians argue that they would lose a valuable source of information if contacts with pharmaceutical representatives were banned and perceive their behavior regarding prescription drugs as motivated mainly by drug performance data. However, physician knowledge and beliefs about selected drugs appear to more closely match the advertising claims of the respective pharmaceutical companies. (11) In addition, very little data distributed by pharmaceutical companies provides information about important scientific progress, and some of it fails to comply with FDA regulations. (12)

During this decade, a number of changes have occurred regarding the way pharmaceutical companies are allowed to interact with physicians. (13) Hearings conducted by the U.S. Senate Labor and Human Resources Committee prompted the American Medical Association as well as numerous specialties to adopt guidelines that better define an acceptable relationship between physicians and the pharmaceutical industry. (2, 14) Table 20.1 outlines these guidelines, of which textbooks, modest meals, and medical equipment are acceptable if they serve a bona fide educational function and ultimately benefit patients. Subsidies to underwrite the costs

of CME conferences or scientific meetings that contribute to the improvement of patient care are permissible. In addition, scholarships or other special funds that permit physicians in training to attend carefully selected educational conferences are considered permissible as long as the recipients are selected by the academic or training institution. On the other hand, acceptance of cash or individual gifts that do *not* benefit patients, such as trips and subsidies for medical educational conferences at which physicians are not speakers, are strongly discouraged. The AMA Council on Ethical and Judicial Affairs has also recommended that physicians should not accept free samples of drugs and other gifts for personal or family use because they do not improve the care that patients receive. When accepting gifts from industry, physicians should be cognizant that patients generally consider pharmaceutical gifts more influential and less appropriate than do their physicians. (15) The acceptance of even small gifts has been documented to affect clinical judgment and heightens the perception (reality) of a conflict of interest. (14) Future guidelines will need to expand and exemplify what are deemed to be "acceptable" gifts, and in so doing, consider the potentially different viewpoints of patients and their providers. Common sense should always prevail. No gifts should be accepted if there are subsequently "strings attached." Always pose the questions "would I be willing to have this arrangement generally known?" and "what would the public or my patients think of this arrangement?", prior to making decisions regarding the acceptance of gifts. (16, 17)

Notes

1 American College of Emergency Physicians. Code of ethics for emergency physicians. *Ann Emerg Med* 1997;30:365–72.
2 American Medical Association. *Code of Medical Ethics: Current Opinions with Annotations.* Chicago: American Medical Association, 1997, p.105.

3 Fakes, RW. Doctors and the drug industry. *BMJ* 1986;293:1170–1.

4 Orlowski, JP, Wateska L. The effects of pharmaceutical firm enticements on physician prescribing patterns. *Chest* 1992;102:270–3.

5 Rawlins MD. Doctors and the drug makers. *Lancet* 1984;2:276–8.

6 Relman AS. Economic incentives in clinical investigation. *N Engl J Med* 1989;320(14):933–4.

7 Chren MM, Landefeld S, Murray TH. Doctors, drug companies, and gifts. *JAMA* 1989;262:3448–51.

8 Noble RC. Physicians and the pharmaceutical industry: an alliance with unhealthy aspects. *Perspect Biol Med* 1993;36:376–94.

9 Heber A. Drug companies and doctors: a troubling alliance. *Psychiatr Resid Newsl* 1993;17(1):1–2.

10 McKinney WP, Schniedermayer MD, Lurie N, Simpson DE, et al. Attitudes of internal medicine faculty and residents toward professional interaction with pharmaceutical sales representatives. *JAMA* 1990;264:1693–7.

11 Avorn J, Chen M, Hartley R. Scientific versus commercial sources of influence on the prescribing behavior of physicians. *Am J Med* 1982;73:4–8.

12 Thompson DF. Understanding financial conflicts of interest. *N Engl J Med* 1993;329:573–6.

13 American College of Physicians. Physicians and the pharmaceutical industry. *Ann Intern Med* 1990;112:624–6.

14 American College of Physicians. *Ethics Manual. Fourth Edition. Ann Intern Med* 1998;128:576–94.

15 Gibbons RV, Landry FJ, Blouch DL, et al. A comparison of physicians' and patients' attitudes toward pharmaceutical industry gifts. *J Gen Intern Med* 1998;13:151–4.

16 Fakes RW. Doctors and the drug industry. *BMJ* 1986;293:1170–1.

17 The relationship between physicians and the pharmaceutical industry. A report of the Royal College of Physicians. *J R Coll Physicians Lond* 1986;20:235–42.

COMMENTARY

Carson Strong

As the case points out, gift-giving from drug companies to physicians is widespread. Practicing physicians, residents, interns, and even medical students receive gifts. In a survey of chief residents of emergency medicine programs in the United States, Reeder and colleagues found that pharmaceutical companies distributed gifts in at least 90 percent of responding programs. (1) Hodges surveyed residents, interns, and medical students at seven hospitals affiliated with a psychiatry residency program and learned that the average number of gifts per respondent during a one-year period was 22. (2)

A variety of gifts are given, and they range in value. Relatively inexpensive gifts include pens, note pads, key chains, and pocket flashlights. Drug companies often distribute gifts at conferences, such as tote bags and travel alarm clocks, as well as free dinners and accommodation. Other gifts include tickets to entertainment, airplane tickets, cash, textbooks, and journals. More lavish gifts include free trips to conferences at resort locations. Academic departments and professional organizations also receive gifts, including research grants, symposia, noon conference lunches, books, and journals.

Several arguments can be given against physicians accepting such gifts. First, accepting them might influence physicians' prescribing decisions. If that happens, decisions might not be based on objective judgments about the patient's interests. This argument is supported by considering the psychology of gift giving and receiving. As discussed by Chren and coauthors, accepting a personal gift is accepting the initiation or reinforcement of a relationship between the giver and recipient. (3) Accepting a gift typically creates in the receiver a set of sentiments including a sense of indebtedness to the giver. This sense of indebtedness typically involves a feeling that one is obligated to be grateful and to reciprocate in some way. These sentiments might consciously or unconsciously affect the recipient's behavior, and if prescribing decisions are influenced by gifts so that a patient receives a drug that is less effective or more expensive than a drug that otherwise would have been prescribed, then the patient's interests are harmed and the principle of nonmaleficence is violated. (4)

Second, patients' trust in their physicians can be undermined when gift-giving creates the appearance of a conflict of interest. Data relevant to this argument can be found in a study by Blake and Early. (5) They conducted a survey in the waiting rooms of two family practice centers, with 486 subjects completing the study questionnaire. One part of the survey asked whether the respondent believed it is all right for physicians to accept certain gifts. It was found that 48 percent disapproved of physicians receiving free dinners, 44 percent disapproved their receiving free baby formula for their own children, and 33 percent disapproved their being given payments for conference expenses. Fifty-four percent of respondents believed that drug company gifts sometimes influence a physician's prescribing of medications, and an additional 16 percent believed that such influence *frequently* occurs. Given these results, the argument that patients' trust in physicians might be undermined should be taken seriously.

A third argument is that the cost of gifts is ultimately passed to patients in the form of higher medicine prices. According to a report of the U.S. Senate Labor and Human Resources Committee, American drug companies spent at least $5 billion on marketing in 1989. (6) A 1987 survey of the 25 largest drug companies revealed that expenditures for marketing were approximately equal to those for research and development. (4) The Senate report also contained results from a survey of 18 major pharmaceutical companies showing that the firms spent $165 million on symposia and gifts in 1988. (6)

Perhaps the main argument physicians give in support of accepting gifts is the claim that gifts do not influence their prescribing decisions. This view – that they are immune from influence – is widespread among physicians. In Hodges's survey of psychiatry residents, interns, and medical students, 56 percent (41/73) of respondents stated that receiving gifts would have no impact on their prescribing. (2)

Additional empirical data are available to help assess the above arguments. A study by Orlowski and Wateska examined changes in the prescribing patterns of physicians after they were given all-expense-paid trips for two to resort hotels to attend symposia sponsored by pharmaceutical companies. (7) Two such symposia were studied, each of which focused on a new drug. One was a new intravenous antibiotic, referred to as Drug A, and the conference for it was held at a luxury hotel on the west coast. The other drug was a new cardiovascular medicine, referred to as Drug B, and the symposium for it was held at an island resort in the Caribbean. The hospital at which prescribing patterns were studied was the Cleveland Clinic Foundation Hospital. For each conference, ten physicians from the Cleveland Clinic Foundation attended. Hospital pharmacy records were used to track the prescribing patterns of the two drugs before and after the conferences. During the one-year period following the conference on Drug A, the average quantity of Drug A used per month was 272 units, compared to 81 units per month during the year preceding the conference. Moreover, the increase in this hospital could not be accounted for by a general increase in use of the drug; over the 2-year period, usage of the drug increased 3.5-fold nationwide, compared to 10-fold at the Cleveland Clinic Foundation Hospital. Study of Drug B yielded similar results; the monthly average increased from 34 to 87 units before and after the symposium. During the 2-year period, Drug B usage nationwide increased approximately 3-fold, compared to 4.5-fold at the hospital, a statistically significant difference. Although this study does not prove that the increased use of the drugs at the Cleveland Clinic Foundation Hospital was a result of the free trips, it strongly suggests that possibility.

According to a survey by McKinney and colleagues, some physicians acknowledge that gifts can influence them. (8) These investigators distributed questionnaires to residents in three internal medicine residency programs. Among respondents who believed that gifts can compromise physician decisions, 57 percent (84/147) believed that a gift of $50 or more could result in such compromise.

In analyzing the ethics of drug company gifts, it will be helpful to distinguish between gifts to individuals and gifts to educational programs such as academic departments. Given this distinction, five main views concerning the ethics of drug company gifts can be identified. To explore the question of what policies should be followed, I shall try to point out the pros and cons of these main views.

1 All gifts are acceptable.
2 Some gifts to individuals and some gifts to educational programs are acceptable.
3 No gifts to individuals and some gifts to educational programs are acceptable.
4 Some gifts to individuals and no gifts to educational programs are acceptable.
5 No gifts are acceptable.

To consider the pros and cons, let us begin with views 1 and 5, which are the least restrictive and most restrictive of the five views, respectively. A serious problem with view 1 is revealed by the study of Orlowski and Wateska discussed above. (7) Their data suggest that expensive gifts like trips to vacation resorts can influence physician's prescribing decisions. Based on this consideration, the view that *all* gifts are acceptable should be rejected.

In opposition to view 5, it can be argued that some gifts to educational programs are ethically acceptable. In particular, if a gift can be handled in such a way that it does not constitute a gift to any individual, then the psychology of gift receiving by individuals would not come into play. An example of such a gift might be a grant to help cover the costs of a conference. With this sort of gift, individual residents and faculty presumably would be less likely to develop a feeling that they should reciprocate. If that is so, then it seems unlikely that prescribing would be compromised. Moreover, a positive argument in support of such gifts is that they have educational value. These considerations support the rejection of view 5.

This argument against view 5 also applies to view 4, which holds that gifts to educational pro-

grams are unacceptable. If some gifts to educational programs are acceptable, then we should reject view 4 as well.

An example of view 2 is the position taken by the Council on Ethical and Judicial Affairs of the American Medical Association. (9) It holds that gifts of minimal value are ethically permissible provided they are related to the physician's work; examples would be pens and note pads. It also holds that other gifts are acceptable if they are not of substantial value and serve an educational function, such as textbooks and modest meals. Examples of gifts that are not acceptable, according to the AMA, are payments for the costs of travel, lodging, or other personal expenses of physicians who are attending conferences or meetings. Other professional organizations have put forward versions of view 2. (10) In response to this view, it can be argued that even minor gifts to individuals are not acceptable, based on several considerations. First, the assumption that minor gifts do not influence behavior can be challenged, and to date there have been no studies to examine this question. Second, even if some gifts are too minor to influence physicians, the problem of distinguishing them from gifts that can influence would be difficult. A straightforward way to resolve this problem is for physicians not to accept any gifts from pharmaceutical companies. Third, even minor gifts might create a perception by patients that physicians have a conflict of interest. If there is a perception of conflict, trust in the physician can be undermined. Maintaining the patient's trust is too important to risk losing it by accepting even minor gifts.

The above considerations support view 3, which holds that some gifts to educational programs but no gifts to individuals are ethically acceptable. This view suggests that we should strive to change the culture of medicine with regard to receiving gifts from pharmaceutical companies. The end toward which we should aim is a culture in which physicians do not accept gifts from drug companies, regardless of the value of the gift.

According to the view being defended, it is

justifiable for educational and professional organizations to accept gifts, provided the gifts are handled in a manner that attempts to avoid unacceptable influence of the gifts on the prescribing behavior of individual physicians. Examples of guidelines that would help insulate such gifts from individuals include the following. First, if the gift ultimately is passed to an individual, such as a trip for a resident to attend a conference, then the relationship between the drug company and the recipient should be made as indirect as possible. This implies that the selection of the recipient should be made by the educational institution, not the drug company. Also, the gift should not transparently be a gift to an individual, as would be the case if only one resident were interested in attending a particular conference, and the drug company's representative makes the gift with that resident in mind. Second, if the gift is a grant to support a conference or lecture, the content of the educational activity should be decided by the educational institution, not the drug company. Third, when the gift supports a conference with speakers, selection of speakers and those invited to attend should be made by the educational institution.

Changing the culture of medicine in this regard probably would be difficult, especially given the fact that some major medical organizations like the AMA support the acceptance of modest gifts. Ongoing debate will be necessary to raise awareness about and further explore this issue.

Notes

1 Reeder M, Dougherty J, White LJ. Pharmaceutical representatives and emergency medicine residents: a national survey. *Ann Emerg Med* 1993;22:1593–6.
2 Hodges B. Interactions with the pharmaceutical industry: experiences and attitudes of psychiatry residents, interns and clerks. *Can Med Assoc J* 1995;153:553–9.
3 Chren M-M, Landefeld CS, Murray TH. Doctors, drug companies, and gifts. *JAMA* 1989;262:3448–51.
4 Margolis LH. The ethics of accepting gifts from pharmaceutical companies. *Pediatrics* 1991;88:1233–7.
5 Blake RL Jr, Early EK. Patients' attitudes about gifts to physicians from pharmaceutical companies. *J Am Board Fam Pract* 1995;8:457–64.
6 Randall T. Kennedy hearings say no more free lunch – or much else – from drug firms. *JAMA* 1991;265:440, 442.
7 Orlowski JP, Wateska L. The effects of pharmaceutical firm enticements on physician prescribing patterns. *Chest* 1991;102:270–3.
8 McKinney WP, et al. Attitudes of internal medicine faculty and residents toward professional interaction with pharmaceutical sales representatives. *JAMA* 1990;264:1693–7.
9 American Medical Association, Council on Ethical and Judicial Affairs. Gifts to physicians from industry. *JAMA* 1991;265:501.
10 American College of Physicians. Physicians and the pharmaceutical industry. *Ann Intern Med* 1990;112:624–6.

DISCUSSION QUESTIONS

Section 6. Making waves: questioning authority and the status quo

1 What is the trainee's responsibility if he or she believes the attending physician has made an error in judgment?
2 What should he or she do when a technical error seems to have been made? What options are open?
3 Trainees become bound to their colleagues, teachers, and institutions, to what extent does integrity require an active questioning of those with whom you are associated?
4 When should a trainee be willing to accept the title "doctor?"
5 Should obfuscation regarding a trainee's status, even if promulgated by authority, be sanctioned? What do patients have a right to know?
7 In a professional environment of maximum competition and stress, what principles should determine relationships among colleagues?

Perceiving misconduct and whistle-blowing: observing peers or superiors commit an act deemed unethical

Professional regulation and self-regulation are essential ingredients in medicine. This regulation requires monitoring, not only of one's self, but also of one's peers. The responsibility to report risks that colleagues and other health professionals may pose to the public lies in the obligation to prevent serious foreseeable harm. Since disclosing often comes with considerable personal cost, how vigilant should trainees be expected to be in disclosing such information? If, for example, trainees perceive professionals abusing drugs or alcohol, how should this be handled? If they are part of a team where patients are mistreated, is there a way to improve that situation? If they are asked to cover up a mistake that has been made, what are the options? When, if ever, is it appropriate to step in and take action?

The power imbalance between supervisors and trainees that makes perceived misconduct and whistle-blowing so complicated also exerts a powerful force in the area of clinical research. How should authorship be determined? How should coauthors, consultation, mentoring, editing, etc. be expressed? What are the obligations of students? Of supervisors? When should trainees challenge or report misconduct?

21

Abusing alcohol or drugs

CASE

"Whistle-blowers take a lot of heat – particularly when you are a nobody"

As a resident, I worked for a while with a pediatric intensivist who was an incredibly bright doctor. He was Board certified in both pediatric intensive care and anesthesia. His anesthesia privileges gave him wide access to drugs, and it was known that this doctor had a cocaine habit. One day he came to work wired out of his mind. We were doing rounds and all I could think of was how to protect the patients? He was far beyond being able to carry out his responsibilities and in his drug-induced state was exposing patients to terrible risk. At the same time, I thought whistle-blowers take a lot of heat, particularly when you are a nobody.

Later, I learned the chief resident reported this doctor to the chief of the department. He went into rehabilitation and now he practices at another hospital in another state.

CASE

"Missing drugs"

As a resident in anesthesiology, I was assigned for the first few months to an attending who would be my direct supervisor. I learned a lot from her and I still use a method of case write-up that she taught me. Sometimes, however, I thought she behaved oddly; for example, I would find her sitting with her legs crossed in an awkward position and she would jump up quickly when she saw me. Once when a drug was not accounted for she said "I

gave it to a patient, but forgot to enter it into the chart." I had a vague sense of unease about the missing drugs, but brushed aside my concerns.

When I returned some months later from an assignment at another hospital she was absent. I asked about her and was told "She's in rehab." It was discovered that she had a heplock under her ankle sock through which she administered drugs.

CASE

"I found the attending overdosed and unconscious"

When I was an anesthesiologist resident one of our attendings was thought to be cold, even mean at times, although even his sternest detractors had to acknowledge him as a serious professional, admired for his knowledge and skill. As part of our duties as residents, we were responsible, by turn, for the daily tallies regarding all the drugs used. He would sometimes offer to do this task for the residents. None of the other attendings ever took over these duties. One day I was in the locker room when I heard a loud thump from one of the stalls. When I went to investigate I found the attending overdosed and unconscious. He was resuscitated and revealed that he had been using narcotics for 10 years. All that time he used a particular drug and was so skilled at titrating that he knew exactly the amount to inject. On this one occasion he had switched to another, more potent, narcotic with the near fatal consequences. Is there, or should there be, an institutional or professional responsibility to reveal this kind of history to future patients?

COMMENTARY

Rosamond Rhodes

The resident in the first case thinks "whistle-blowers take a lot of heat, particularly when you are a nobody." Unfortunately, the resident is right. Although a few instances of blatant inappropriate behavior are addressed, for the most part, misconduct is ignored. Although venues for employee grievances and hearing complaints about misconduct and harassment can now be found in many institutions, they are seldom used. In sum, medicine has failed to create an effective mechanism for addressing unethical behavior. In describing disturbing cases of clinical misconduct, physician-ethicist Joel Frader criticizes "the routinization of 'looking the other way' and our own complicity in tolerating unethical behavior." He points at

doctors who frankly coerce patients or family members into accepting unwanted treatment; situations where doctors and scientists blatantly violate institutional policies regarding peer scrutiny and protection of human subjects; situations where the organization of treatment teams and services brutally exploits trainees and simultaneously compromises mundane and exotic aspects of patient care. (1)

In other words, clinicians have learned to systematically avert their eyes and to be unresponsive to serious peer misconduct. And the residents in all three of the cases in this chapter have already mastered this silent curriculum. Largely, that is because medical institutions regard whistle-blowers as enemies and punishes them.

Constance Holden reported on some of the personal costs to faculty members who blow the whistle on colleagues. (2) Whistle-blowers are ostracized, pressured to drop allegations, and threatened with counter allegations. They lose desirable assignments, have their research support reduced, and their promotions and raises denied. Their contracts are not renewed, and they are fired. (3) If faculty members are at such risk,

the peril for a resident must be far greater, and everyone knows it.

Clearly, the abuse of narcotics by physicians can be harmful to themselves, to their patients, and to the professionals who work with them and rely upon their performance and reports. Clearly the behavior should be stopped. But stopping the behavior requires authority, authorities cannot act until they know about a problem, and everyone is reluctant to inform because of concern about the consequences.

It is important to notice that two sets of consequences are typically considered by reluctant witnesses to drug abuse. There are worries about the personal consequences for the informant and concerns about the consequences for the physician who is using drugs. Any policy that is to encourage reporting so that drug abuse can be addressed has to take account of both sorts of considerations. Senior physicians, residents, medical students, and other health professionals are moved by complex reasons: they want the misconduct to stop because they appreciate the danger, they also need to feel safe in blowing the whistle, and they also need to be assured that the drug-abusing physician will be helped rather than harmed, or at least not harmed more than is deserved because they do not want to be responsible for doing more harm than good, especially to a peer.

Any recourse to legal mechanisms for addressing the drug abuse would involve criminal charges against the drug-abusing physician and the prospect of meting out punishment because the drug use is illegal in our society and its appropriation in these cases is theft. The legal approach, however, is problematic. It makes the subject of a misconduct hearing into "the accused" who must then be protected with all of the safeguards accorded a defendant in a criminal case. Adjudicating misconduct within a legal framework starts with a presumption of innocence and leaves those who raise the charges with the burden of proof. It also involves the legal standard of proof, which is much too high, and the risk of severe punishments that are so high that few doctors would want them imposed on a fellow physician.

An alternative to the legal route would involve medicine policing itself. As these cases and the recent literature suggest, medicine as a profession has been reluctant to take on this role with a sincere commitment to doing the job well. Yet, medicine is a profession with an acknowledged fiduciary relationship. As such, it has a definite responsibility to all patients and potential patients to assure that its practitioners and institutions are trustworthy. Rather than turning a blind eye or sweeping misdeeds under the rug, medicine has to uncover misconduct and address it so that patients can feel assured that incidents of misconduct will be remarkably uncommon and that the rare occurrences will be quickly uncovered and speedily addressed. From the perspective of medicine, physicians' behavior should be like the comportment of Caesar's wife. Instead of worrying about the slim possibility of punishing an innocent, medicine should aim at assuring that physicians' behavior does not even appear immoral. (4) Furthermore, as a self-policing profession focused on assuring the trustworthiness of physicians and medical institutions, medicine's primary concerns should be scrutiny and remediation, in that order. If medicine could make itself into a profession that pays serious attention to oversight, the threat of punishment would play a coercive role and it should be imposed only in the most egregious cases or after corrective measures had not succeeded in altering the behavior.

To affect such a change in the status quo, the incentives for addressing problematic behavior have to be changed. From the institutional responses that have been reported we should know that the whistle-blower is seen as the enemy from within. That attitude leads to attacks on whistle-blowers and a protective defense of culprits. If the institutional incentives could be changed and the whistle-blower could come to be seen as the valued friend of the institution, appropriate reactions would be more likely.

The point of this observation is that medical institutions operate in a political environment. And the aim of a political system should be to manipulate the natural and artificial incentives that move individuals so that they behave in socially desirable ways. The current arrangement of incentives works at cross purposes to the social good. They "censure rather than encourage" whistle-blowing behavior. (5) Individuals in medicine are now coerced to do what they should not, to conceal rather than disclose misconduct, to ignore misconduct as long as possible (e.g., until an attending is found overdosed and unconscious), and to silence or discredit whistle-blowers. The solution to this problem lies, first, in recognizing the structure of the predicament and, then, in addressing it effectively. In this situation, a change in incentives is required and such a change can only be effected by a significant force from outside the system.

Unfortunately, no one is prepared to create and empower the coercive structure that could effect the necessary transformation of incentives. But existing accreditation agencies could be authorized to take on an expanded role in preventing academic and clinical misconduct. If they demonstrated the will to investigate institutions and to seriously punish the institutions for tolerating unacceptable behavior of clinicians, and if the threatened sanctions against the institutions were sufficiently severe, the balance of incentives could be realigned to overcome those that incline institutions to turn blind eyes toward clinician misconduct.

People are reluctant to give up any measure of control over their own behavior. Physicians, in particular, fiercely resist limitations on their liberty. They need to open their eyes and recognize that their present independence is only an illusion. In an environment where doctors are constrained to conceal or accommodate behavior that they find dangerous or profoundly objectionable, they are not free. To recognize this fact of contemporary institutional life we need only to recall that in at least two of our cases the drug abuse was suspected for some time. Nothing was done because the inclination to report the suspicious behavior was silenced by the suppressive environment. Political philosophy can point the way to a more far-sighted approach and teach the lesson that empowering an overseeing authority can be liberty enhancing. By forceful policing from powerful extra-institutional review, medicine stands its best chance of becoming free to confront and constrain professional misconduct.

Notes

1 Frader JE. Aspects of ethics consultation. *Theor Med* 1992;13:31–44.
2 Holden C. Whistleblower woes. *Science* 1996;271:35.
3 Glazer MP, Glazer PM. *The Whistleblowers: Exposing Corruption in Government and Industry.* Basic Books Inc, New York, 1989.
4 Driver J. Caesar's wife: on the moral significance of appearing good. *J Phil* 1992;89(7):331–43.
5 Poon P. Legal protection for the scientific misconduct whistleblower. *J Law, Med Ethics* 1995;23:88–95.

COMMENTARY

Neal Cohen

The cases presented in this chapter provide descriptions of some of the problems associated with drug use and abuse by health care workers. Alcohol and drug use are serious and unfortunately common problems for health care providers. Abuse of controlled substances is more frequent in physicians than it is in the general population. Alcoholism and illicit drug use are also prevalent.

The frequency of drug and alcohol use is probably due to a number of factors. First, health care providers experience high levels of stress accompanying their professional roles and responsibilities. Physicians are expected to cure patients, relieve their pain and suffering and treat their physical and psychological problems. Expectations are high and the room for error small. The physician is expected to have answers to every question a patient might pose and to be able to diagnose and treat the most complex clinical problems. In response to the pressure associated with these responsibilities, some physicians turn to controlled drugs that they know have effectively treated patients' anxiety, pain, or suffering. Others choose alcohol or illicit drugs. Second, controlled substances are more accessible to physicians, nurses, and other health care providers than they are to the lay public. Physicians and nurses can get narcotics, other analgesics and sedatives easily without raising any question from their coworkers. Anesthesiologists in particular handle narcotics and other controlled substances on a daily basis. They administer them to almost every patient to whom they provide care. They also observe the therapeutic effects of the drugs as part of their routine practice.

No matter what drugs they abuse those who begin down this path find it difficult to stop. The drugs or alcohol usually do relieve the tensions associated with the responsibilities of a clinical practice. Many physicians who became dependent on narcotics, in particular describe the initial experience as incredibly comforting, often making them feel "at ease" for the first time in their professional lives. Some experience an immediate dependence, psychologically if not physically.

Physicians and nurses who become habitual drug users find creative ways to obtain the drugs and to hide their use and abuse. Some will pretend to administer drugs to patients, recording the administration in the patient's medical record. They will then sequester the drugs for their own use. Others have carefully removed narcotics from closed ampules using a variety of creative techniques, replacing the drug with saline. When the vial is subsequently used by another physician or nurse, little question would be raised if the patient did not respond appropriately to the drug. Since there is significant patient variability in dosage and clinical response, it is not unusual for some patients to require larger doses of narcotics or other analgesics than others do.

The identification of the physician who uses alcohol or drugs is difficult. Physicians are often very clever at disguising their addiction. Professional colleagues and family members are also very trusting and rarely recognize even very obvious signs of addiction. In fact, even when found lethargic or comatose, addicted physicians will often be able to convince colleagues that they are suffering from the flu, sleep deprivation, or some other problem that is influencing their behavior.

The findings associated with alcohol or drug use also differ. Alcohol is often easier to identify. Although some physicians can restrict their alcohol use to nonworking hours, many consume alcohol in sufficient quantity that it impairs their judgment, slows response time, and interferes with appropriate patient care. Unlike other drugs, alcohol abuse can be somewhat easier to recognize, since the user often smells of alcohol, no matter how he or she tries to mask the use.

The abuse of narcotics or other controlled drugs is harder to recognize. In most cases of narcotic abuse, the physician's behavior is minimally affected. Impairment in judgment or altered response is rarely a recognized sign of narcotic use. In some cases behavior will change, often because of concern about being "found," rather than because of mistakes in clinical management or inappropriate patient care. Sometimes patient management will change in subtle ways. For example, for the anesthesiologist, use of narcotics as part of the anesthetic management will increase. In other cases, narcotic losses will be noted either by the person who distributes them or by the pharmacy.

The physician who is using cocaine or other illicit drugs will also frequently demonstrate physical manifestations of the drug abuse. When clinical responsibilities are not being appropriately addressed, patient protection becomes paramount. If a house officer identifies a physician who is unable to fulfill responsibilities, again, the resident should report the findings to a superior, either the chief resident or chief of the clinical department. The cause for the bizarre behavior requires evaluation, even if subsequent monitoring does not confirm illicit drug use.

Identification of the physician using prescription drugs, such as morphine, fentanyl, other narcotics, or sedatives is actually more difficult. As two of the cases defined, drug overdose or inappropriate accounting of drugs are more frequent indicators of prescription drug abuse than is change in behavior. Many physicians are able to function remarkably well despite huge drug habits. They become very creative at identifying ways to obtain the drugs and administer them to themselves with little indication of the abuse to the colleagues. As a result, although the case "Missing drugs" suggests that odd behavior is a manifestation of narcotic use, even in that case, drug accounting was the key to identification of the addiction.

When a resident or student is confronted with an attending physician who is either intoxicated or physically or emotionally impaired and unable to fulfill responsibilities, the subordinate should report the findings to a supervisor. In some situations, other providers may be aware of the impairment, but have not reported it because of concern for the welfare of their colleague. Even if others object, if drug or alcohol abuse is suspected, it should be reported to the department chair or chief of the clinical service as soon as it is suspected. When doing so, a careful description of the findings or situation that warranted the report should be provided, so that the supervisor can determine how to most appropriately intervene.

Because of the serious personal and professional consequences of drug use, any colleague who suspects abuse from another physician has a responsibility to carefully define the reason for concern and report it to a superior. When a physician changes the pattern of administration of drugs or begins to report drug losses, the possibility of abuse should be considered. In the case of the anesthesiologist who overdosed on drugs, a review of the drug administration patterns for that physician versus his or her peers might have been a first indication of a potential problem.

When a colleague is suspected of drug or alcohol use, the primary responsibility is to protect patients. At the same time, assistance and support should be provided to the individual. As a result of increased awareness of drug and alcohol use in physicians, most hospitals have established mechanisms for initiating an evaluation process. Many hospitals and departments have created "well-being" committees which have the responsibility for defining ways to respond to allegations and to identify resources available to physicians in need of help. Many such committees will initiate an "intervention" in which a group of colleagues will confront the individual with the allegations and require evaluation by a drug or alcohol treatment program. Voluntary evaluation is desired, but if the individual refuses to voluntarily undergo assessments, mandatory evaluation can be required to maintain clinical privileges. The evaluation process, once initiated is relatively consistent from one program to another. The physician suspected of drug or alcohol use is interrogated about their behavior and potential drug use. Drug testing is also required. If there is sufficient evidence of drug use, whether acknowledged or not, the individual is required to undergo inpatient evaluation. The goal of the entire process is to identify the risky behavior and seek rehabilitation. The cases in this chapter raise a number of questions related to identification and notification of potential drug or alcohol use. First, as a result of the acknowledgment of the risk of drug and alcohol use, the whistle-blower is not at significant risk. In fact, the responsibility of reporting far outweighs the risk to the person doing so. For the majority of reports, drug or alcohol use has been confirmed. In the minority of cases, when no abuse is identified, no record is made of the allegations and no report is provided to the Medical Licensing Board. When the allegations are founded, a report to the Medical Board is required. In most states, the Medical Board has a

diversion program to provide rehabilitation, counseling, and guidance. After completion of a mandatory diversion program, in most states, a physician can maintain his or her medical license, although often on a probationary status for some postrehabilitation period of time. Careful ongoing monitoring is required to ensure compliance with the rehabilitation program.

Despite improved monitoring and rehabilitation services, some physicians who abuse drugs or alcohol will return to their former use after initially successfully completing a rehabilitation program. For many of these physicians, ongoing monitoring identifies the recidivism. Repeated use of drugs and alcohol does jeopardize one's license, although return to a diversion program can often result in long-term rehabilitative success.

For some physicians, returning to the environment in which their drug use began is impossible. For example, some anesthesiologists find it very difficult to return to an anesthesia practice after undergoing rehabilitation for drug abuse. The easy access to drugs and the need to utilize the drugs daily as part of their clinical practice is too inviting. As a result, some anesthesiologists as well as other specialists who routinely administer narcotics will change specialty to decrease access and improve the likelihood of successful rehabilitation.

Although these cases identify the problems a resident or student might have in interacting with an attending physician, the possibility of personal drug use and abuse must also be considered. When confronted with the stresses of a clinical practice and the expectations of flawless behavior, each physician is at risk for drug and alcohol abuse. One's personal risk cannot be overestimated. When the stresses of training and clinical practice become too great, each physician should seek professional assistance to minimize the risk of personal drug abuse and other potential consequences.

These cases raise another very important issue that is of relevance to every health care worker. As mentioned earlier in this discussion, physicians are subjected to enormous stresses as part of their work. The responsibility to the patient is an enormous one. They must deal with difficult clinical problems thoughtfully, effectively, and without mistake. At the same time, the physician–patient relationship is a special one, and one that differs from any other interaction. Patients confide in their physicians in ways they will not with others, even spouses, or other close relatives or friends. The impact of this responsibility on the physician cannot be underestimated. Not only does the physician have to help the patient deal with important personal and health-related issues, but the physician is also not able to discuss some aspects of these difficult challenges with others in order to protect patient confidentiality. There are few outlets to deal with these often stressful situations.

The responsibility not only takes a great deal of professional time, but it also impacts family and personal time. As a result personal relationships can be strained. The physician is often caught in a bind between commitment to the patient and to all other responsibilities.

The impact of these responsibilities should be acknowledged by each physician and their professional colleagues. When an individual appears to be having difficulty dealing with a specific issue or the stresses imposed by these clinical responsibilities, help should be offered. At the same time, if a colleague identifies behaviors that are unusual, inappropriate or interfere with clinical judgment or patient care, the problem must be addressed, preferably before a physician seeks alcohol or drugs as a solution.

A variety of methods are available to assist a physician who is stressed, troubled, or whose care is compromised. Most hospitals (or departments) now have physician well-being committees. Members of these committees can identify resources for the physician to seek help. The committees provide confidential review and counsel. Each physician should find out what resources are available and take advantage of them whenever a problem is identified. By doing so with the earliest sign of distress, it might be possible to prevent the problems from progressing and potentially prevent another physician from retreating to drugs or alcohol to deal with the stresses and responsibilities of clinical practice.

22

Mistreating patients: nasty, rude or hostile behavior toward patients

CASE

"The patient had been verbally assaulted"

On my medical rotation there was a Black patient who was an IV drug user. The resident was exasperated about her failure to comply and lashed out at the woman by saying that her 13-year-old daughter should be searched when she came to see her mother because she was probably bringing in drugs. I was horrified and felt that the patient had been verbally assaulted, but I didn't know what to do about it.

CASE

"Stop bothering us"

As a student I was asked to work up an elderly man with all sorts of pains, including back pain. He had severe arthritis and had been in and out of the hospital many times. He was obviously somewhat depressed and feeling his pain terribly. As we spoke, he almost warned me, "No one believes me, I am in terrible pain." I had just opened the door to his room to present as the resident came by, when the resident shouted out in a very loud offensive way, as though deliberately trying to make sure the patient heard, "Well, tell me, is this patient's pain legitimate or not?" I felt miserable because I knew the patient's pain from his own perspective was "legitimate." But, of course, there was nothing the orthopedic surgeon was going to be able to do and therefore as far as he was concerned it wasn't "legitimate." In his mind if it couldn't be fixed by surgery it didn't count and he

was really saying to the patient, "Stop bothering us." As a student I felt totally inadequate, caught between trying to remain professionally respectful and witnessing a patient verbally assaulted.

CASE

"The unknowing widow"

I remember as a medical student when a patient died and efforts to find the family were unsuccessful. The patient's spouse appeared on the floor and I recognized her. I went looking for the house staff and found the senior resident, along with the junior resident, huddled in the on-call room. I told them the deceased's wife was nearby and could be notified. They told me to quickly come into the room and shut the door. I said "Someone has to tell her what has happened." They advised me to stay with them so I wouldn't have to break the news. I could see they were hiding in order to avoid having to confront the widow. I didn't know what to do. I didn't think it should fall on me to tell her what happened, but I felt terrible that she was wandering around the floor ignorant of her husband's death.

CASE

"The patient's wishes were ignored"

I was a medical student on a surgery rotation when a patient was admitted to hospital for a sigmoid resection. Two years before he had executed an advance directive, naming his only living relative, a nephew, as his decision-maker should he become incapacitated. His advance directive stated that he never wanted CPR or intubation if it was necessary to prolong his life. However, he did not state in his advance directive that he did not want any form of medical therapy, including even basic treatments such as antibiotics or IV fluids.

Seven days following surgery the patient developed acute respiratory distress secondary to pneumonia, which was rapidly advancing to sepsis. His nephew, who held his uncle's power of attorney for health care, was contacted and agreed to the intubation, but only with the understanding that it would be for a few days while his uncle recovered from his temporary pneumonia.

Despite aggressive intervention, days turned into weeks and the patient remained intubated. The resident taking care of the patient spoke with the nephew. Feeling obligated to carry out his uncle's wishes, and quoting his uncle's verbal and written directive, the nephew instructed that the ET tube be removed at once. The other residents were all in favor of terminating life-support measures; however the attending physician vetoed extubating the patient. He felt that the patient was within days of being extubated because he was showing signs of improvement. However, the patient continued to fail the weaning parameters with several trials of continuous position airway pressure (CPAP).

The dispute was taken to the ethics committee for consultation where a compromise was reached. It was decided, with the nephew's agreement, that a 2-week trial would be instituted. If at the end of 2 weeks the patient was unable to survive without a ventilator, the life support would be withdrawn. At the end of the 2 weeks, continued attempts were made to wean the patient from the ventilator with no success. However, the attending refused to extubate the patient. A week later, at the end of my surgery rotation and 3 weeks after the ethics committee meeting, the attending was still ignoring the terms of the compromise.

I felt the patient had taken the correct steps by giving explicit verbal and written directives – all to no avail. His wishes were ignored by the health care team. I felt in his case treatment was really mistreatment, but what could I have done?

COMMENTARY

Ben Rich

"The patient has been verbally assaulted"

This case presents at least two concerns for the medical student: (1) what, if anything, should he or she say to the patient who has been the target of this unwarranted rebuke? and (2) how, if at all, should the student confront the resident about the inappropriate behavior? Before addressing either of these questions, however, a few background points should be made.

Presumably the patient is participating in a drug rehabilitation program and is having difficulty complying with its strictures. She may have another medical condition that is the reason for her hospitalization, but we do not know and hence cannot factor it into our analysis of the case. Our society, including the medical community, is still in conflict as to whether or not addiction and alcoholism are genuine diseases or disorders, or whether they are nothing more than antisocial and self-destructive behaviors engaged in by individuals who lack sufficient impulse control. Those clinicians who are in the latter camp are much more likely to fail in their ethical responsibility to provide empathic care to such patients. Indeed, the more hard line among them may even fail to recognize that their insensitive behavior toward them is unacceptable.

The resident in this case is clearly failing to fulfill his or her responsibility not only to provide compassionate and respectful care to the patient, but also in the mentoring role to the medical student. While there may be some remote possibility that if confronted by the student at an appropriate time the resident might recognize his or her failures in this regard, it is more reasonable for the medical student to anticipate resistance if not hostility when the subject is broached. To acknowledge this, however, is not to suggest that the student should simply keep quiet and remind him or herself that not all role models in medicine or any other profession are positive.

Initially, I suggested that this situation presents the medical student with a two-fold task. The first is to apologize to the patient for the rudeness of the resident. This should be done in a manner that does not gratuitously denigrate the resident, but at the same time does not make excuses for the resident to which he or she may not be entitled, e.g., the resident was stressed out from overwork, or the resident is going through a difficult time right now. It should be made clear to the patient that she has a right to expect respectful and courteous treatment from all health care professionals, and that when she receives anything less than that she should not hesitate to report such incidents to the attending physician and/or the institution's patient representative.

The second task is for the medical student to express his or her concern directly to the resident. Indeed, the student could indicate that the resident should apologize to the patient, and provide the resident with an opportunity to do so, but that if the resident refuses then the student will do so on behalf of the treatment team, as well as relate to the attending physician that one of his or her patients has received less than courteous care from a resident.

I am not oblivious to the awkwardness of the situation for the student. There will be, as the student indicates, a strong temptation to say nothing and not make waves with superiors in the chain of command. Moral courage will be required to act in the manner I have suggested. However, the capacity to demonstrate moral courage is one of the hallmarks of any professional.

"Stop bothering us"

This case presents us with an example of one of the most neglected and maligned groups of patients in the health care system – elderly victims of chronic, nonmalignant pain. Studies indicate that if the patient, in addition to being elderly, were also a woman, poor, and an ethnic minority, she would be still more likely to have her pain discounted by health care professionals. Despite the fact that from its Hippocratic origins medicine has recognized the relief of pain and suffering arising from illness as one of its core values, modern medicine has notoriously undertreated pain, particularly that of the chronic, nonmalignant variety.

Very often such patients report pain levels that seem to be inconsistent with the physical findings. The response of too many health care professionals has been to discount the patient's reports of pain or to advise the patient that medicine has nothing to offer and they will simply need to learn to live with it. The assumption, of course, is that since the patient's reports of pain are exaggerated, their burden will actually not be all that great.

The fact of the matter is that pain is a subjective experience. The International Association for the Study of Pain (IASP) defines pain as "an unpleasant sensory and emotional experience which we primarily associate with tissue damage or describe in terms of such damage, or both." The clear implication of this definition is that the relationship between pain and tissue damage is neither uniform nor constant. Indeed, chronic pain such as this patient reports, although clearly attributable in significant part to severe arthritis, may occur in the absence of any explanatory organic processes.

Insult is added to injury for many victims of chronic nonmalignant pain precisely because, as the orthopedic resident suggests, that which cannot be alleviated through surgical intervention lacks any clinical legitimacy. Those who suffer from moderate to severe chronic nonmalignant pain that does not respond to traditional medical or surgical interventions are a constant and irritating reminder to health care professionals of the limits of medicine and the need for compassionate clinicians to refrain from discrediting and ultimately abandoning such patients by suggesting that they have nothing to offer.

The student, whose role at this point is much more that of learner than caregiver, should carefully question residents and attendings about the most appropriate way to care for these patients. If sensitive and appropriate responses are not forthcoming, the student may wish to look further into the resources of the local or regional health care system for services or clinics that specialize in chronic pain. Finally, the student should trust his or her feelings and refuse to model the insensitive behaviors of these mentors. Chronic pain is perhaps the most glaring contemporary example of instances in which the prevailing custom and practice among health care professionals lags far behind what state-of-the-art care and treatment has to offer. State medical licensing boards have begun to recognize this disturbing fact and responded by promulgating clinical practice guidelines for pain management, as has the Federation of State Medical Licensing Boards. Undertreated pain does not simply diminish a patient's quality of life; it can impair healing, result in repeated and unnecessary hospitalizations, and in the most extreme cases, actually shorten a patient's life. According to current guidelines in many states, the resident's behavior toward this patient could be construed as unprofessional conduct that is a basis for disciplinary action. The emerging standard of care requires that the responsible professional either promptly and effectively assesses and manages the patient's pain, or transfers the care of the patient to another professional who can and will do so.

"The unknowing widow"

One has to wonder what sort of an institution this case arises in, that there is not a single nurse on the floor who would approach and offer assistance to the spouse. Of course the primary responsibility for informing her of the death of her husband is that of the senior physician who is readily available and has been involved in the care of the patient. The responsibility of the nurse would be to page that physician and insist that he or she come and talk with the wife.

Recent studies that have revealed the manifold deficiencies in end-of-life care in the United States highlight the extremely poor performance of health care professionals in general, and physicians in particular, in breaking bad news to patients and/or family. While "breaking bad news" is a phrase that usually refers to a terminal diagnosis or the unresponsiveness of a life-threatening condition to therapeutic measures, it may also apply, as here, to an unwillingness or inability of the responsible caregivers to sensitively communicate with family members the fact that a patient has died. Both the American Board of Internal Medicine in its 1996 report *Caring for the Dying: Promoting Physician Competency*, and the American Medical Association's Education for Physicians on End-of-Life Care (EPEC) Project, developed in 1998, have identified "breaking bad news" as one of the core or essential competencies that every physician who cares for dying patients must possess.

In the case under consideration, attending physician faculty have failed to instruct and mentor the senior resident in this competency, not only how to do it sensitively yet effectively, but also its cardinal importance. Moreover, the senior resident is demonstrating a lack of professional maturity that seriously calls into question his or her readiness to move from the residency program to the next level of responsibility in patient care. In the minutes and hours, even days after a patient's death, the professional responsibility of the caregivers immediately shifts to the next of kin. While nurses, pastoral counselors, and social workers also have a role in the bereavement process, it comes after the responsible physician has initiated the process by which the deceased patient's loved ones have been apprised of not only the fact of the patient's death but also the surrounding clinical circumstances. They will, in all likelihood, have questions and concerns which they will want to express that can best, and perhaps only be answered by the physician most immediately involved in the patient's care.

There are also institutional implications in the behavior of these two residents. In the increasingly competitive environment in which hospitals must operate, and given the concerns that managed care has engendered in the general public, patient and family satisfaction with the care provided, which relates not only to *what* is provided but also *how* it is provided, has become a focus of senior hospital administrators. Furthermore, the Joint Commission for the Accreditation of Health Care Organizations (JCAHO) has begun to pay increased attention to the quality of end-of-life care which patients receive. The wife of this deceased patient is being treated in a manner that is likely to engender disappointment, frustration, and perhaps ultimately, hostility. A competent hospital administrator would neither condone nor tolerate such treatment of a patient's family by a member of the medical or nursing staff.

If the situation were such that the responsible physician or physicians were truly unavailable within a reasonable period of time to speak with the spouse, then it would fall upon someone who was available, the medical student or a senior nurse, to inform the wife that her husband had died. The longer she is in the dark, the more difficult it will be for her when she is finally told. The student, who at least understands what needs to be done in the situation, whether or not he or she knows the best way to go about it, should not avoid this task simply because in an ideal world someone else would undertake what is truly their responsibility.

"The patient's wishes were ignored"

The attending physician in this case is not only violating a fundamental principle of medical ethics, respect for patient autonomy, but also, in all probability, the law of the jurisdiction. Advance directive legislation – statutes recognizing the authority of living wills and durable powers of attorney for health care – have been adopted in every state primarily because neither health care professionals nor the courts were willing to give sufficient credence to the prior oral directives of presently incompetent or unconscious patients. Unfortunately, as the report of the SUPPORT principal investigators revealed in 1995, there are still too many physicians, including attendings at academic medical centers, who disregard advance directives and other reliable indicators of patient preferences with impunity. This cavalier attitude that advance directives need only be followed when the treatment team agrees with them continues to be modeled as appropriate behavior, particularly in medical and surgical intensive care units.

This case is an extreme one in that it presents a complete breakdown in institutional structures that should exist as checks and balances on inappropriate physician behaviors. If this case were to come to the attention of a JCAHO survey team, it would constitute a glaring instance of noncompliance with prevailing practice guidelines and accreditation standards. The institutional ethics committee is also derelict in its responsibility to follow-up on its case consultation.

The ethical and legal responsibility of the attending physician in this case is clear and unequivocal – accede to the demands of the patient's designated surrogate decision-maker or transfer the care of the patient to another physician who will. The attending has no moral or legal authority to hold this patient hostage to his or her own preferences for continued treatment. Anyone involved in the care of this patient – residents, medical students, nurses, or the patient's family – can and should refer the matter back to the ethics committee and/or to senior hospital administration. This is clearly not a case in which the surrogate is insisting upon demonstrably inappropriate, unethical, or illegal action or inaction on the part of the health care providers or the institution. Even if there were such concerns, the appropriate response is not to ignore the surrogate, but to invoke the jurisdiction of the court to review the case and resolve the dispute.

The violation of prevailing ethical standards is so flagrant in this case that it actually places both the attending and the institution in legal jeopardy. Such litigation can arise at the initiation of frustrated or angry family members, or in response to subsequent efforts on the part of the physician and the institution to secure payment for the treatment for which there was no consent.

COMMENTARY

Tod Chambers

Seeking truth from power

These cases represent one of the most common features of the moral life of medical students during their clinical years. The writer of "Stop bothering us" encapsulates this in stating, "As a student I felt totally inadequate, caught between trying to remain professionally respectful and witnessing a patient verbally assaulted." This statement captures students' feelings of being both a witness to events and a collaborator in those events. Being forced to act as a witness to immoral events is clearly a feature in all of these cases, and it also represents the powerlessness that students often feel during their clinical years. Medical students are marginal figures within the ethos of the clinical environment and due to this status they are frequently acutely self-conscious of the moral dimensions of medical care. Students often have more time to spend becoming acquainted with patients and, by doing so, can have a better understanding of problems from the patient's point of view. But I believe that the fact that medical students are forced to be witnesses to injustices does not completely reveal why cases of patient abuse are so disturbing to many students. The student's telling observation of feeling caught "trying to remain professionally respect-

ful" reveals the way in which students are aware of themselves as being – or at least perceived as being – a part of the group carrying out actions. It is this sense of being both a powerless witness *and* an unwilling collaborator in causing the pain of others that explains the particular anguish felt by medical students. In "The unknowing widow," the medical student expresses what has come to be a common sentiment among others: "I didn't know what to do. I didn't think it should fall on me to tell her what happened, but I felt terrible that she was wandering around the floor ignorant of her husband's death." In "The patient's wishes were ignored," the writer feels certain of what should have been done but concludes, "what could I have done?" And in "The patient had been verbally assaulted," the writer states, "I was horrified and felt that the patient had been verbally assaulted, but I didn't know what to do about it." If one feels as if one is simply a witness to events then there truly is no sense of final responsibility but these students feel as if they are both witnesses and collaborators, both outside of the action and within the action. In the end, they seem to be tragic figures, unable to act yet feeling responsible for these actions.

But what path can a medical student take? Medical students are keenly aware that they are at the bottom of the hospital hierarchy. Yet they are also aware that they are a part of that hierarchy and therefore do share a degree of moral responsibility for actions that occur around them. Although it is an aspect of the American ethos to distrust hierarchies, they can serve a vital function in areas like medical education where degrees of knowledge and skill have profound consequences for people's lives. Perhaps the first thing to learn within a medical setting is to "work the hierarchy." I have often noticed that students get in trouble in situations where they do not go through the proper channels of the hierarchy, that is, jumping over levels. For example, if in the case "The patient had been verbally assaulted" the medical student had immediately called the attending physician without first speaking directly to the resident, this would result in strong condemnation by the residents and the attending as well. Often students are labelled as "not team players," when they do not heed the power hierarchy within a teaching hospital. One of the advantages of "working the hierarchy" is that when done properly there are always levels of authority to which one can appeal – from intern to resident to chief resident to attending to clerkship director. This does not mean that one will escape criticism by those challenged but following a proper chain of appeal can result in lessening this sense of challenge. In the case "The patient's wishes were ignored," I must confess that I am not exactly sure why the attending physician has not agreed to the compromise reached; it seems a case that is far more the result of a deficient hospital.

The coin of the realm within the teaching environment is knowledge. It is one of the reasons that physicians often think of teaching hospitals as exciting places in which to work. There is a phrase, which I have been told has its roots in the Quaker tradition, that I believe provides guidance for medical students: "Speaking truth to power." The phrase suggests a person lacking genuine political power forcing those with such power to an awareness of the truth of a condition. I think this can be an appealing guide for medical students, for within an academic environment, truth should itself bestow power. Regardless of a physician's standing within a hospital, if a procedure is shown to be futile as a form of treatment, one expects the physician to stop performing that procedure. Of course, this represents an idealized view of the way knowledge is used in the medical environment. Medical knowledge because of its fundamental uncertainty can be used as a weapon against those lower in the hierarchy. Medical students and residents can furnish many examples where a physician has drawn upon "my clinical experience" to silence a debate. Nevertheless it is an ideal of academic environments that the truth holds a special status and should be used in the service of patients. One of the virtues of a teaching environment for the practice of medicine is the checks and balances that exist when one must teach as one is treating. A virtuous clinician encourages students to challenge the knowledge claims, but a challenge assumes that in these cases the clinicians are virtuous.

Because of the essential educational goals of a teaching hospital (that is, a hierarchy based upon degrees of knowledge and skill), a medical student normally should feel comfortable in requesting justification for actions. I have heard many students reveal that they use the normal student–teacher relationship to bring forth moral issues that concern them. When done in a genuinely open manner this is a highly effective technique. Perhaps the phrase for medical students (or any in the medical hierarchy) should be "Seeking truth from power."

As in all pursuits one must be open to having one's opinion changed by others. In many of the cases, there are points in the accounts where as an outside reader I find myself questioning the validity of the author's statements. In "Stop bothering us," the student makes many assumptions about the actions of the resident I think we may wish to challenge. The author states that "as far as he was concerned it [the patient's pain] wasn't 'legitimate.' In his mind if it couldn't be fixed by surgery it didn't count and he was really saying to the patient, 'Stop bothering us.' " Is this true? How does the author know this? What would the resident say if the student asked about the case at a later time? Did the resident truly wish to offend the patient? Similarly in "The unknowing widow," the student makes a series of assumptions that the residents "were hiding in order to avoid having to confront the widow." Once again, is this true? How does the student know this? Is it not possible that an attending has told them that he or she wishes to give the news to the patient's spouse? In both cases, if the residents were unable to justify their actions as anything but anger or cowardice, then the student has done a great service in having them acknowledge the reasons for their actions.

There is one fact that no one in the hierarchy can ignore and that is the student's feelings towards these events. In "The patient had been verbally assaulted," the student "was horrified"; in "Stop bothering us," the student "felt miserable"; and in "The unknowing widow," the student "felt terrible." It is possible to get in a strong disagreement over the facts but no one can disprove your feelings. One of the truths that can be spoken to is whether one's perception of the events is valid and thereby whether one's feelings are warranted. But in any event, the feelings themselves can be the source of conversation, that is, they are truths that cannot be ignored.

It is of course central to remember that each of these cases concerns the abuse of a patient. Patients, regardless of how difficult or how hateful they may be, must always be treated with respect. If there are any events that warrant speaking truth to power it is those in which another person is being abused. Once one is sure of the facts, this is one situation where challenging those in power will not be regretted. For a number of years, I led student ethics conferences with a physician colleague, Robert Winter, and when a case was clearly an issue of patient abuse, he would advise students that there is always a place to express what he referred to as "righteous indignation." Although he was sensitive to the precarious place of medical students in a teaching hospital, he always argued that few people (when the truth is recognized) do not respect others when they stand forth and claim that they question the morality of an action.

23

Covering up

To acknowledge?

CASE

"The camouflaged patient"

I was on a surgical rotation and the patient was an elderly woman who had developed a severe postoperative infection after undergoing a cholecystostomy. The surgical residents were terrorized as to what the attending physicians would say on rounds. In an attempt to camouflage the patient's condition, the residents staged a scene in which they propped her up with pillows and put a breakfast tray in front of her to make her look better than she really was.

CASE

"Didn't you write that order?"

A very sick patient on the cardiac care unit was waiting for a heart transplant. Hospital routine was such that, beginning on Thursday, residents or interns on call left the care of their patients to others over the weekend, often during critical periods of hospitalization. As an intern, it fell to me to cover this particular cardiac patient for another intern on his weekend off.

Before he signed out, the intern stated his concern that despite high doses of potassium the patient's level remained low. Because there was no apparent renal insufficiency, I decided to increase the potassium dose and scheduled a dose of 3 times a day, assuming it would be monitored in my

absence. The next morning the level was normal, so I continued him on that dose.

When I returned after the weekend the patient's name was not on the list. I asked "What happened?" and was told that the patient had become septic and had been taken to the operating room to remove an indwelling catheter. Lab tests revealed such a high level of potassium in his blood that the patient had to be dialyzed. Although he survived the operation, the patient died later that night. One of the fellows said, "Didn't you write that order for potassium?" I was stunned. I checked the records and he was right. I wish someone had seen my error and said something earlier. Nothing further was ever mentioned. In medicine there seems to be an unspoken agreement not to discuss each other's mistakes.

CASE

"What should they have been told?"

During my surgery rotation a patient had undergone cancer surgery (for which the surgeon was guardedly optimistic), and was deemed stable enough to continue his recovery at home. In preparation for this, our intern on the service began to remove dressings, drains, and the triple-lumen catheter in the patient's neck. Although standard protocol for catheter removal prescribes that the patient be supine, our intern, also being new (and likely in a hurry) removed the catheter while the patient was seated in his chair. Approximately 30 seconds after removal of the catheter, the patient had a seizure and suffered a cardiac arrest. After a long resuscitation effort spanning about 20 minutes, the patient was revived, but had suffered a massive anoxic event that left him on the respirator without any discernible activity in the cerebral cortex by EEG.

Although there was considerable debate over whether the intern acted negligently, or was the proximate cause of death, none of this information was discussed with the devastated family. What, if anything, should they have been told?

CASE

"I knew the damage was iatrogenic"

I was a third year medical student on oncology rotation, when a classmate told me that he and his intern had admitted an oncology patient for routine chemotherapy. The patient was to be hydrated overnight and receive chemotherapy in the morning. In preparation the preceding evening, the order was written to give the patient 300 cc of normal saline per hour, and the student dutifully inserted the line into the reservoir situated beneath the skin in the patient's chest. Subsequently, my classmate discovered that the port in the patient's chest was part of an Omaya reservoir which had been placed in the patient's brain and the 300 cc of fluid had been directed into his brain. I asked my colleague who he had told of the incident and he said "no one." Since I now knew that any damage the patient suffered was iatrogenic, what was my responsibility in the matter? Should I check on the patient to determine if he had been harmed? Should I check to see if there was any notice in the chart? Should I inform the attending as to what happened?

CASE

"Boxed kidneys"

An incident that stands out in my medical rotation still troubles me. A patient was given contrast (for imaging) and the team forgot to take steps before administering the contrast to protect his kidneys. We were told by the intern, accompanied by nervous laughter, that we had "boxed" his kidneys. There was no attempt to acknowledge the mistake to the patient. I was especially surprised because this was a patient who had been in the hospital a long time, he was well liked and had formed attachments with the medical team. I pressed the question, "When are we going to tell him?" and was answered with the rebuke, "Oh shut up!" No one wanted to talk about this sad result any more.

CASE

"By not telling am I an accomplice?"

The third day of my internship in internal medicine in Holland, I went with an 80-year-old patient who needed a colonoscopy. During the procedure it became obvious that the scope could only penetrate the colon with great difficulty. The colon was very weak and the sides of the intestine made penetration difficult. The patient was in a great deal of pain and became very restless. He was given more anesthetic and the scope was tried several more times but the scope did not penetrate the colon far enough. After about half an hour the nursing staff thought the test should be stopped because the scope was not going into the colon. However, the physician wanted to continue. After another try the staff again told the physician to stop. Nevertheless, he continued. Suddenly the patient's abdomen became very hard, his eyes rolled back in his head. The scope showed a perforation on the monitor and the patient's heart had stopped. Resuscitation was attempted but without result. The patient's wife was called and told that her husband had died during the test. She was not informed of the perforation.

Two "shoulds" are clear to me: the physician should have stopped the procedure and the family should have been told about the specifics of the patient's death. By not telling am I an accomplice, not legally but morally?

COMMENTARY

Thomas A. Cavanaugh

In the following reflections on selected cases, I propose a number of general rules concerning the disclosure of iatrogenic harm. In the case of "The camouflaged patient," we are told of "terrorized" surgical residents who so fear the reaction of their attending physicians to a severe postoperative infection in an elderly patient that they make the patient appear healthier than they know her to be in the hope of deceiving the attending physicians. This exemplifies one problem found in medical education: the honest admission of error is not given a sufficient place. Why are the residents so terrorized of the attending physicians? Medical educators should create a learning environment within which errors are acknowledged and prevented. In its failure to accommodate the admission of error, medical education loses the opportunity of learning from error, one of the best teachers. Institutions of medical education need to create environments open to and supportive of admissions of error.

Regardless of the terror of the residents, their act of camouflaging the patient is seriously wrong, for at least two reasons. First, such an act is a positive act of deception, undertaken in the hope of misleading the attending physicians. As an act of deception, it is comparable to telling a lie in contrast to not saying anything. Just as we reasonably consider lying more objectionable than not saying anything, so also, actively deceiving the attending physicians is worse than not telling the physicians of the infection. (Of course, this is not to say that not telling the physicians is acceptable, only that it would not be as bad as attempting to deceive them.) Generally speaking, acts of deception are wrong; clearly, this act falls into that category. Moreover, residents do have an affirmative obligation to disclose patients' conditions to their attending physicians; accordingly, deceiving the attending physicians is especially egregious.

Second, deceiving the attending physicians can only worsen the patient's condition. If the attending physicians are unaware of the existence and severity of the infection, it is likely that the patient will not be cared for properly. If the residents' ruse works, it does so at the cost of jeopardizing the patient's health. This is to add injury to the original insult. More specifically, this act violates one's obligation as a physician to care for patients. Disclosure is at least as obligatory as providing the care of the patient that depends upon disclosure. When one needs to disclose an error to remedy it or to prevent further harm to the patient's health, one's obligation to disclose correlates in strength and derives from one's obligation to care for the patient.

In the case entitled "By not telling am I an accomplice?," during a colonoscopy an intern witnesses a physician, whom she portrays as overly aggressive, perforate the patient's colon. Such a perforation can be thought of as an error or as an avoidable complication. This leads to the death of the patient. The patient's wife is not told of the cause of death. The intern wonders if she is morally an accomplice in not disclosing this to the wife.

In cases in which one witnesses iatrogenic harm, one's role relative to the patient should structure what one does. The physician performing the colonoscopy has the primary responsibility to disclose the cause of death to the wife, for the care of the patient was entrusted to him. The intern should encourage the physician to disclose. Before doing so, it would not be appropriate for the intern to talk about the case with the wife. However, if the physician who performed the colonoscopy does not disclose the perforation after being encouraged to do so, then, depending upon his or her role vis-à-vis the patient, it may be appropriate for the intern to speak to the wife, to give her some sense of how her husband died. For example, if this patient was under the intern's care for a period of time or if the intern had referred the patient for the colonoscopy, then the intern would have a more than passing obligation to disclose. However, if the intern was acting merely as an escort for the patient and had had no relationship or history with the patient that led up to the colonoscopy, then the intern would have a much less significant obligation to tell the wife. For one's obligation to disclose errors and complications and the events surrounding medical care does not derive its strength merely from one's role as witness. Rather, this obligation derives from one's role as one entrusted with the care of patients. The most significant obligation to disclose concerns what one does in the care of one's own patients; next, comes one's obligation to disclose what others do in the care of one's own patients (e.g., those to whom one has referred a patient); finally, one should encourage other caregivers to disclose errors one witnesses and support them when they do so.

In the case entitled "I knew the damage was iatrogenic," a third year medical student learns of an error made by a fellow medical student who has told no one else. The student told of the error asks what course of action to take. The medical student who committed the error should tell the intern so that it can be discerned whether any harm did result and, if so, measures can be taken to remedy the harm and to prevent further harm. The student who has learned of this error should encourage and help his or her colleague to tell the intern. This case, like that of the terrorized residents, indicates the need in medical education for instruction on what to do when one commits or learns of an error as a medical student. To fail to guide students with principles for disclosure and to fail to give them room within which to disclose without punitive reactions is to fail to educate.

In the case entitled "Boxed kidneys," a patient's kidneys are not protected from a dye employed during imaging. A student on rotation learns of this from the intern and asks when the patient will be told. The student is told to "shut up." (Here, one again sees medical education failing to find a proper place for error.) The student is – appropriately, given one's primary obli-

gation to one's own patients – especially surprised that this patient is not told of the error as the patient was "well liked and had formed attachments with the medical team." Clearly, the intern does have an obligation to let the patient know that damage to his kidneys was caused by the failure to protect them during imaging. This obligation is even more pronounced due to the extended relationship that these caregivers have with this patient. It is not clear from this case that the student has a similar obligation, as it seems that the student was only tangentially involved in the care of the patient. In pressing the question of disclosure, the student has acted well and is rightly surprised and disappointed by the intern's and the medical team's unwillingness to disclose.

Finally, the case entitled "What should they have been told?" tells of a new and rushed intern removing the catheter of a patient seated in a chair instead of while the patient was supine, in accordance with standard procedure. Within 30 seconds of removing the catheter, the patient – who was being discharged for recovery at home – suffered a seizure and cardiac arrest. The patient was revived and placed on a respirator, but showed no brain activity. The patient was withdrawn from the respirator and died. "Although there was considerable debate over whether the intern acted negligently, or was the proximate cause of death, none of this information was discussed with the devastated family." The medical student asks "what, if anything, should the devastated family be told?" This case highlights one significant epistemological problem surrounding error: how can one be certain that the removal of the catheter – conceding that it was an error – led to the patient's death and was not merely correlated to the patient's death? Sometimes, such a question may merely be an attempt to deny the reality of error and the need for disclosure. Nonetheless, many times the question is legitimate, and cannot be dismissed as a mere rationalization for avoiding the discomfort of disclosure. Uncertainty surrounds medical care generally and the occurrence and outcome of error specifically. Given the fact of ambiguity, how ought one to act in the face of opacity concerning whether an error occurred or whether an error caused harm? What degree of certitude must one have to justify or obligate one's speaking with the family or patient concerning the untoward event? One approach attractive for its frankness would be to hold that amongst what one would disclose would be one's own lack of certitude concerning the occurrence of an error; or, the lack of certainty one has that an error harmed. Some might legitimately think that this approach is too officious and that in order to avoid causing unnecessary fear, anger, and anxiety, one need not, indeed, ought not to talk to patients about ambiguous cases in which error may not have occurred or may not have resulted in harm. The ethical principles governing disclosure of unclear cases of error and of clear errors' at times of ambiguous causal relations to harm remain as opaque as our knowledge of error and of its causality of harm sometimes is.

COMMENTARY

Marli Huijer

In none of these cases is the question of how to acknowledge medical failures directly addressed. Instead, the interns, residents, and medical specialist are all preoccupied with covering up their mistakes for their colleagues, superiors, or patients. The cases are formulated as descriptions of a situation, as if these are the facts of medical life. Only in the last paragraph do the authors express a doubt or a moral question: "What was my responsibility?" "By not telling am I an accomplice?" "No one wanted to talk about this sad result any more."

In these carefully worded conclusions, the ethical dilemmas of the interns become known. They seem to condemn the covering up of medical failures, but at the same time they express an inability and unwillingness to act in accordance with this condemnation. The cases raise questions like: Why is it so difficult for interns and physicians to acknowledge mistakes? What causes their silence? Why do interns not follow their intuitive moral instincts that people should be honest about failures and mistakes? Are there other ways to deal with medical failures?

Several conclusions can be drawn from these cases:

1 Interns are very upset about failures, and even more upset about the silence regarding failures.

2 Interns and residents themselves do not acknowledge mistakes.

3 Medical students are taught to "shut up," and let failures pass.

4 Medical students experience the silence as an ethical dilemma. Being witness they feel guilty and responsible, but they do not see any opportunities to act in accordance with the honesty they value and have learned to value.

During internship, students are regularly exposed to medical failures. Of the 500 cases that Dutch interns presented in the last 4 years in our clinical ethics teaching seminars, 16% concerned medical failures. The first notable issue is that students in general turn out to be very upset about their supervisors making mistakes. The students enter their clinical years with trust in medicine and physicians. This confidence is shaken when they perceive that even the most talented physician is fallible. As a consequence, they have to face their own fallibility. The knowledge that their own well-intentioned acts can cause the death of patients is not easy to accept.

The second notable aspect in the discussions with students is their indignation with regard to dishonesty about medical failures. In this phase of education, they are all convinced of the value of honesty and truth-telling. Physicians who are not honest with colleagues or patients are condemned. The students refuse to identify with these physicians.

However, when asked what they tell a patient who has to be subjected to a second blood sample because of the intern's inattention, most of them shift their opinion slightly. If honesty would lead to the patient becoming angry they prefer to cover up the failure and tell the patient the supervisor recommended an extra test. Confessing one's failures to the patient is valued as the highest moral standard, but as soon as this value conflicts with the patient's best interest, the students are no longer certain if honesty is best.

In the case examples the interns also wrestle with the general moral obligation of honesty. They are troubled by the dishonesty of fellow interns, residents, and supervisors. The student who asked when the team was going to tell the patient his kidneys were not protected and therefore "boxed" was told to shut up. His frustration can be heard in the words, "No one wanted to talk about this sad result any more." The intern to whom a classmate told he made a mistake which caused damage to the patient's brain, does not seem very happy with this knowledge: "Since I now knew that any damage the patient suffered was iatrogenic, what was my responsibility?" His idea of honesty obligates him to check if there is any notice in the chart, and to inform the attending about what happened. His loyalty to his classmate keeps him from doing this.

The questions at the end of the case are rhetorical: everybody knows they *should* be answered positively but *are not*. The "shoulds" are clear, as the Dutch intern in the last case states. Physicians *should* be honest about their failures, and interns who witness dishonesty *should* assume responsibility. Asking rhetorical questions is a way to avoid answers. In this way, we as readers also become accomplices: we are not expected to have an answer to these questions.

Why is it so difficult to be honest and open about failures? One of the most prominent reasons is the anxiety of students and residents about receiving negative evaluations. An example is given in the first case, in which the student observed how the residents were terrorized about what the attendings would say regarding a postoperative infection. Failures by students and

residents are often not uncovered because they fear reprisals. "Chronic evaluation pressures encourage students and residents to cover up rather than to explore mistakes," Bickel states, "thus a 'conspiracy of silence' develops." (1) The intern who keeps silence will enter the conspiracy, and this can bring her certain advantages. One of our students once told me she had witnessed a surgical failure that caused the death of a patient. When she asked the surgeon as to what had happened, he acknowledged his failure. In addition, he told her he would be grateful if she would not discuss his failure with others. She agreed. The physician rewarded her silence by making her internship a very valuable experience. Nevertheless, she felt bad about it.

A second reason for covering up failures is the powerlessness of interns, residents, and sometimes even of supervisors. Interns who want to be open encounter all kinds of resistance. In the case examples, the resistance to honesty consists of the supervisors' reluctance to pay much attention to the interns' failures, the loyalty expected by colleagues who confess their failures to each other, the unspoken agreement in medicine not to discuss each other's mistakes, or the team's rebuke, "Oh shut up!" Although the students would like to discuss the mistakes with their supervisors, their classmates, and with the patients, they are unable to break the rule of silence.

A third reason for covering up is to be found in the so-called "hidden curriculum," that is, the informal curriculum, composed of messages transmitted that are primarily concerned with replicating the culture of medicine. (2) In this curriculum, messages are transmitted that may be in direct conflict with ethical standards touted in formal courses and conversation. The informal message that it is probably better for a relative not to know her husband died of a badly performed colonoscopy is in conflict with the ethical standard of truth-telling. Also in the third case, the informal message that it is not a good idea to tell the family their relative died of an intern's negligence, is in conflict with this same truth-telling standard.

The truth of the ethical standard is questioned by the informal messages. The result can be a progressive decline of moral reasoning: The student accepts the informal message as the best message, and tries to stop worrying about the values and rules taught in the formal courses. In this process the students' perception of what is going on alters. (2) Maybe it is better not to tell the relatives? As questioned in the case, "What, if anything, should they have been told?" If all physicians have agreed not to discuss each other's mistakes, does that not indicate a stronger obligation than the formal standard of truth-telling?

A last reason for covering up seems to be that interns do not feel responsible for the failures they make or witness. In our ethics course, the students usually fall silent when asked about their own failures. They try to cover up by saying that they are not in the position to actually make failures. And if they occasionally would make a mistake, their supervisors are the ones who are held responsible. The intern who increased the potassium dose sighs "I wish someone had seen my error and said something earlier." He knew he was the one who was morally responsible, but it would be easier if he could pass the buck to someone higher up the decision ladder.

All these reasons for covering up do not prevent students from having personal and ethical dilemmas. In a study by Charon and Fox, students who were unable to stop ethically dubious actions or to extricate themselves from them, reported extreme guilt about these failings. (3) Like survivors of a disaster, the students can feel guilty for things they cannot help. Not being honest with patients or their relatives about failures can increase their sense of guilt and shame. "By not telling am I an accomplice, not legally but morally?" asked the intern who participated in the colonoscopy. Part of this shame can be ascribed to the students' belief that physicians ought to be perfect. But another part has to be ascribed to an experienced discrepancy between what they have learned as humans and students and what they see and do in practice.

What can we learn from these cases? It is clear that one of the interns is unhappy with what happened and with the ways the physicians involved reacted. All their questions and statements express a desire for greater openness regarding medical failings. They are conscious that covering up prevents them from discussing and learning from their own failures and the failures of others. Students who have been able to discuss failures openly with the supervisors, experience this as beneficial. Interns need supervisors who are prepared to discuss mistakes openly and teach trainees how to deal with them properly. Students know the ethical standard of truth-telling, but it is in practice that they have to learn how to respond to the failures – which they most certainly will make.

A proposal for these kinds of discussions has been formulated by Novack et al. (4) with the suggestion that discussions in protected settings be organized into five topic areas:

1 What was the nature of my mistake?
2 What are the beliefs about the mistake?
3 What emotions did I experience in the aftermath of the mistake?
4 How did I cope with the mistake?
5 What changes did I make in my practice as a result of the mistake?

In an ethical sense, the discussion could be extended with topics such as: Are there moral reasons to keep silent with colleagues, patients, or relatives regarding the failings? Do these reasons outweigh the standard of truth-telling? How far do I go in cooperating with wrongdoing?

If students are given the opportunity to openly discuss failures with their supervisors, they can learn how an ethical value, such as truth-telling, can be brought into practice. In this way, trainees learn to transform their feelings of guilt and shame into an ability to be honest about failures, to learn from them, and to better carry the responsibility of being a physician.

Notes

1 Bickel J. Summaries of Break-out Sessions. Conference Proceedings of the AAMC Conference on Students' and Residents' Ethical and Professional
   Development. *Acad Med* 1996;71:634–40.
2 Hafferty FW, Franks R. The hidden curriculum, ethics
   teaching, and the structure of medical education.
   Acad Med 1994;69:861–70.
3 Charon R, Fox C. Critiques and remedies: medical
   students call for change in ethics teachings. *JAMA*
   1995;274:767, 771.
4 Novack DH, Suchman AL, Clark W, Epstein RM,
   Najberg E. Calibrating the physician. Personal awareness and effective patient care. *JAMA* 1997;278:502–9.

To intervene?

CASE

"Does anyone have a problem with this?"

My first clerkship was surgery and one of my first
cases involved a patient who had been on a respirator for about a week with only minimal slow-wave
activity by EEG. With great difficulty, the family
came to terms with the attending physician's suggestion that he be taken off the ventilator. They felt
that his wish would be "not to live like that,"
though he had never been explicit about any end-
of-life decisions.

While the family waited, our entire medical team
gathered to oversee what we expected would be
the patient's quiet death. Morphine was administered in quantities deemed sufficient to make the
patient "comfortable" (this had been discussed
and approved by the family). The patient was then
extubated. Unexpectedly, he started to breath
strongly, if noisily and laboriously due to his pro-
fuse oropharyngeal secretions. More morphine was
administered, despite the lack of any evident pain
or distress. No change was observed.

At this point the attending physician asked those
present "Does anyone have a problem with what I

am doing?" Although not articulated, his intent was
clear – to euthanize the patient. He did not leave to
consult again with the family about the patient's
condition. I remember feeling uncomfortable, but
sympathetic toward the attending, and unable to
think of a coherent objection.

The doctor repeatedly administered large doses
of morphine while expressing concerns that the
patient's survival would further upset the family
who was prepared for his death. The doctor persis-
ted in administering boluses of the drug despite a
nurse's objection that this would "look bad." The
physician stated that he would "take full responsibility." After a dose sufficient to "kill you and me
ten times over" the attending left to explain the
patient's stubborn refusal to die to his family. Approximately 12 hours later, the patient expired.

CASE

"No one stopped him"

During an internship, I, along with several residents, was observing a patient undergoing a mas-
tectomy. Even to my relatively inexperienced eye,
the surgeon in his carelessness appeared to be
spreading metastatic cells throughout the woman's
body. I glanced around for a sign to indicate that
others were as alarmed as I was; but I detected
nothing. After the operation was completed, the
residents privately confirmed my own worst fears
regarding the surgeon's dismal performance and
blatant lack of skill. Yet, nothing was said and no
one stopped him. The residents predicted that the
patient would be dead within a year.

COMMENTARY

Neal Cohen

The two cases included in this chapter represent
clinical situations in which the attending physician's judgment or skill was questioned. Each

case raises a number of issues related not only to the responsibility for reporting the physician, but also concerns about informed consent, active euthanasia, and credentialing.

In the first case "Does anyone have a problem with this?," the attending responded to a difficult situation inappropriately. When patients have no likelihood of meaningful recovery and the patient or the patient's surrogate requests that life-sustaining efforts be withdrawn, the physician has a responsibility to consult with the patient, review clinical options and potential outcomes and discuss plans for further care. If the physician and patient differ in their opinion about the management options or outcome, the assistance of another provider, an ethics committee or other neutral party may be required both to clarify the facts associated with the case and to separate the factual issues from subjective responses to them. If the patient and physician cannot resolve any areas of disagreement, the physician can help the patient find another provider to assist with further care. The physician is not obligated to provide care that he or she thinks is inappropriate or not medically indicated. Although the physician cannot abandon a patient, he or she can transfer care to another qualified provider.

From an ethical perspective, witholding or withdrawing support are similar. If the clinical management is not helping the patient and will not alter the outcome, it does not have to be continued. It is not uncommon for the physician to try a therapy and evaluate the patient's response to it. If the treatment is not working, however, it should not be continued, simply because it was initiated. For example, if a patient is hypertensive, blood pressure-lowering medications will be administered to the patient. If the patient's blood pressure is not controlled with the initial therapy, either another drug will be added or a new drug substituted for the first. The initial therapy would not be continued just because it had been started. The same approach should be taken when evaluating the need for and response to end of life care. If a patient has respiratory failure and needs mechanical ventilatory support, it should be initiated. If the patient's lung disease does not improve despite appropriate care, the ventilator may no longer be appropriate, since it will not reverse the disease process.

Withdrawal of support is not, however, the same as withdrawal of care, nor active euthanasia. When a decision is made to withdraw support, the specific interventions that are to be withheld must be clearly defined. All other routine measures of care should continue to be provided. At the same time, patient comfort should be assured. For patients weaned from ventilation support, pain, discomfort, and respiratory distress can and should be treated with analgesics and sedatives. The goal of the treatment is to minimize the patient's discomfort and distress. If the analgesics and sedatives also depress the patient's venalatory drive, that "second effect" is an accepted consequence of appropriate management. In this case, however, the physician chose to administer morphine for no additional therapeutic benefit to the patient. Once the patient's pain and discomfort were adequately treated, the additional morphine was not required and should not have been administered. Although the attending physician was willing to "take full responsibility," the interventions were not clinically, nor ethically appropriate.

The nurse, student, or house officer did have a responsibility to state an objection. If the physician continued to administer the drugs, the administration of the drugs should have been documented in the medical record, including the doses administered. The student is not expected to intervene and it would be inappropriate for the student to confront the physician or interfere with the patient's care. If the student were asked to administer drugs or provide other therapy that the student felt was not medically indicated, the student himself or herself could not be mandated to provide the treatment. If, on the other hand, the student identified questions about the physician's management, the case should be reviewed as part of the department's quality review.

A retrospective review of the record as part of a quality assurance program would define the clinical decision making including the drug doses and goals of therapy, and provide a forum to discuss whether the physician acted inappropriately or unethically. In the case of a patient death, the case would also be discussed as part of the review of all hospital deaths.

The second case "No one stopped him" identifies another way in which inappropriate management is often ignored. In this case, a number of observers privately questioned the skill of the surgeon. While the intern may have been inexperienced, she was able to identify some questionable surgical techniques that were subsequently verified by the resident. During the procedure, the intern could have asked about the surgical approach, seeking education, rather than validation of the surgeon's skills. At the same time, it would be difficult and inappropriate for the student to recommend a surgical approach to an attending physician. In this case, as is true in the first case, retrospective review of the surgical procedure and outcome should have been performed as part of a quality assurance program. In addition, the intern or residents have an obligation to inform the chief of the surgical service of their concerns and ask that the surgeon's management be evaluated by another experienced clinician.

These cases raise two additional issues. The first case emphasizes the importance of the informed consent process and the elements of informed consent. In this clinical case, the attending physician described some of the management changes that would occur during withdrawal of mechanical ventilation. If the physician had indicated that narcotics would be administered, he had not defined the reasons for the administration of the medication or the therapeutic goals. The physician should have indicated why the morphine would be administered and that it would not be provided to end the patient's life, but to ensure the patient's comfort. As part of the informed consent process, the physician

could not ensure a time of death, nor could the physician guarantee to the family that the patient's respiratory pattern would not be labored or that they might not witness some unusual motion or respiratory patterns. The case therefore emphasizes the importance of the informed consent process. It should include a careful description for the patient or family of the clinical assessment and therapeutic options. The discussion should also provide a description of the benefits, risks, and alternatives of each therapy and a recommendation. The rationale for the recommended approach should also be provided. As part of any informed consent process, but particularly during the withdrawal of support, the physician should describe what interventions will no longer be provided and a rationale for why each will be withheld.

The second case also raises questions about the credentialing process. Once a physician applies to the medical staff of a hospital, he or she requests specific privileges based on training and experience. The credentialing process includes an assessment of the specific skills associated with the privileges requested with documentation that the individual practitioner has the skill to define each of the contested procedure care. After obtaining temporary privileges, the physician must undergo proctoring by another credentialed physician to verify that he or she has the clinical skills and judgment appropriate for the requested privileges. While in some cases the proctoring is subjective, credentials committees generally require an objective assessment of skills and completion of a minimum number of procedures to confirm that the physician has the skills necessary for the privileges requested. Once privileges are approved, recredentialing is required for every member of the medical staff, usually every year or two. Although proctoring is rarely required with recredentialing, some form of validation of the quality of care is required, such as review of departmental quality assurance committee reports and morbidity and mortality review. The individual requesting recredentialing must also report any malpractice claims. A review of the National Practitioner Database will also reveal any reports of substandard care.

COMMENTARY

Bethany Spielman

Like many moral problems in medical education, "Does anyone have a problem with this?" and "No one stopped him" must be analyzed at two levels. The first level focuses on the responsibilities of physicians (either residents or attendings – and sometimes both). At that level, students wonder, "Was the physician wrong to do what he or she did?" The second level involves the responsibilities of students within the medical education hierarchy. At that level, students wonder, "What is my responsibility as a student to respond when I see moral lapses in physicians' treatment of patients?"

In these brief comments, I will devote little space to the physician-centered question and more space to the second, student-focused question. This second level of analysis differs from the first because the social location of medical students as underlings in the medical hierarchy is unlike that of physicians. The student's situation in these cases is like that of a subordinate in a nonmedical context who must decide whether to speak up or remain silent. But the subordinate here is not witnessing the typical boss's misstep. Rather, the medical student is witnessing acts by a superior that may hasten the death of a patient. (1)

What was the physician's responsibility?

The first level of inquiry focuses on physician responsibilities. There is, of course, a vast and complex ethical literature on voluntary and involuntary euthanasia and terminal sedation that could inform analysis of the physician's responsi-

bilities in the first case. (2) Nevertheless, the basic (though complex) concepts of intention, proportionality, causation, and consent can probably provide a sufficient foundation for a reasonably productive student discussion. Such a discussion will likely lead to the conclusion that the first physician's attempted involuntary euthanasia wronged the patient. In the second case, no complex set of constructs is required to determine that the surgeon's act was both seriously harmful and morally unjustified. Analysis of the harm to the patient and potential harm to future patients will comprise most of the comparatively straightforward assessment of the second physician's responsibility.

What is my responsibility as a student?

The second level of inquiry focuses on student responsibilities. The case examples illustrate a student problem that occurs with some frequency: whether to "speak up." (3) When medical students witness a physician behaving in an ill-considered manner that may hasten a patient's death, the students can be likened to bystanders in an emergency situation. Social scientists have analyzed bystander intervention in such situations. Their research suggests that the process of bystander intervention consists of five steps: (1) noticing that something is wrong, (2) deciding that the event is an emergency (one that, without relatively quick intervention, will result in significant harm), (3) deciding the degree of one's personal responsibility, (4) deciding the specific mode of intervention, and (5) implementing the intervention. (4) Discussion of the student dilemmas can be organized around these steps. (5)

Noticing that something is wrong
The students in "Does anyone have a problem with this?" and "No one stopped him" did notice something problematic about the course of events (the first step in the process of bystander intervention). That is why the first student felt "uncomfortable" and the second, "alarmed."

Additionally, the physician in the first case asked, "Does anyone have a problem?" and stated, "[I'll] take full responsibility" – cues that he thought something could be wrong.

Deciding that the event is an emergency
The student in the first case said "[I was] unable to think of a coherent objection." I will focus here on the "coherent thinking" aspect of the remark. The student may have been unsure whether a patient with such minimal brain function and who was reported to have "not wanted to live like that" could be harmed by a hastened death. The clarity of the student's thinking was not enhanced by the nurse's comment, "It looks bad." Part of the reason the student could not decide whether the event was an emergency was that he or she had not thought in a nuanced way ("coherently") about the kind of harm being done to the patient. (6)

The student in the second case was also uncertain about whether to interpret the situation as an emergency (step 2). "I glanced around for a sign to indicate that others were as alarmed as I was; but I detected nothing." At each of the steps in the process of intervening in an emergency situation, a bystander's response can easily be inhibited by the presence of others. The inhibiting effect of "others" is no doubt exaggerated when the individuals are students and the other bystanders – residents – are both more experienced and higher on the medical hierarchy than they are. (7)

The student in "No one stopped him" learned after the surgery though, that the situation should have been interpreted as an emergency. When the student "glanced around for a sign" and "detected nothing" he or she thought the "nothing" from the residents meant, "Nothing is wrong." But the residents themselves knew that something was, in fact, very wrong. While the medical student was still struggling with whether to define the situation as an emergency (step 2), the residents had already decided on a response of calculated silence (step 4).

Determining one's degree of personal responsibility
The third step in bystander intervention is determining one's degree of personal responsibility. Does a student who fails to intervene or protest "share" some responsibility for the wrongdoing? Wouldn't speaking up be going above and beyond the call of a student's duty? Could it even be wrong to speak up when residents don't? The first physician gave mixed signals, first asking witnesses if they objected (implying that they might feel some moral responsibility for the attempted euthanasia), then claiming that he would "take full responsibility" (implying that they should assume no responsibility).

Careful analysis of the issue of personal responsibility, however, requires consideration of the student's relationship to the patient, the causal link (if any) between the potential intervention and the prevention or reduction of harm to the patient (and others), and the likely consequences of intervening for the student. Someone is considered a "bad Samaritan," for example, if he or she

1 stands in no "special relationship" to the endangered party
2 omits to do something which could have been done without unreasonable cost or risk, and
3 as a result of which the other party suffers harm or an increased degree of harm. (8)

But such an individual could be a "minimally decent Samaritan" if he or she went to some negligible trouble to aid the endangered party. (9) Alternatively, if the individual is not a stranger, but a medical student who has been involved in the care of the patient and should be learning to be a caring physician, the standards for "minimally decent Samaritanism" might be considerably higher. (10)

Choosing a mode of intervention
The fourth step in bystander intervention is choosing an action that might reasonably be expected to prevent or stop the harm, prevent its recurrence, or rectify it in some way. The first student said "I [was] unable to think of a coher-

ent objection." But, with the advantage of hind-sight, it should be clear that the possibilities for student action in that case range from, "I'm not sure" (whether I have a problem with what you are doing) to seconding the nurse's "I think it looks bad," to "Stop! That's wrong and I'll turn you in to the authorities!" In the second case, the range of possibilities is equally broad, from "How does this technique prevent the spread of cancer cells?" to "That will kill the patient, and I'll tell the family!"

If no reasonable student response has even an outside chance of making a positive difference for the patient, analysis can proceed to the "dirty hands" problem. (11) Is it morally worthwhile to make some kind of symbolic gesture, even if it won't affect the outcome? If so, what kind of gesture and for what reason? But, assuming that there is some student response that might make a positive difference, analysis should proceed to the fifth step of the bystander intervention process.

Implementing the intervention
The fifth step in the process is implementing the intervention. Although implementing a plan to speak up to the attending physician is not nearly as complex as, say, implementing a plan to "blow the whistle," it still requires students to make choices. James Dwyer highlights some consider-ations about how to "speak up:"

The question of when students should speak up cannot be completely separated from the question of how students should speak up . . . Students need very little cause or justification for asking about . . . a particular procedure . . . The phrasing and tone of what they say is more than a matter of style. Insofar as different ways of speaking up express different sensitivities, these ways are of ethical significance. (12)

In light of Dwyer's observations, the first stu-dent's expectations for himself or herself – to formulate "a coherent objection" before speaking – seem unnecessarily high. A question, even a poorly formulated question, would have been quite appropriate and perhaps even welcome.

Concluding thoughts

Whether to speak up when a patient's death is being hastened by a physician who is acting in an ill-considered manner is a dilemma that many medical students are likely to face. It is among the "speaking up" situations in which silence can have profound consequences – for patients, for families, for medical students, and for the caring physicians those students hope to become.

Students' responsibilities in these situations are often underestimated. The comparatively limited scope of student authority, power, and expertise should not, however, be allowed to crowd out the reality that effective student action is often poss-ible, and occasionally even morally required.

Notes

1 I will assume here, for the sake of analysis, that the facts as they appear in the case are accurate and complete enough for a fair assessment of the partici-pants' acts (an assumption I do not make in student ethics case conferences).
2 A brief and useful discussion of resemblances be-tween terminal sedation and involuntary euthanasia can be found in: Orentlicher D. The Supreme Court and physician-assisted suicide: rejecting suicide but embracing euthanasia. *N Engl J Med* 1997;337:1236–9.
3 Christakis DA, Feudtner C. Ethics in a short white coat: the ethical dilemmas that medical students confront. *Acad Med* 1993;68:249–54. Feudtner C, Christakis DA. Making the rounds: the ethical devel-opment of medical students in the context of clinical rotations. *Hastings Cent Rep* 1994;24:6–12. Dwyer J. *Primum nom tacere*: an ethics of speaking up. *Hasti-ngs Cent Rep* 1994;24:13–18.
4 Latane B, Darley JM. *The Unresponsive Bystander: Why Doesn't He Help?* Appleton–Century Crofts, New York, 1970.
5 I am not suggesting that the case discussion should proceed point by point along the lines of analysis in the literature cited in this commentary, but rather that the "leader" of such a discussion should be familiar with the literature and have its key points in

mind as directions for student discussion. Clinical ethics teaching should proceed as a "workshop," described well in: Chambers TS. No Nazis, no space aliens, no slippery slopes and other rules of thumb for clinical ethics teaching. *J Med Humanit* 1995;16:189–200.

6   See Feinberg J. *The Moral Limits of the Criminal Law: Harm to Others.* Oxford University Press, New York, 1984. Feinberg's work is helpful, although one must be careful to use only the distinctions that help clarify the student's problem.

7   Latane B, Darley JM. *The Unresponsive Bystander: Why Doesn't He Help?* Appleton–Century Crofts, New York, 1970, p.41. They comment on the social determinants of bystanders' perceptions of emergencies: "Occasionally the reactions of others provide false information as to the true state of their feelings – and this may be especially likely in a potential emergency. If each member of a group is trying to appear calm and not overreact . . . each other member, in looking to him for guidance, may be misled into thinking that he is not concerned. Looking at the apparent impassivity and lack of reaction of the others, each individual is led to believe that nothing really is wrong."

8   Feinberg J. *The Moral Limits of the Criminal Law: Harm to Others.* Oxford University Press, New York, 1984, pp.126–86.

9   The term "minimally decent Samaritan" is borrowed from Thomson J. A defense of abortion. *Philos Publ Aff* 1971;1:47.

10   Dwyer J. *Primum nom tacere*: an ethics of speaking up. *Hastings Cent Rep* 1994;24:16. On the connection between speaking up and learning to care, he observes: "It would be somewhat misleading to say that students need to act in those situations so that they will learn to be caring physicians. It is more accurate to say that they need to act in those situations so that they will not learn to be uncaring physicians."

11   Childress JF. Disassociation from evil: the case of human fetal tissue transplantation research. *Soc Resp: Bus Journ, Law, Med* 1990;16:32–49. Hill TE. Symbolic protest and calculated silence. *Phil Pub Aff* 1979;9:83–102.

12   Dwyer J. *Primum nom tacere*: an ethics of speaking up. *Hastings Cent Rep* 1994;24:17.

COMMENTARY

Akira Akabayashi

These cases remind me of a couple of unforgettable scenes when I was training to be a chief resident in the mid 1980s, at a general hospital with 400 beds in a rural area. I was in charge of two first-year residents and one second-year resident, and together we covered 100 beds in the department of internal medicine. Life on the ward was hectic, as this was the only hospital in the area.

A first-year resident A, who was in charge of a terminal female cancer patient with hepatoma in her 60s, was facing the first experience of a patient's death as an attendant physician. Her breathing became weaker and weaker and her blood pressure started to drop. The patient seemed to be dying peacefully, without pain or distress, consistent with the last stages of hepatic coma. A couple of days before, I had instructed him about how to tell when she had passed from coma into death by checking corneal reflex, heart beat and respiration, and then to give the precise time of death to the patient's family. On that day, her husband, children, and relatives were with her, waiting for her last moments. The patient almost stopped breathing and her ECG monitor became flat. Suddenly, the resident started cardiac massage and asked a nurse to prepare adrenalin for intracardiac injection. I was a bit upset and after a few seconds, whispered to him not to do any more. In response, the resident answered "But Dr. Akabayashi, it is a physician's duty to do everything possible! I must do this." He performed the injection and continued cardiac massage despite my instructions to the contrary. After several minutes of attempted resuscitation, one of the family members firmly requested, "Doctor, please stop." Then I held the resident's arm and made him stop the massage.

The second scene concerned a male patient in his 70s with terminal pulmonary emphysema. He had been unconscious and on a respirator with a tracheostomy for more than 2 months. The attending physician was a second-year resident B. Because of malnutrition, hypoalbuminaemia, and long time bed-rest, his face was awkwardly edematous, and according to his family, he looked like a totally different person. The patient had been aggressively treated every time he developed respiratory or urinary infections. However, the nursing staff felt uncomfortable with the treatment plan the resident had instigated. Since B was in his second year, and was a competent practitioner, he did not need the detail of the treatment regimen to be intimately supervised. (Here I mean, the choice of drugs, content of infusion, and the setting of respirator.) One day, after a general round with the director of the department, I suggested to him that he should talk with the patient's family, and discuss and reassess the patient's future treatment plan. I also expressed my opinion that the treatment should be less aggressive. In response, B replied, "But Dr. Akabayashi, the patient does not have any malignant disease!" The treatment was continued as before, and the patient died about 3 months later.

In both situations, there was no strong obligation for me to intervene with the residents' decision, to change their actions, because their acts were not illegal, nor could they be considered to be acts of misconduct, although it could be said that they prolonged life in an inappropriate way. As the ideals of hospice or palliative care gradually prevail in Japan, we may see such situations less frequently. However, other dilemmas about ending life have entered the public arena. It would be worth noting a recent prominent mercy killing case in Japan. In this case, a physician infused potassium chloride (KCl) to a terminally ill patient without the patient's consent. (1)

The mercy killing case in Japan differs in several important ways from the case study "Does anyone have a problem with this?" The drug infused was not KCl but morphine. Moreover, a team was involved with the decision, not physician alone. The case study probably falls within

the legal gray-zone protected by the doctrine of "double effect." Such was not the case in the Japanese mercy killing incident. However, if the drug used had not been KCl but morphine or other kinds of sedatives, the Japanese physician would probably not have been brought before the court because it would be difficult to prove his intent to kill the patient.

In both cases, the physician's statement "I will take full responsibility" is significant. In the Japanese case, this sentence reveals that the physician's action was traditionally paternalistic and the relationship among members of the care team (particularly the doctor–nurse relationship) was not a cooperative one. However, it should also be noted that in legal terms, in both countries physicians have the final responsibility for the medical treatment they have carried out. Therefore, those who are liable are the physicians who actually performed the medical treatment, even if a team of carers were involved. The way in which these legal responsibilities can be shared among doctors, nurses, and co-medical workers should be an issue for discussion in both countries. In the case "Does anyone have a problem with this?," there are also some problems with the decision from a medical point of view. I think there were good medical grounds for the physician to have tried weaning and/or an apnoea test (disconnecting the respirator for a short period in order to confirm loss of voluntary breathing) before extubation.

When to intervene as a doctor in training?

In considering the cases under discussion, I can think of only two situations when intervention by a physician in training is permissible, or moreover required. First, when an action of a colleague (including nurses, and other co-medical staff) is clearly violating the law, for example, infusing KCl. Secondly, when an act is apparently against established hospital policy. Those policies are usually in written form, such as a manual for care for Jehovah's Witness patients, or procedural

guidelines regarding how to withdraw life-sustaining treatments.

Physicians are required to be loyal to colleagues. This obligation may conflict with the
duty to disclose information about the actions of
peers. The case "No one stopped him" particularly raises issues about how to manage negative
information that affects colleagues and patients.
(2) Beauchamp and Childress state that

A wall of silence frequently surrounds medical malpractice, particularly when the patient is unaware of the
malpractice and members of the treatment team or
consultants are aware of it . . . silence in a circumstance
of malpractice is morally indefensible . . . It is sometimes equally indefensible to fail to defend a colleague
when his or her truthfulness eventuates in a malpractice
suit or dismissal from a position. (2)

In some cases, it is indeed a moral duty to disclose a colleague's malpractice to others. That is,
it is morally required to blow the whistle. However, it is sometimes equally difficult to protect
colleagues from dismissal and collegial indifference.

Are there any other situations where physicians
in training can intervene with their colleagues'
actions if they have deep reservations about
them? Alas, the answer is "No" since such situations may be either legally ambiguous, or may
be a reflection of the preferences (including religious belief) of the physician in training. In the
first case, no one can say with certainty that the
action taken was legally (and morally) incorrect.
In the latter cases, there is the risk that one person may impose subjective beliefs upon another,
without respect for the physician's decisions.

In such situations, especially in a legally ambiguous case, what a physician in training can do
is to initiate discussion with his or her colleagues.
At the same time, they can discuss what are the
best interests of the patient. This, I believe, is vital
to effective clinical training. During the training
period, young physicians need to learn the technical skills necessary to treat patients. But this is
only part of medical training. They also need to

learn skills that will enable them to resolve the
complicated problems of medical practice.

Medical training is still a kind of apprenticeship. However, the center of decision making has
shifted from the physician alone to include patients and their other carers. This tendency will
increase opportunities for young physicians to
initiate discussion. This, in turn, may elucidate
further hidden problems medical professionals
have to tackle more seriously. Moreover, medical
professionals should take the initiative in assessing legally ambiguous cases before they are
brought to court. Such problems seem universal,
as a recent case demonstrates. (3)

Notes

1 Yokohama District Court Case (1995).
   On 13 April 1991, a 34-year-old physician gave an
   intravenous injection of 20 ml of potassium chloride
   (KCl) solution without dilution to a terminally ill 58-
   year-old man, a cancer patient at Tokai University
   Hospital, Kanagawa, Japan. The patient died 3.5
   minutes later.
   By the beginning of April 1991, the patient had
   developed multiple myeloma and renal failure, and
   was suffering from severe pain and convulsions. On
   the morning of 13 April, the patient became comatose, and the physician withdrew intravenous feeding
   tubes, following the family's request. His family
   repeatedly asked the physician to withdraw all treatments. On the evening of 13 April 1991, after repeated
   requests by the family for medical action to ease the
   patient's suffering as quickly as possible, the physician injected him with two kinds of tranquilizers at
   about a 1-hour interval. Thereafter he decided to give
   the patient intravenous injections of KCl solution.
   The physician told a nurse in the same ward who
   strongly disagreed with his intended action: "I will
   take full responsibility." In the end, the physician
   acted without a request from the patient, and without
   his consent.
   On 25 April 1991 the physician was dismissed as a
   disciplinary measure. Meanwhile, the Kanagawa
   Prefectural Police Headquarters forwarded police
   initiated proceedings regarding suspected murder.

On 28 March 1995 the Chief judge of the Yokohama District Court described the four new legal requirements for "physician-assisted voluntary euthanasia." The conditions set by the district court were: (1) The patient must be suffering from unbearable physical pain; (2) the patient's death must be unavoidable and imminent; (3) every possible palliative treatment and care to ease the patient's physical pain and suffering must have been provided, and no alternatives must be available; and (4) the patient must have expressed a clear and voluntary desire to have his or her life shortened. It was concluded that in this case the physician's action only fulfilled the second requirement. Therefore, he was found guilty of homicide, sentenced to two years imprisonment, and given a suspended sentence. Hoshino K. Euthanasia: current problems in Japan. *Camb Q Healthc Ethics* 1993;2:45–7. Hoshino K. Euthanasia in Japan: update. *Camb Q Healthc Ethics* 1996;5:144.

2 Beauchamp TL, Childress JF. *Principles of Biomedical Ethics, 4th edn.* Oxford University Press, New York, 1994, pp. 404–6. Beauchamp and Childress described this issue as follows:

Incompetent or unscrupulous health care professionals present additional problems about veracity. The AMA Principles of Medical Ethics require disclosure of information in order to preserve trust between the public and the medical profession: "A physician shall deal honestly with patients and colleagues, and strive to expose those physicians deficient in character or competence, or who engage in fraud or deception." Exposes by fellow physicians are, however, uncommon. Bonds of professional loyalty, accented in the Hippocratic and collegial traditions of medical ethics, present a formidable barrier, but this sociological fact does not excuse failures to expose serious deficiencies. Often disclosures are essential to preserve institutional or public trust, as well as the confidence of professional colleagues.

3 Anonymous. A piece of my mind. It's over, Debbie. *JAMA* 1988;259(2):272.

24

Misrepresenting research

"Was I a coward?"

As an intern I felt privileged to have the opportunity to work in the laboratory of a chief researcher in an area of particular interest to me. At a professional meeting the researcher, who was also head of the lab, presented the results of a study with which I was familiar in a way that I thought inaccurately inflated the potential benefits of the findings. I was aware that the work had been written up and was being submitted for publication. Challenging the researcher's interpretation would be, in my opinion, an act of professional suicide. I also assumed that future attempts to duplicate the results would either prove or disprove the conclusions presented. Was this assumption enough to justify my inaction, or was I just a coward?

CASE

"A faculty member listed his name as first author"

My medical school program involved a special curriculum that required students to write a thesis in a health-related field. As it turned out, my work received acclaim beyond the academic requirements. I was invited to do a presentation at a professional conference and I wrote a paper that was accepted for publication. A faculty member, who had played an important advisory role, listed his name as first author. I felt angry and betrayed but didn't know whether to make an issue of it or not.

CASE

"Unethical author attribution"

I am an MD/Ph.D. student and work as a research assistant for the director of a division of the school of medicine who is an MD. He assigned me to research a certain topic and gave me no guidelines or guidance as to how to do it. Nevertheless, I did the research and wrote it up. My supervisor liked the report and said that he thought it was so good that "I would like to offer you the opportunity to publish it and list you as the primary author." Some bells went off when he so grandly offered to let me author the report for which I had done 100 percent of the research and writing. I consulted some other people in the field and they said that as long as I was the primary author, it was legitimate for him to list himself as secondary author if he did some editing later. After editing the abstract only, he emailed his revisions to me and in a note at the bottom he asked me what I thought of his revised author order. His name was first, mine second, and the name of his girlfriend (who had no part in this research or its revision) was third. I was shocked by what seemed to be a case of unethical author attribution and confronted him asking why he changed the order when we had agreed that I was primary author. He said that he had put in several hours of work. I reminded him that I had put in 150 hours of work on that project and he agreed to change it back so that my name was first. I sent him a written message noting my surprise at seeing a third name on the article. He did not respond to that. Supposedly, as it stands now, I am listed as primary author and he is second. I don't know if there is still a third author name or not. Since that time he has even asked the "third author" in front of me if she has read the article, confirming my suspicion that she has had no part in its editing. The problem is that even though my boss has agreed to put my name first (twice now), I do not know what will happen when he finally submits the article for publication.

COMMENTARY

Akira Akabayashi

Contemporary researchers' competence in the biomedical sciences fields has come to be judged by new criteria. These criteria exercise great influence on their appointments and promotions, criteria such as publications and letters of recommendation from other well-known researchers. In the case of clinical medicine, those who hope for promotion have also to demonstrate their clinical competence. As far as scientific papers are concerned, being named as a first author is of great importance, since the first author receives far more credit than the second or subsequent authors. Therefore the question of who will be named as an author, and the ordering of attribution, has become a critical issue among scientists, especially in the area of natural science as well as medicine.

The International Committee of Medical Journal Editors (known as the Vancouver Group) has produced a document entitled *Uniform Requirements for Manuscripts Submitted to Biomedical Journals.* (1) In its revised fourth edition, it prescribes who should be considered to be an author of a paper. However, when discussing the order of the authorship, the guidelines are somewhat unclear, stating only that attribution should be a "joint decision" by the coauthors. This statement does not really account for the power dynamics that are often found in research teams. Those who are in superior positions might use their

positions unfairly, as is illustrated by the cases presented.

Scientific misconduct has been a topic of great interest everywhere. The number of papers related to this issue listed in Medline, for example, have dramatically increased since the late 1980s. (2) Besides problems related to attribution, fabrication, falsification, plagiarism, interpretation or judgment of data, as illustrated in the case "Was I a coward?" are similarly serious issues about scientific fraud that have evoked widespread commentary.

Cultural perspectives

I would like to discuss the issue of attribution from a cultural perspective. Recently, Feters and Elwyn compared the numbers of authors per original article by Japanese and non-Japanese research groups in two qualitatively similar medical journals, namely *Circulation Research* and *Japanese Circulation Research* during three different years. (3) They found that in each year there were 2–3 more Japanese authors per original article in *Japanese Circulation Research* than in *Circulation Research*. They suggested that there were intercultural variations in crediting authorship, attributing them to the Japanese group-ethics, the role of professors in conducting research, and the funding system. They concluded that "the movement to credit only those who deserve authorship is noble, though the assessment of legitimate authorship is a cultural, not a scientific judgment."

The most influential factors relating to their findings are the differences in the funding, appointment, and promotion systems between the two countries. In the U.S., the requirements for funding by bodies like the NIH are firstly, the feasibility and scientific significance of research, and secondly the competence of the applicant as judged by their last several years' publications. The grant application sheets are huge, often as thick as a monograph. In Japan, a grant application form from the Ministry of Education,

Science, Sports, and Culture is relatively simple, and a young researcher in reality cannot apply for a grant of more than $40 000 per year. These applications are, of course, peer reviewed. However, in a small country like Japan, there are a limited number of researchers, who know each other, and therefore they try and distribute money equitably.

When considering the way appointments are made, in the U.S., a tenure track researcher must publish a certain number of papers to achieve tenure, while in Japan, appointments are usually tenured automatically from the level of assistant professor, and salaries are guaranteed until retirement, regardless of accomplishments in research. There are good and bad things to be said about both of these systems. For example, in the American system, competitive efforts produce highly scientifically-evaluated papers. However relatively short and quickly developed papers are also produced in great numbers. The rush to publish does not enable researchers to focus on areas that will take a long period to come to fruition. Also the pressure to publish means that there is frequent opportunity for acts of scientific misconduct such as fabrication, falsification, and misinterpretation of data. Fundamental to the differences between the two systems is the difference in the value of having large numbers of papers published and the value of being a first author. (4)

What should we do when confronted by unethical practices?

In returning to the case studies, it is important to ask the question, what can students do when they feel uncomfortable about their supervisor's acts? One thing they can do, after talking to the immediate supervisor, is to consult with a research ethics committee, or to go directly to the general supervisor or the dean. This is considered to be an act of internal, personal whistle-blowing. (5) As a first step, it is a moral requirement to address the immediate supervisor, and then exhaust all the internal resources within the institution that deal with complaints of this kind. If no satisfaction can be found using these methods, then the student has several options. First, she may take the misdemeanor outside the institution concerned (an act of public whistle-blowing). Secondly, she can dissociate herself from the publication or action, and thirdly, actually follow the publication order given by the supervisor. The third alternative may seem to be overly submissive. However, at institutions where whistle-blowers are not protected, even if their cause is just, this is the only way to avoid professional suicide.

Regarding the case "Unethical author attribution," adding the girlfriend's name, who has no relation with the research is an extreme example of an unethical practice. A less extreme, but still highly problematic situation may arise more frequently, whereby a supervisor may pressure a researcher to include another person who has not worked directly on the project. Although this is a kind of coercion, it is a situation where it often pays to think through the options with great care.

It is my view that 150 hours of work on a project (suppose the researcher in question worked for 10 hours per day, which means he spent 15 days altogether) is not enough to perform a full research experiment from the onset. Although the student asserted that the supervisor did not give any guidelines or guidance for the research, these relatively short hours of work tempt me to suspect that there was enough previous research, including a pilot study, that enabled the student to obtain successful data in such a short time. The amount of time spent puts the student in a weaker position when making his case. This assertion is also valid in the case of "A faculty member listed his name as first author." It is hard for me to imagine that an inexperienced medical student could complete all the processes pertinent to research, including actually writing the paper. The contribution by relatively inexperienced researchers needs to be carefully assessed.

How can we then judge contributions to research papers? This is a problem relating to professional ethics that modern scientists have to address. They need to achieve some kind of consensus on this issue, in order to alleviate the problems demonstrated in the case studies, and discussed in this chapter. Values and norms in different cultures may also influence the kinds of decisions that are made. International societies of scientists need to further develop tools to solve possible conflicts, balancing the objectivity of science with cultural values.

Notes

1 International Committee of Medical Journal Editors. Uniform requirements for manuscripts submitted to biomedical journals. *JAMA* 1993;269(17):2282–6.
2 In a search of database Medline using the keywords "Scientific Misconduct," 108 articles (including letters and commentaries) were found for the period 1985–1990, 587 for 1991–1995, 263 for 1996–1999.
3 Fetters MD, Elwyn TS. Assessment of authorship depends on culture. *BMJ* 1997;315:747.
4 I am indebted for their discussion concerning this section to Drs Todd S. Elwyn at University of Hawaii, Honolulu and Michael D. Fetters at University of Michigan, Ann Arbor.
5 Whistle-blowing has often been discussed in the arena of business ethics. It can be classified into (1) internal vs. external; (2) personal vs. impersonal; and (3) governmental vs. private-sector whistle-blowing. DeGeorge has proposed five conditions for whistle-blowing to be morally justifiable, permissible, and morally obligatory. In his analysis he focuses on nongovernmental, impersonal, external whistle-blowing, the motivation for which is moral, rather than for revenge. The five conditions are: (1) there is a serious and considerable harm to the public; (2) the whistle-blower should report to the immediate superior; (3) the whistle-blower should exhaust the internal procedures and possibilities within the firm; (4) the whistle-blower must have accessible, documented evidence that would convince a reasonable, impartial observer; (5) the whistle-blower must have good reasons to believe that by going public the necessary changes will be brought about. (1) to (3) are

conditions for morally permissible whistle-blowing, (4) and (5) are conditions for morally required whistle-blowing.
DeGeorge RT. *Business Ethics, 3rd edn.* Macmillan Publishing Co., New York, 1989, pp.200–16.

COMMENTARY

Charles Weijer

My mentor at Dalhousie University, Nuala Kenny, greets each incoming class of medical students with the caution that "you are already becoming the doctor you are going to be." Sound advice. The same might be said to clinician-investigators in training: "the way you deal with ethical dilemmas today shapes the sort of scientist you will be tomorrow." Few begin a scientific career with the intent of becoming unscrupulous; those who have become so, got that way because of the sorts of choices they make along the way. These three cases illustrate well just how difficult are the dilemmas that routinely face clinician-investigators in training. Questions of honesty and allocation of credit do not arise in isolation, but are mired in a real-world tangle of relationships, hierarchy, and uncertain consequences.

Dealing with these questions requires that the clinician-investigator in training be knowledgeable about the norms that govern the conduct of science and embody the virtues of a good scientist. The former provides the tools needed to make the right choice; the latter provides the inclination to actually make it. The emphasis in the scientific integrity literature is on the articulation of precise guidance for particular cases. Too little attention, in my opinion, has been given to the character traits of the good scientist.

A good scientist strives to embody a number of virtues (this is an incomplete listing, to be sure):
- The good scientist is *objective*: she seeks truth about the physical, psychological or social world.

- She is *skeptical*: she evaluates critically received wisdom and the findings of others.
- She is *honest* about her work, even if findings differ from those expected or challenge her own theory.
- She is *fastidious* in the way she conducts her work, always being careful to follow a reproducible method, and record and report results accurately.
- She has *humility* before her subject matter and her colleagues.
- Finally, she has the *courage* to dare to be right, to admit when she is wrong, and to do the right thing, especially when it is hard or unpopular to do so.

No one is born with these virtues intact; rather you must strive in the choices faced in your own personal and professional life to make these virtues your own. A single decision to tell the truth, rather than withhold it, is an *honest act*. Someone who consistently chooses to tell the truth, is an *honest person*.

The three cases presented challenge us to live out these virtues in the choices we make in daily life. Two of the cases touch on issues of authorship – in my experience, the most common issue faced by clinician-investigators in training. In the standard scientific paper, credit is allocated in one of three places: the list of authors, acknowledgements, and references. Authorship receives the most attention because here the stakes are highest. Authorship on peer-reviewed papers is the yardstick by which scientists are measured and the rewards in science, including fellowships, grants, promotion, and even prestige, are distributed. Detailed guidance exists for the question as to whether one should be included in the list of authors or not. The International Committee of Medical Journal Editors authoritatively set out three necessary conditions for authorship:

Authorship credit should be based only on substantial contributions to (a) conception and design, or analysis and interpretation of data; and to (b) drafting the article or revising it critically for important intellectual content; and on (c) final approval of the version to be pub-

lished. Conditions (a), (b), and (c) must all be met. (1) Importantly, they go on to say that ''[p]articipation solely in the acquisition of funding or the collection of data does not justify authorship. General supervision of the research group is not sufficient for authorship.'' (1)

The title of the case ''Unethical author attribution'' is accurate. The student was given by the supervisor ''no guidelines or guidance'' as to how to approach the topic, and she did ''100 percent of the research and writing.'' The supervisor's only contribution, according to the narrative, was to edit the abstract. Thus, the supervisor fails to meet two of the three conditions for authorship: he did not make a substantial contribution to the study's design or analysis, and he did not draft or revise the article for important intellectual content. The supervisor should, therefore, withdraw his name as an author on the paper. The supervisor's act of making his partner, who had nothing whatsoever to do with the work, an author strains belief. So-called ''gift authorship'' is widely recognized as an immoral act. The authors of *On Being a Scientist: Responsible Conduct in Research* rightly observe that

[o]ccasionally a name is included in a list of authors even though that person had little or nothing to do with the content of a paper. Such ''honorary authors'' dilute the credit due the people who actually did the work, inflate the credentials of those so ''honored,'' and make the proper allocation of credit more difficult. (2)

The other authorship case, ''A faculty member listed his name as first author,'' is more difficult. We are told nothing of the research, but are informed that the student made ''a presentation at a professional conference'' and ''wrote a paper that was accepted for publication.'' Of the supervisor's role, we are only told that he ''played an important advisory role.'' The answer to the dilemma posed depends on the nature of that advisory role. As the authors of *On Being a Scientist* point out

If a senior researcher has defined and put a project into motion and a junior researcher is invited to join in, major credit may go to the senior researcher, even if at the moment of discovery the senior researcher is not present. (2)

The student, in this case, must reflect carefully on the role the supervisor actually played. Did the supervisor pick the topic for research? Is the topic part of a research plan developed by the supervisor? Did the supervisor provide the student with key direction as to how to go about answering the study question? If so (provided the conditions for authorship listed above are fulfilled), the supervisor does qualify to be an author on the paper. The question as to the ordering of authors is perhaps even more uncertain.

No definitive guidance exists as to the proper ordering of authors on a paper. This is at least in part due to the fact that the norms for differing scientific disciplines diverge. In some fields, authors are listed from those who made the greatest contribution to those who made the least. In other fields, the senior author is listed last rather than first. In yet other fields, authors are listed alphabetically. Because of this variation in practice, coauthors should agree up-front on criteria for ordering of authors. The final ordering for a particular paper is best discussed early, rather than late, in the preparation of the manuscript and, if at all possible, in person. The subject is, in my experience, too delicate for email discussions.

The case, "Was I a coward?," raises another issue, namely, the accurate reporting of research results. The success of the scientific enterprise depends on a foundation of trust. Researchers, and ultimately the community at large, must be able to depend on the scientist to accurately and dispassionately report her research findings. Indeed, there is a well acknowledged obligation in the publication of scientific results to "[l]ink the conclusions with the goals of the study but avoid unqualified statements and conclusions not completely supported by the data." (1) Failures to meet this obligation fall along a spectrum from unbridled (and irresponsible) enthusiasm to outright falsification, that is, changing or misrepresenting data or results. The consequences of such actions can be serious. Patients may be harmed by ineffective or unsafe treatments, scarce funds are squandered, and, ultimately, trust in science as a whole is diminished. With increasing frequency, institutions, funding agencies, and governments are taking action against scientists who fail to report research results accurately.

In each of the cases, the power imbalance that exists between investigators in training and senior researchers complicates the situation in which the students find themselves. Students often depend on the supervisor for favorable evaluations, letters of recommendation, help getting a job, and a salary. This relationship confers a variety of obligations upon each party. Most important, though, is the supervisor's duty not to abuse the power imbalance to her own advantage. The student and the supervisor should both strive to maintain an open dialogue about the proper conduct of science. The institution has an important role to play in encouraging a healthy learning environment. When disputes do occur, a mechanism should exist to arbitrate them. Since students are particularly vulnerable in such disputes, the institution has an obligation to protect them from undeserved harm. Clinician-investigators in training would be wise to ensure that their institution has such policies and procedures in place, and, if not, to advocate for their adoption.

The decision whether to challenge authorship claims or report misconduct, despite potentially adverse consequences, requires both humility and courage. The student should carefully examine the facts, seek the advice of others more experienced, and be open to the possibility that she is misreading the situation. If false authorship claims or misconduct are apparent, however, the student must have the courage to face the supervisor and, if necessary, report misconduct to institutional authorities. While one of the cases refers to the risks of acting as "professional suicide," the risks of not acting are often at least as great. Regret for not having done the right thing may be hard to shake, and your reputation – a scientist's most valued possession – may be tarnished by being included on a publication with an inflated list of authors or, worse yet, falsified or fabricated results. When a supervisor errs, it reflects poorly on her; when you fail to act, it reflects poorly upon you. In the end, it comes down to the question: What sort of scientist do you want to become?

Notes

1 International Committee of Medical Journal Editors. Uniform requirements for manuscripts submitted to biomedical journals. *N Engl J Med* 1997;336:309–15.
2 Committee on Science, Engineering, and Public Policy. *On Being a Scientist: Responsible Conduct in Research, 2nd edn.* National Academy Press, Washington, DC, 1995.

DISCUSSION QUESTIONS

Section 7. Perceiving misconduct and whistle-blowing: observing peers or superiors commit an act deemed unethical

1 In your role as a professional-in-training, what does fidelity to medicine mean? with colleagues? with patients?
2 What is your responsibility if you believe a doctor is practicing substandard medicine?
3 Where is the line to be drawn between loyalty to colleagues and loyalty to the patient? What factors weigh in the balance?
4 Should you inform superiors of mistakes made by your peers?
5 What is your obligation if you know that a patient is aware of a colleague's derogatory reference to him or her? Should you try to smooth things over, to cover for the colleague, or confront them? In the presence of the patient?
6 Morality requires a reasonable degree of action on behalf of others, but does it, or when might it, also extend to heroic self-sacrifice? How can the two be distinguished?
7 Would you risk your future for the sake of a moral principle? Any moral principle or just a few?
8 Rather than a motivation to protect others, some whistle-blowers are motivated by a desire for revenge for perceived injustices. What difference, if any, do intentions make?
9 Taking into account that some people are just natural renegades, do you tend to see whistle-blowers as troublemakers or as heroes or heroines?
10 What are some effective means organizations could create to minimize the need for whistle-blowing?
11 If you have reason to believe a research report is erroneous, do you have a responsibility to try to see that it is corrected? If you do come forward and your efforts are not successful, what should you do next?
12 What constitutes legitimate authorship on a research paper?

Epilogue: Using this book

One physician-educator we interviewed for the book concluded,

Currently ward ethics issues are handled, when they are handled at all, on an ad hoc basis. The message is that these issues are not that important. The situation must change but it will not change overnight and it will not change without ruffling feathers.

Even if some feather-ruffling is inevitable, given any institution's natural resistance to change, there are still a number of ways in which training dilemmas such as those described in this book could be identified and addressed. Our recommendations can be summarized in three categories: education, reporting, and organizational responsibility.

Education

Educational opportunities can range from occasions as informal as brown bag lunches to ward ethics cases incorporated as an integral part of the curriculum itself. The latter might take the form of:

1 *Ward ethics rounds.* Once a week the various services could devote one of their rounds to ward ethics dilemmas. During these sessions trainees present cases and participate in a forum on how best to address the issues generated on this particular service. For example, the intern who complained of her discomfort in being given an order to deliver devastating news to a patient with whom she had had no previous contact, would

have the opportunity to discuss her own feelings and response. Although she complied, she believed that her inexperience was instrumental in causing the patient additional pain. Describing her experience at a ward ethics round would not only address the needs of the individual intern, but also offer an educational opportunity for the team to discuss how to deliver bad news.

2 *Ward ethics student seminars.* Small groups of 8–10 trainees could be scheduled every 2 or 3 weeks for the purpose of bringing their own cases for discussion. Rules would include: no names mentioned of offending pesons and no finger-pointing. The purpose of these sessions would be not only for airing issues, but to place emphasis on identifying alternative ways of dealing with their ethical problems.

Beyond simply articulating the problems, the discussion should aim at finding answers to questions such as: "What are some of the different options that could have been tried?" and "How could that alternative be put into action the next time a similar situation arises?" An open and unfettered exchange of experiences and ideas is only possible in the protection and comfort of a "judgment-free zone." For this reason, the seminars should be led by a neutral ombudsman, someone not in the immediate medical hierarchy or in a position to make evaluations.

3 *Faculty workshops.* Senior physicians who hold teaching positions should be made aware of and become sensitive to the special dilemmas of trainees. Concentrated efforts should be made to reach directors of residency programs within an insitution. Workshops may last, for example, for half a day and take cognizance of several of the categories of cases identified in our taxonomy. The faculty would then be more comfortable raising training ethics issues as part of their ward rounds.

Realistically, unless awareness of these issues, and appropriate ways of dealing with them, is fully recognized as part of the skills required for physicians in teaching positions, progress is impossible. And if the institutional merit system does not reward physicians for taking ward ethics seriously, these issues will never command attention or be considered of sufficient importance to warrant the time and energy of senior physicians.

Reporting

There is no way that discussion of issues in this book will be fruitful unless they occur in an environment of open and nonconfrontational dialogue. Airing of the issues, however therapeutic and informative, is not always sufficient. There are times when action must be taken. This requires serious efforts to establish mechanisms for reporting and responding. Responsible institutions will establish some safe way of reporting based upon an agreed-upon process of reporting and intervention. Sometimes this process might take the form of a single individual within the institution identified as the "point person" to whom trainess could refer the dilemmas they face today without recourse or guidance.

We are also fond of the idea of a ward ethics committee, similar to the ethics committees which, since the early 1980s, have evolved within healthcare institutions for the purposes of addressing ethical dilemmas involving patient treatment. Ward ethics committees would focus on ethical issues in training and might offer consultation when the need arises, policy development for departments with training programs, and take the initiative in developing education activities surrounding ward ethics issues. Committee membership would be interdisciplinary representing clinical faculty, house staff, medical students, hospital and medical school administration, etc.

Organizational responsibility

Institutional expectations must include not only the recognition of the importance of these issues but the commitment to address them. Without firm and on-going institutional support the most vulnerable members, i.e. trainees, will remain at considerable risk. Furthermore, there is a danger of professional hypocrisy in any system that proclaims a dedication to the goal of producing humane and compassionate physicians while allowing institutionalized behaviors that undermine that effort.

Healing is sometimes referred to as a "sacred task" because of the mysterious way in which human beings impact upon one another. This interaction is no less healing, or harmful, between the powerful and the powerless in a medical training hierarchy as between patient and physician. There can be no true healing environment in the presence of the conflicts and crises recounted in the stories told here. Clearly, organizational responsibility requires creating and enforcing clear policies that there will be zero tolerance for the sorts of behaviors brought to light by our self-descibed "bottom feeders."

Glossary

The following terms appear regularly in cases and commentaries. Terms used once only are defined in the text where they appear.

Attending: A fully trained physician who oversees and retains the ultimate authority and accountability regarding the management of the patient's care.

Chief resident: Selected based on experience and demonstrated ability, the chief resident provides supervision, direction, and education to house staff as well as managing the schedule.

Clerkship: A clinical experience for 3rd or 4th year medical students in a specific specialty or location.

Code: Performing advance cardiac life-support procedure.

Consultant: In the British system a consultant is a fully trained physician or surgeon, the equivalent of an attending. In the United States a consultant is generally a board certified subspecialist asked to give advice on or to manage a specific patient problem.

Extern: A visiting medical student participating in a rotation at an institution other than one affiliated with his or her own medical program.

Fellowship: A course of training following completion of a specialty residence.

House staff, house officer: Interns, residents, and fellows are collectively referred to as the house staff, their responsibility is to provide patient care under faculty supervision.

Internship: First year of residency training.

Junior doctor: A British term describing the training grades from house officer to senior registrar.

Residency: A course of post graduate study for physicians in a specific specialty.

Rotation: Although usually reserved for resident postgraduate training, a rotation is similar to the medical student clerkship in that it refers to a clinical experience in a specific specialty or location.

Rounds: A team, usually composed of house staff, medical students, nurses, and other members of the health care team (e.g. pharmacist, social worker, bioethicist), frequently including a senior member of the medical staff, go around to visit each patient. The patient may or may not be examined but at minimum will have some communication with the team.

Senior registrar: The British equivalent of a chief resident, an advanced resident, usually in the final year of training who is responsible for the performance of all the residents in the specialty area.

Staff physician: An attending physician who is on staff at the hospital.

Sub Intern (or Sub I): Usually a 4th year medical student, or clerk, who is doing clinical work under the supervision of a resident.

Teaching hospital: A hospital affiliated with a medical school that has a teaching program for medical students, interns, or residents.

Index